Genetics of Substance Use

Michael M. Vanyukov
Editor

Genetics of Substance Use

Research and Clinical Aspects

Springer

Editor
Michael M. Vanyukov
Departments of Pharmaceutical Sciences, Psychiatry, and Human Genetics
University of Pittsburgh
Pittsburgh, PA, USA

ISBN 978-3-030-95349-2 ISBN 978-3-030-95350-8 (eBook)
https://doi.org/10.1007/978-3-030-95350-8

This Springer imprint is published by the registered company Springer Nature Switzerland AG
The registered company address is: Gewerbestrasse 11, 6330 Cham, Switzerland

Preface

Research in the genetics of substance use has progressed from early family and adoption studies and attempts to relate phenotypic variation to simple genetic markers, to phenotypic variance component analysis in biometric genetic research, and to whole genome approaches and epigenetic mechanisms of gene expression. Promising findings have been obtained on this path, some later rejected, some worth continued pursuit. Many unresolved questions remain, pertaining to the genetic analysis of complex traits in humans in general, to behavioral problems, to genetic studies specifically in substance use and addiction, as well as to translation of research results.

This book is intended to fill in a gap in the discourse concerning genetic studies in psychoactive substance use. Although the empirical literature in this area is abundant, and reviews on various aspects of genetic research have been published, there have been no books, to our knowledge, that systematically address this field in its current state. Moreover, in the last few years, the field of genetic analysis and related methodologies have undergone substantial changes. Insofar as substance use and liability to substance addiction are complex behavioral traits, many of the considerations and conclusions from substance use research can be extended to such traits in general, particularly psychological and psychiatric. Nonetheless, the focus of the book is unique. It covers the entire span of research in the human genetics of substance use, from phenotyping to mechanisms to biometric and molecular genetic approaches, authored by experts in respective fields.

The book has three sections, besides this Introduction, and eight chapters in total. The first section deals with the traits and phenotypes that are the targets of genetic research in substance use and addiction. The first chapter in that section, by Kirisci and Vanyukov, considers the problems and their possible solutions in the phenotypic characteristics that the society and the professionals deal with specifically in characterizing substance use, both categorically and as continuous traits, on the background of historic and secular changes. The second chapter, by Butelman and Kreek, reviews data on the neurobiology of substance use, including key contributors to the development of substance use and addiction in general as well as those pertaining to specific groups of substances. The third chapter, by Tarter and Reynolds, provides a psychological perspective on the etiology of substance use and addiction. The second section explicates the methods and results of biometric genetic studies of variation in the risk for addiction. This section includes chapters by Neale and co-authors on twin methodology, and by Stallings and co-authors on family and adoption studies in substance use. The third section reviews research in gene mapping and epigenetics. The chapter by Terwilliger covers the general problems in gene mapping that pertain to substance use and other complex traits, and the chapter by Maher details linkage and association research in this area. Finally, the chapter by Lax and co-authors presents results of epigenomic research in substance use/addiction. In each chapter, the progress and remaining lacunae in the respective area of research are summarized.

It is expected that the book will allow professionals, such as psychiatrists, psychologists, and substance abuse specialists, as well as other interested readers to update and expand their knowledge in an important component of biomedical research. It is hoped that this information will help positive development in solving one of the most persistent medical and societal problems, misuse of psychoactive substances.

Pittsburgh, PA, USA Michael M. Vanyukov

Acknowledgment

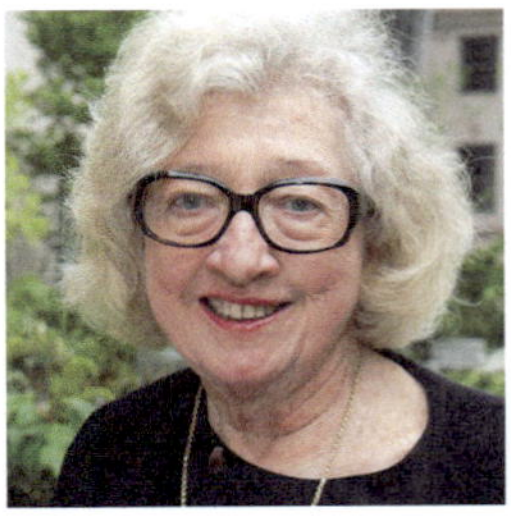

We acknowledge and celebrate the life of Mary Jeanne Kreek, MD, who was a leader in the field of the biology of substance use disorders and their treatment.

Contents

Contributors

Daniel Bustamante Integrative Life Sciences – Virginia Institute for Psychiatric and Behavioral Genetics, Richmond, VA, USA

Eduardo R. Butelman Laboratory on the Biology of Addictive Diseases, The Rockefeller University, New York, NY, USA

Maia J. Frieser Department of Psychology and Neuroscience, University of Colorado, Boulder, Boulder, CO, USA

Institute for Behavioral Genetics, University of Colorado, Boulder, Boulder, CO, USA

Nathan A. Gillespie Department of Psychiatry, Virginia Institute for Psychiatric and Behaviour Genetics, Virginia Commonwealth University, Richmond, VA, USA

QIMR Berghofer Medical Research Institute, Brisbane, QLD, Australia

Kyle R. Kent Department of Psychology and Neuroscience, University of Colorado, Boulder, Boulder, CO, USA

Levent Kirisci Departments of Pharmaceutical Sciences and Psychiatry, University of Pittsburgh, Pittsburgh, PA, USA

Mary Jeanne Kreek Laboratory on the Biology of Addictive Diseases, The Rockefeller University, New York, NY, USA

Elad Lax Department of Molecular Biology, Ariel University, Ariel, Israel

Brion Maher Department of Mental Health, Johns Hopkins Bloomberg School of Public Health, Baltimore, MD, USA

Michael C. Neale Department of Psychiatry, Virginia Institute for Psychiatric and Behaviour Genetics, Virginia Commonwealth University, Richmond, VA, USA

Maureen D. Reynolds Pharmaceutical Sciences, University of Pittsburgh School of Pharmacy, Pittsburgh, PA, USA

Michael C. Stallings Department of Psychology and Neuroscience, University of Colorado, Boulder, Boulder, CO, USA

Institute for Behavioral Genetics, University of Colorado, Boulder, Boulder, CO, USA

Moshe Szyf Department of Pharmacology and Therapeutics, McGill University, Montreal, QC, Canada

Ralph E. Tarter Department of Pharmaceutical Sciences, School of Pharmacy, University of Pittsburgh, Pittsburgh, PA, USA

Joseph D. Terwilliger Columbia University – Department of Psychiatry, Gertrude H. Sergievsky Center, Department of Genetics and Development, New York, NY, USA

New York State Psychiatric Institute – Division of Medical Genetics, New York, NY, USA

Michael M. Vanyukov Departments of Pharmaceutical Sciences, Psychiatry, and Human Genetics, University of Pittsburgh, Pittsburgh, PA, USA

Gal Yadid Faculty of Life Sciences & The Gonda Brain Research Center, Bar-Ilan University, Ramat-Gan, Israel

Yi Zhou Daniel Virginia Institute for Psychiatric and Behavioral Genetics, Virginia Commonwealth University, Richmond, VA, USA

Part I

Substance Use: Traits and Phenotypes

1 Substance Use: Disorders and Continuous Traits

Levent Kirisci and Michael M. Vanyukov

Introduction: Traits and Genes

Genetics as pertains to human organisms deals with two related types of causality, often conflated. One is due to the genes' (specific segments of DNA) being at the inception of the biological processes, determining the *structure and function* of other biomolecules by encoding information for building and deconstructing them. This type of causes, call it type 1, is detected by biochemical and physiological research tracing the paths from the physiological function to its organ, tissue, and cell mechanics and to constituent biomolecules and the genes encoding them. The rate of the mechanistic processes and whether they occur at a particular point of pre- and postnatal development depend on the environmental input, including a possibility of a lethal one. Thus the genes determine the *norm of reaction* of the organism [1]—i.e., the distribution of all possible phenotypic values for a particular trait in an *individual* for all possible environmental conditions. Inasmuch as the norm of reaction under a set of environmental conditions includes a disorder (or even does not include a normal health status), it is the type 1 causes that are etiological.

Due to mutations that occur in the reproductive tissue, pass to the gametes, and are not incompatible with life of the future offspring, a gene may have several variants (alleles), giving rise to genetic polymorphisms in the population. These mutations, via type 1 causality, may result in structural/functional changes—e.g., when a mutation in a gene changes the amino acid sequence of the respective protein, which would correspond to a different norm of reaction rather than being neutral. Not all mutations cause those changes. The genetic code is degenerate, the term indicating that more than one coding DNA unit, a codon, a triplet of nucleotides, corresponds to a particular amino acid: there are 64 combinations of the nucleotides in the triplets, 61 of which correspond to an amino acid, but only 20 amino acids. A substitution of a nucleotide in the third position of a triplet may be inconsequential: e.g., all four possible triplets that have cytosine and thymine in the first and second positions, respectively, code for the same amino acid, lysine (the numbers of such possible synonyms vary from two to four for different amino acids). When a mutation causes a functional change, however, a gene's polymorphism may also contribute to the causes of *populational variation* in the biomolecules and, conse-

L. Kirisci (✉)
Departments of Pharmaceutical Sciences and Psychiatry, University of Pittsburgh, Pittsburgh, PA, USA
e-mail: levent@pitt.edu

M. M. Vanyukov
Departments of Pharmaceutical Sciences, Psychiatry, and Human Genetics, University of Pittsburgh, Pittsburgh, PA, USA
e-mail: mmv@pitt.edu

M. M. Vanyukov (ed.), *Genetics of Substance Use*, https://doi.org/10.1007/978-3-030-95350-8_1

quently, *may* contribute to *variation in* diverse *traits* of the organisms—from gene products to complex behaviors. This contribution is type 2 of genetic causality. This type of causes is detected statistically at the population level.

The aldehyde dehydrogenase 2 (AlDH2) gene story is especially illustrative of the differences between the two types of causality. The *ALDH2* gene, located in the long arm of chromosome 12, encodes the polypeptide sequence of that enzyme—regardless of the individual or the population. The gene is polymorphic, encoding different versions of the AlDH2 enzyme protein. The enzyme in the liver metabolizes acetaldehyde, ethanol's toxic derivative, into much less harmful acetic acid (acetate) that is then utilized by the organism. Inasmuch as the subjective experience of drinking is influenced by alcohol's noxious effect, the *ALDH2* gene *may* thus also play a role in the variation in the risk for alcoholism (alcohol use disorder, AUD), as it indeed does in the East Asian populations. In a significant proportion of these populations (e.g., Japanese), this enzyme is inactive, coded by a mutant allele of the *ALDH2* gene (*ALDH2**2). The absence of the AlDH2 activity causes an aversive response to alcohol, thus decreasing the risk for AUD [2–4].

Therefore, that physiological response influences *behavior*, decreasing the possibility of developing a pattern of excessive *alcohol use despite negative consequences* that, according to the current psychiatric classification [5], largely constitutes the disorder. In the Caucasian populations, however, there is no effect of the *ALDH2* gene on *variation* in alcohol-related behavior and thus alcohol use disorder (AUD) risk, because the *ALDH2**2 allele is absent there, while the rest of the existing allelic variants of that gene are not known to be related to strong physiological effects [6]. Hence, a gene's being a type 1 cause does not necessarily mean its being type 2 cause. To be sure, the enzyme itself as well as the gene encoding that enzyme remain part of the organismic response to alcohol and thus of alcoholism's etiology regardless of the *ALDH2* polymorphism.

Moreover, a finding that a polymorphism accounts for a proportion of phenotypic variance (ostensibly a type 2 cause) does not necessary mean that the gene, in which this polymorphism is located, is type 1 cause: the polymorphism may be only linked to the actual causal one, due to their being inherited together because of relatively close localization on the same chromosome. Alternatively, an associated polymorphism may be located in a different and less obvious than originally thought gene. For instance, the polymorphism associated with risk for alcoholism that was assigned to the dopamine D2 receptor gene (*DRD2*) [7] was later shown to be located in a different nearby gene, *ANKK1*, downstream from *DRD2* [8, 9]. Moreover, this association finding is still dubious 30 years after it was first reported [10]. The *DRD2* gene is likely mechanistically related to the organismic response to psychoactive substances, considering that the receptor is an integral part of neurobiology, but that does not mean that there should be *DRD2* polymorphisms contributing to variation in risk for using substances or becoming addicted. As discussed in this monograph by Terwilliger on the example of lactase persistency [11], the mutation may be far from the gene whose product it influences.

Importantly, most genetic research—from biometric genetics employing data on relatives (twins, adoptees, etc.) to genome-wide association studies—deals with type 2 causality, the contribution of genetic variation to phenotypic variability of traits, including risks for disorders. As noted long ago [12], when a genetic polymorphism does not appreciably contribute to variation in disorder risk on the background of all other sources of phenotypic variation (i.e., the phenotypic difference between respective genotypes is not significant), purely genetic studies are unable to discover the related type 1 etiological—structural/functional—mechanism (in that population) that does, in fact, exist.

The differences between the two types of genetic causes may seem trivial and obvious, but their conflation leads to major errors and misdirection of research effort. The lack of a trait's association with a particular gene, whether true or by error, can be wrongly taken as a proof of the *mechanistic* irrelevance of that gene and its product. However, a gene's *encoding* an element of the trait's development/manifestation mechanisms (as opposed to the trait's *variation* causes) does not necessarily entail the existence of polymorphisms in that gene that are capable of contributing to the trait's heritability (a proportion of the trait's variance that is due to genetic variation) with an effect that is detectable in genetic association studies. In fact, the lack of the detectable impact of a gene on phenotypic variation may mean that functional variation in that gene is strongly selected against because of a vital role of the gene's functioning in a specific range. This is why genes' strong effects on variation in disorder risk, as in the risks for so-called genetic diseases, are relatively rare. In contrast, individual genes' contributions to variation in "complex" traits, including risks for psychiatric disorders where there is no clear division between the ailment and the norm, are small. In other words, for complex (i.e., most non-Mendelian) traits, existing variants of a gene are not related to considerable phenotypic differences: the average phenotypic values (risks) of the carriers of different genotypes for that polymorphism are very similar.

It follows that the genes' necessary involvement in a trait's development/manifestation (there is no other program for that development but genetic) does not necessarily entail even a significant heritability of the trait (a proportion of phenotypic variance that is due to genetic variation). Nonetheless, estimates of heritability, based usually on biometric genetic (e.g., twin) studies, are often misinterpreted as *mechanistic* genetic effects ("influence") *on the trait or a phenotype* rather than on phenotypic variation, e.g., that "disorders have [or do not have] a considerable genetic component" or "the risk of a particular psychiatric disorder is [or is not] under a degree of genetic influence, and to some extent allow us to quantify the degree of this influence" [13]. From that, the confusion extends into "debate… as to whether these genes are involved at all," exactly the error discussed in the above paragraph. The expectation of "progressing to a deeper understanding of the biology of psychiatric disorder, moving from genetic variant, to gene, to the neurons and neuronal circuitry associated with the disorder" [13] is flawed because it results from the conflation of the two types of causality, mechanistic vs. statistical. It has been noted [14] that this confusion, a leap from understanding that the genes underlie mechanistically any trait to the conclusion that there must be actionable etiologically relevant variation in genes, persists even among professional geneticists. If a genetic polymorphism accounts for a proportion of trait variance, the respective locus may have some mechanistic involvement in the trait—unless, as it often happens, this polymorphism is a marker of another, functional, polymorphism, or the association is spurious.

Large proportions of complex traits' heritabilities remain unaccounted for by known genetic polymorphisms. Nevertheless, that so-called "missing" (or "hidden") heritability should not have been a reason for geneticists to be "flummoxed" [15] as they should have expected that—because of a large number of genetic and non-genetic variables, interacting among themselves and the environment, on the very long way from the genome to a complex trait, such as risk for addiction. Even if the genetic variance in disorder risk (i.e., heritability) were fully accounted for by concrete genetic variants, and, as it is for many monogenic disorders, that variance were due to very large genetic effects, it might not bring us closer to solving the related health problem. For instance, despite the knowledge of such mechanisms, prevention and treatment of monogenic disorders remain the exceptions, not the rule.

For complex *disorders* such as addiction, the situation is further complicated by the difficulty in assigning an "etiological" role to an allele associated with risk increase. Such a role implies an *abnormality*, which is hardly applicable to something that is present at virtually the same level in unaffected individuals, barely changing average risk (as indicated by the small effect sizes of genetic associations) and thus by itself quite "normal." This militates against deriving disease causation from an association—e.g., as in the "reward deficiency syndrome" [16]. This designation was based on ascribing a causal role to a single polymorphism in a gene that, as noted above, was probably misidentified as *DRD2* [9] and thus interpreted as a "dysfunction" of the dopaminergic system, in numerous behavioral disorders from various substance addictions to attention deficit hyperactivity disorder, obesity, and Tourette's syndrome. Indeed, while it is tempting to identify a singular cause, genetic or otherwise, of a range of complex human behaviors, caution is needed when such data are presented. All behavioral traits, including their extreme values often designated as disorders, have ultimately the same foundation, the brain, and thus share sources of variation in the brain function as contributors to these traits' variances, including common variation mechanisms in risks for behavioral/psychiatric disorders. Nonetheless, these variants do not amount to a *defect* rendering, e.g., substance use disorder a "genetic disease."

The small genetic effects also rule out a gene-related "corrective" action, whatever it might be, especially considering the high possibility of inadvertent consequences thereof, as recently exemplified by the potentially shortened life expectancy of the babies whose genomes were edited in order to make them HIV-resistant [17]. Moreover, the "risk" allele for one disorder outcome may "flip-flop" into a *resistance* (e.g., "protective") allele for another unwanted outcome (e.g., [18, 19]) or under different sets of genetic and non-genetic conditions (epistasis and gene-environment interaction). The genes have many pleiotropic effects in numerous systems of the organism. At least 90% of the genes that have so far been found to be associated with any traits (in an analysis of 4155 genome-wide association scan [GWAS] results from 295 studies) are associated with multiple traits [20]. This further complicates any manipulations with genes, particularly their permanent editing as opposed to transient changes in expression. Obviously, the expression effects are mediated by the genes' products, and the above considerations pertain to those products as well.

The *ALDH2* example of a strong genetic effect on behavioral variation, particularly on psychoactive substance use that is the subject of this monograph, is rather unique. Behavior is the domain that tops the hierarchy of biological organization, functionally far removed from DNA and gene products. Behavior is determined by the entire complexity of mechanisms from genes through bio/neurochemistry and the structure and physiology of the nervous system and the entire organism, with the environmental inputs at all levels, from RNA gene expression to conscious behavioral decisions. All these mechanisms are nonuniform among the individuals in the population, giving rise to behavioral variation. With so many sources of variation, behavioral traits are continuous rather than discrete/categorical.

While supporting the existence of the individual organism as a biological unit by addressing its needs, behavior in humans as social animals is also an essential part of human sociality. Behavioral traits, like all others, evolve via direct Darwinian selection of individual phenotypes. At the same time, the society, which is composed of those phenotypes, is an active component of selection mechanisms, being itself an important part of human environment. Among numerous other influences, this involves the society's establishing *limits* to the phenotypic ranges of behavioral traits, in various ways encouraging or, more often, discouraging their extremes. The ends of the distribution of a behavioral trait in humans as a social species, *statistically* far deviating from the mode, have often been perceived/classified as behavioral deviance and suppressed via those limits, thus also maintaining their low frequency. As humans are not eusocial animals (those with hard-wired social roles like communal bees), these limits themselves undergo changes that arise and unfold at a rate that is often much higher than that of the evolutionary changes of underlying biological mechanisms.

While a selection factor, the societal contribution also does not always serve to augment adaptation. As noted by Darwin [21, p. 99],

> [t]he judgment of the community will generally be guided by some rude experience of what is best in the long run for all the members; but this judgment will not rarely err from ignorance and from weak powers of reasoning. Hence the strangest customs and superstitions, in complete opposition to the true welfare and happiness of mankind, have become all-powerful throughout the world.

On the other hand, asymmetric societal restrictions on certain phenotypes, which are at an extreme of a behavioral trait's distribution and related to harming oneself or others, may and often do have straightforward benefits. For instance, while aggression has had diverse functions in humans (e.g., corresponding to its eight "recognized principal forms" [22, p. 242]), individual aggression is often discouraged in human societies, as is the existence of non-sanctioned aggressive/violent groups. Where extreme behavioral phenotypes are detected, the society attempts to approach them from the moral/legal (codified morality) and/or medical aspects, with respective tools that vary across time and populations.

Substance use is one of the many human behavioral traits that in their upper extreme manifestations present multiplicity of problems, both social and personal, sometimes incompatible with life. Both moral and medical aspects of the societal approach to these problems, often in a conflicting fashion, have been applied to them and are reflected in the related trait and extreme phenotype definitions. The latter are continually changing—not necessarily for the better from either individual or social viewpoints. These definitions are critical for identifying and analyzing appropriate variables, influencing causal inference and thus their practical utility. That particularly concerns genetic variables applied in the analysis of substance use. This chapter reviews concepts and phenotypic characteristics involved in this research area, provides alternative perspectives, and finishes with a statistical case analysis of the content of the most commonly used phenotypic formulation pertaining to substance use, the symptoms of substance use disorder.

Substance Use and Substance Use Disorder

Substance Use Initiation and Gateway/"Staging" Hypothesis/Theory

Psychoactive substances are frequently viewed from the perspective of a ready analogy with other environmental factors that are related to health problems as causal agents. That is exemplified by the use of the "epidemic" terminology that is common for infectious diseases but unique among mental disorders to which addictions are assigned. Since drugs are also related to human agents, their suppliers, the "war on drugs" has been fought with engagement of actual armed forces, let alone law enforcement. Interdiction, however, including its milder forms such as age limitations for alcohol, nicotine products, and now marijuana in the states where it is legalized, is needed only inasmuch as there is demand for these substances.

It would thus seem logical to focus on what creates that demand, in order to prevent its harmful consequences. Interdiction, to be sure, addresses supply instead. To a large degree, this is due to the domination of the attractively simple idea that barring supply, particularly that of the illicit substances whose use precedes the development of the most severe effects of substance use, can preclude that development. After rescinding the 18th Amendment, when support for this idea had been undermined, it was regained in a new form by reviewing the users of the so-called hard drugs, heroin and cocaine, and the substances they *have used before* arriving to those drugs.

Psychoactive substance *use* is usually initiated with substances that are licit—typically (in the USA) tobacco and alcohol or increasingly socially acceptable marijuana—then proceeding, *if ever*, to the "harder" ones (i.e., illicit, more difficult to obtain, less socially acceptable, more difficult to administer, and perceived as more dangerous). Unsurprisingly, "hard-drug" users have thus typically used "softer" substances, particularly cannabis. This observation, while neglecting the fact that the majority of marijuana, alcohol, or tobacco users never start using hard drugs, has given rise to a common *post hoc ergo propter hoc* logical error, inferring causality from a temporal sequence, i.e., that use of softer substances causes use of harder drugs. Since the 1970s, owing mainly to works of Denise Kandel [23] and colleagues [24–30], this has been represented by the "gateway theory" (GT). The 1930s predecessor of the GT, the "stepping-stone theory," despite lacking empirical evidence and thus being ideological rather than scientific, was even more categorical in its deterministic claim of drug use progression. In turn, the latter was akin to the "road to ruin" of a century before, which road was due to the *Gin Lane*'s "pernicious effects of British Spirits" [31], dramatically depicted by William Hogarth's engravings—in contrast to the "health and gladness" of the *Beer Street*.

The GT uses the term "stages" for the consecutive initiation of use of various substances—when the sequence of initiation complies with the "gateway" template (generally, from licit to illicit substances). The numerous exceptions to that template, including its reversals, are dismissed as "errors" [23] and the like. The "stages" are defined in a circular fashion: a stage is reached when a certain substance is used but the substance is used when a certain stage is reached. This renders the "stages" identical with substances and implies no mechanism underlying this presumably developmental sequence, in contrast to the common notion of biological developmental stages.

When attempting to avoid straightforward causal statements, the GT nonetheless implies causality by conditioning "later" (harder substance) "stages" on passing through the earlier (softer) ones [32]. Obviously, without specified causal connections, the concept of "gateway" is opaque and its meaning is unclear, and so it has remained for a long time (e.g., "[t]he notion of a Gateway drug itself is vague" by Kandel's own admission [27, p. 7]). Originally, the queueing of the substances tried, the essence of the GT, was explained by a brief cautious sentence, "[t]hese sequences are probably culturally determined" [24].

More recently, however, the GT proponents have progressed to stronger causal statements, defining the "gateway drug" role of specific substances (alcohol, nicotine, and marijuana [28, 30]) as "a drug that lowers the threshold for addiction to other agents" [28]. This causal mechanism was ostensibly buttressed by the finding that giving *mice* nicotine for a week results in their greater conditional place preference and locomotor response to the combination of nicotine and cocaine [30]. The 7-day nicotine pretreatment almost doubled the effect of cocaine, while the reversal of conditions, i.e., pretreatment by cocaine, had no effect on *nicotine*-induced locomotion. Nonetheless, while the cocaine effect was far from "amplified many times," as D. Kandel later claimed in her interview [33], it is unclear what the latter experiment proves. Nicotine, according to the same study, has no effect on murine locomotion, in contrast to cocaine; hence it could not be "amplified" by cocaine pretreatment. More importantly, the synergism of nicotine and cocaine after nicotine pretreatment in mice has little to do with "addictive behavior" that the authors allude to. The GT has relevance neither to those data, as it deals with *volitional human* rather than *laboratory murine* behavior, nor to addiction, as the GT does not make claims about substance use beyond the order of its initiation with various substances (which is far from invariant). Buried in the small print of "References and Notes" in Kandel's original *Science* article introducing the GT [23], there is a caveat, never modified, that the "stages" pertain only to substance use initiation rather than progression of involvement and severity.

In other words, the GT has no clinical meaning in humans, while the "staging," its essence, is not an observable behavior in mice. It is also certain that drugs change the organism's response to themselves and to other substances; these changes, however, are not identical to disorder. Addiction is a behavioral pattern of drug pursuit rather than the physiological reaction that, "although it may occur among addicts, … is quite distinct from compulsive drug-seeking behavior" [34, p. 764]. In fact, the data on involvement with various substances contradict expectations that would follow from the GT, with its implied or stated causality and the notion of a "gateway drug." For instance, the overall level of illicit drug use does not depend on access to the purported gateway substances, whether alcohol/tobacco or cannabis, as would be expected if the GH were true. The queuing of substances is often reversed relative to the GT "stages" [35–37], in contrast to any biological staging process. The "gateway" role of alcohol is refuted by the evidence that whereas the aldehyde dehydrogenase deficiency is related to lower rates of drinking, it does not predict lower rates of non-alcohol substance use [38]. Interventions that are not directed at drugs specifically and significantly reduce the risk for use of illicit drugs exert that effect without changing the risk for use of alcohol and marijuana, the supposed "gateway" substances [39].

High phenotypic and genetic correlations between risks for specific drug addictions are parsimoniously accounted for by common mechanisms of variation, whereas any queuing is readily explained by the differential opportunities [40, 41] and behavioral barriers for use of different drugs. For instance, it is much more difficult in the USA to start using substances with heroin injections than with cannabis, which has very low perceived attendant harm, is widely available, and is now decriminalized and legalized in a number of states. Hence, contrary to the gateway theorists' claim that involvement with various classes of drugs "is not opportunistic but follows definite pathways" [42, p. 3], the sequence merely reflects what is accessible at the least personal cost in a particular environment/population, perhaps including the cultural traditions alluded to by D. Kandel [23]. For instance, marijuana is likely to be the first illicit drug offered to the non-initiated person in the USA (but not in Japan, where overall frequency of cannabis use is low [43]) not only because it is likelier to be available than another substance but also because it is likelier to be accepted by a novice than, for instance, intravenous heroin. Once substance use is initiated, however, it may remain under control and be limited to experimentation or episodic/moderate use, or it may proceed to wider and deeper involvement, including that with other substances, and to a behavior described as addiction as well as physiological changes that contribute to maintaining it.

The initiation of use of multiple drugs, if a polydrug career occurs, is thus spread over time. In that case, common risk variation mechanisms are illustrated by the comparison with the sequence of chickenpox and shingles, due to a common cause [44]. Polydrug use is a rule among users [45], contributing to correlations among risks for respective disorders. As determined in biometrical genetic studies, there is low to no substance-specific variance underlying addiction diagnoses [46]—aside from the licit/illicit groupings [47], i.e., those related to the behavioral response to societal norms.

As noted, the GT provides no explanation for drug use behavior, its initiation, or the transitions between the "stages." Interestingly in this connection, the paper by Kandel and Faust [24], published virtually simultaneously with Kandel's *Science* article but with a more detailed literature review, not only presents the same data but also cites, albeit with no discussion, publications preceding their work that do suggest such an explanation. Thus, the 1972 article by Whitehead et al. [48] preempted the entire "gateway" line of reasoning. Namely, it points out that while "[t]he clearest datum that emerges from studies of drug use is that those who use *any* one drug are more likely to use any other drug than those who do not use that drug" (p. 179; emphasis added), the fact that "overwhelming majority of heroin addicts used marijuana prior to heroin… tells us nothing about those who have used marijuana but have not progressed to heroin and other opiates… [n]either does it tell us anything about the etiology of the process of going from marijuana to heroin" (p. 181). The article notes that the association between marijuana and opiate use *among marijuana users* is much weaker and inconsistent among different population groups than that association *among opiate users*. Obviously, since the frequency of opioid use is lower than that of marijuana use, fewer individuals *start* using opioids *in general*—not just using more seldom opioids before marijuana. The authors also observe that the cause for multiple drug use and "multihabituation" may be "socio-legal" and psychological (e.g., promoted by group drug *subculture*) rather than pharmacological. An even more effective interpretation of multiple drug use, mentioned as well only in passing by Kandel and Faust, was provided by Johnston in his 1973 book [49]. He concludes that there exists a "general propensity" (p. 52) to drug use, "a basic personality characteristic which can be described as a propensity to use (or avoid the use of) psychoactive substances" (p. 230).

This viewpoint, consistent with the notion of nonspecific "problem behavior" [50] that was called by Kandel the "fundamental theoretical antithesis" to the GT perspective ([51], p. 68), has received further development based on the long-standing concept of *liability to disorder* developed in human genetics [52], discussed further in this chapter. Although the GT proponents have later claimed that this concept is "complementary" to the GT [28], there are indeed substantial differences between them. One is that the liability perspective, in contrast to GT, does include addictions. To reiterate, the GT only describes the queuing of use initiation for various substances (in some populations) and, nowadays, tries to find support for causality with animal models [28, 53] that are hardly adequate for human substance-related behavior [54]. Another important distinction is that the liability perspective, in contrast to the GT, allows identification of traits and phenotypes pertaining to substance use that are amenable to genetic and other mechanistic research. Tellingly and understandably, the purported GT "stages" have *not* been used as target phenotypes in genetic research.

Human Substance Use Behavior

Substance use is a complex trait in many respects. On its surface, regardless of possible concomitant health problems, it is often an illegal behavior. It is thus by definition beyond the boundaries allowed by the society, which sets limits to the consumption of various substances that are often arbitrary, changeable, and inconsistent. There is no natural pale delimiting legal and illegal substance use. Nonetheless, once established, the societal boundaries determine the behavior barriers that need to be overstepped to engage in illegal substance use, including the use of licit substances (alcohol and nicotine, and marijuana in some states while still completely banned by federal law) before a legal age. In turn, these barriers likely contribute to the well-known association of substance use with antisocial behavior, since different levels of the personal acceptance of social norms are involved in behaviors that comply with or violate those norms. This renders illicit substance and excessive alcohol use an attribute/facet of what is variably termed externalizing psychopathology, disinhibition, and dysregulation [55–59]. As tobacco smoking's social acceptance and prevalence have been decreasing—to the degree that cannabis, classified Schedule I (i.e., illicit according to federal law [60]), is perceived by adolescents as less risky than cigarettes [61]—tobacco smoking's association with psychopathology has been strengthening as well [62]. Moreover, as genetic studies show, the differences in social norms regarding drugs, an *environmental* factor, influence the structure of correlations between risks for addictions to different substances—not only at the phenotypic but also at the *genetic* level, with stronger relationships within than between the groups of disorders based on the substance legality, licit vs. illicit [47].

An important characteristic of substance use is that, outside of pain therapy (and even there an option of a non-addictive treatment does often exist [63]), it is a voluntary behavior that is well known to be multi-system pathogenic and to frequently lead to personal and social degradation. These effects differ across substances and individuals: alcohol, for instance, while addictive and harmful at high consumption levels, has been a food component for millennia. Although less valuable than other nutrients from the purely nutritional viewpoint [64], at moderate consumption levels by adults it has been associated with increased longevity and lower age-related cognitive impairment and morbidity [65, 66]. Abuse of alcohol as an euphoriant rather than a food item is thus akin to abuse of other foods in overeating, a pathogenic extension of a vital behavior. It may result in multiple physiological changes, possibly including transition of brain energy supply from glucose- to alcohol-derived acetate [67]. In contrast, consumption of other addictive substances, particularly illicit ones, is with no nutritional value, purely recreational, in "pursuit of happiness" (a positive affect change) by knowingly and consciously wrong, harmful, and/or excessive means. Even when other benefits are mentioned—e.g., health benefits in arguing for legalization of marijuana—those are of less importance as motivators of use, as attested by proponents of legalization themselves (e.g., [68]).

The legality of substances, which is currently based on contradictory federal and state laws, is an important determinant of drug behavior. The social permissibility of use of various substances varies across populations, cultures, and time. The history of Prohibition in the USA, an important period in the formation of relevant behavioral boundaries, is often used as an argument for drug legalization. This argument, however, is as anachronistic as the recent fad of removing memorials to figures of the short American history and applying contemporary moral standards to personages of 200 years back, whereby Thomas Jefferson becomes little more than a slaver. By those standards, virtually none of the ancient authors should be read any longer, as all of them were slave owners, and Leo Tolstoy, Ivan Turgenev, and Alexander Pushkin should be erased from the pedestals and school curricula as owners of serfs, slaves bound to landowners' estates. To be sure, any event in the past can and should be viewed from the standpoint of the current set of morals—to evaluate whether any progress is achieved. That contemporary set, however, cannot be unconditionally used for retroactive judgment replacing the historic one and should include the requirement of considering both moral failures and achievements of an individual in his own historic context. It is in surpassing the prevailing coterminous morality and reaching for the moral ideal where one's outstanding virtue may be found, not in compliance with the rules of later modernity that themselves may indeed be quite far from that ideal. Neither ideology, nor circumstances, nor methods of Prohibition are applicable to the present.

Second, it has been noted that "Prohibition," the culmination of a century-old temperance movement, is a misnomer [69]. The National Prohibition Act (the official name of the Volstead Act that implemented the 18th Amendment) did not prohibit production for sacramental and medicinal use, and personal alcohol possession, use, stockpiling, and limited home production ("nonintoxicating cider and fruit juices"—the term "nonintoxicating," defined by the Volstead Act as containing less than 0.5% alcohol, was successfully challenged in court). The ban thus was not absolute, as it is now with Schedule I drugs (at least at the federal level). *Third*, while in force, Prohibition did not fail entirely. All the negative consequences of alcohol use sharply decreased immediately after its enactment and did not rise to the prior high levels long after that [70].

Alcohol history is also no argument for legalization because, despite that history's long span, the problems related to alcohol are still rampant. Whereas it could be argued whether cannabis or other drugs should or should not have been originally banned, their legalization would *add* to the existing social and health problems with legal substances rather than alleviate any. It can hardly be expected that lifting drug prohibition barriers would turn the violent criminals and drug dealers into law-abiding citizens. Whereas substance use is a behavior for which the individual is ultimately responsible, legalization is a potent environmental factor directly influencing that behavior by facilitating availability of a psychoactive substance and, indirectly, resulting in changes in societal attitudes and lowering barriers to substance use in general.

As any behavioral excesses by individuals, especially those legally barred, meet societal opprobrium, so do illicit substance abuse, addiction, and their health and social consequences. The deviance of the behavioral cause creates additional complexities in dealing with its effects, raising barriers to users' access to professional help and exacerbated by their involvement with groups where antisocial behavior is normative. On the other hand, within the mainstream society, its negative attitude toward substance use is protective against it. It is likely that the increasingly negative change of the societal attitude to smoking has resulted in its dramatic decrease from the 1960s [32, 71, 72]. The dual status of substance use as a legal and health problem creates additional inconsistencies furthered by both legal contradictions (e.g., between federal and state laws in regard to cannabis and its products) and the specifics of the medical classification of substance use. The latter, pertaining to the diagnostic approach, deserves special attention here, as it concerns the phenotypes that are objects of genetic research.

Diagnoses and Systematics

Humans are fond of categorizing. It must be gratifying when an entity can be put on a certain shelf, even when both are imaginary. As noted by John Stuart Mill [73],

> The tendency was always strong to believe that whatever receives a name must be an entity or being, having an independent existence of its own; and if no real entity answering to the name could be found, men did not for that reason suppose that none existed, but imagined that it was something peculiarly abstruse and mysterious, too high to be an object of sense.

The categorizing tendency, starting with binary categories, probably originates from the times when threats from the phenomena, objects, and persons (groups included) had to be quickly identified, to either eliminate or flee from. As with many evolutionary adaptations, there are both gains and losses associated with that, the former hopefully prevailing for it to be, indeed, an adaptation. It is also possible that what has been an adaptation under one set of conditions turns into its opposite under another. It makes sense to consider the utility of diagnoses and their alternatives as targets of genetic research.

The variety of psychoactive substances, differing in routes of administration, physiological effects, and addictive potential, represents one of the aspects reflected in the nosology. The diagnoses are mostly guided by the versions of two systems, currently the American Psychiatric Association's Diagnostic and Statistical Manual, DSM-5 [5], commonly in the USA, and the World Health Organization's The International Classification of Diseases and Related Health Problems, ICD-11 [74] (the hyphenated numbers following the acronyms correspond to the editions). The substance use disorders are organized by chemical classes and (in the ICD) by pharmacologic modality. The substances, however, are often used concurrently, including those with opposite pharmacological effects, such as depressants and stimulants.

Although diagnoses are substance-specific, i.e., assigned according to the substances used, they are largely based on the same behavioral patterns that are reflected in the application of the same symptoms to substance-specific disorders. All these patterns essentially denote the same phenotype, *persistent use despite various negative consequences*, i.e., the characteristics of behavior rather than of the substances (in fact, mental disorders are generally described as *behavioral patterns* in the DSM). This is one likely reason why these characteristics are highly correlated, indicating a single dimension [75] corresponding to their shared variance.

This is also the justification that has inaccurately been noted as lacking in the analyses of the addiction symptomatology from the latent trait viewpoint [76]. In a simple unidimensional latent trait model, the partial regressions of the symptoms/diagnostic criteria on the latent variable indeed contain respective error terms. That does not mean, contrary to the cited article, that "the distinctive features of each criteria… are actually irrelevant to the model." First, the path coefficients (partial regression coefficients; factor loadings) are different for each criterion. Second, not only are alternative models supposed to be tested in order to arrive, if at all, to that simplest factor analytic model, but those alternatives will include at least testing whether error terms are correlated, implying symptom- or symptom-group-specific sources of variance or absence thereof, in addition to the common variance represented by the factor. Moreover, bi-factor models, as the one presented in this chapter (see the case analysis section below), have been consistently shown to fit well the data where symptoms for various substances, which as a rule are used concurrently [45], are analyzed, reflecting both common (general, non-substance-specific) and substance-specific liabilities [47, 75, 77–79].

We are not taking herein a position in the long-standing dispute regarding whether psychiatric conditions can be properly classified as diseases (e.g., see a collection of arguments relevant to addictions in a special journal issue [80]). Nonetheless, from the standpoint of the amenability of phenotypic definitions to genetic analysis, it is worth noting that even according to the DSM (fourth edition), "no definition adequately specifies precise boundaries for the concept of 'mental disorder'" ([81], p. xxi). The current iteration, DSM-5, has that statement modified into "no definition can capture all aspects of all disorders in the range contained in DSM-5" [5, p. 20], but the definition that follows, that it is a "syndrome" of "clinically significant disturbance," does not clarify the boundary issue either. It may well be that "no definition of which we are aware adequately specifies precise boundaries for the concept of *non*-psychiatric medical disorder either" ([82], p. 1763; emphasis added), but it would be illogical to ignore the problem just because it may exist in other conditions as well.[1]

A distinct objective boundary is absent between the *disorder* and those substance use patterns that do not qualify for a psychiatric diagnosis. This argues against drawing addiction to a "brain disease" [83], in which a person is deprived of choice ("it's not a choice to take the drug" [84]) by "the disruption of the areas of the circuits that enables us to exert free will" [84]. These statements are contradicted, e.g., by the data on opiate-addicted Vietnam veterans, the overwhelming majority of whom were not readdicted upon their return stateside [85, 86]. Far from the inevitability of drug abuse's continuing until death once started, as would be expected for a chronic brain disease, in many cases individuals with addiction—treated as well as without medical treatment—have been capable to wean themselves off drugs and maintain sobriety, termed "maturing out" [87]. This ability, exemplified by high-profile recoveries from long-term addictions to crack cocaine [88] and to opioids [89], is reflected in a statement after a decade of sobriety, explaining the cause of quitting as "[m]aybe it's God; maybe it's our conscience" [89].

The notion of substance addiction as being almost hopelessly refractory may have resulted from clinicians' dealing often with hard cases [90]. For the general population, the lifetime probability of remission from DSM-IV dependence ("finally stopped" having dependence criteria) was estimated at 84% for nicotine, 91% for alcohol, 97% for cannabis, and 99% for cocaine [91]—the high proportions that are contrary to those expected from the "epidemic" perspective or for any chronic diseases. Although the true probabilities may be lower due to the latter survey study's limitations, the figures are sufficiently strong to question the finality of the diagnosis. Importantly, time to remission for half of the cases was much longer for legal substances (26 years for nicotine and 14 years for alcohol, reaching their respective ceiling after 50 years of age) than for illegal drugs (6 years for cannabis and 5 years for cocaine, with respective ceilings at about 40 years of age). This suggests that the stronger legal/social pressure provides an additional incentive to quit, which is consciously acted on.

In addition to the definition/diagnostic problems shared with other mental disorders, addictions also have complexities of their own. For instance, the DSM-5 SUD criteria include withdrawal and tolerance, but not when a substance "is taken solely under appropriate medical supervision" ([5], e.g., opioids, p. 541). Numerous combinations of symptoms correspond to the same categorical diagnosis of SUD with slightly varying small number of categories. The combinations themselves change approximately every decade. For instance, SUD diagnosis according to DSM-5 is positive when any 2 or more out of 11 symptoms are observed in a 12-month period, with hundreds of possible combinations and with 3 possible severity levels based on the number of symptoms reported. In DSM-IV, the prior classification, there were two SUD diagnostic catego-

[1] Without delving into the differences between distributions of continua (of liability—see below) for mental disorder and, e.g., infectious diseases, the former would likely be unimodal and assumed normal (Gaussian) while the latter bimodal (the uninfected, with no disease, and the infected, with some distribution of severity around the mean, from no disorder to its severest form).

ries, abuse and dependence, with no severity levels. Implicitly, however, dependence followed abuse as more severe, because when symptoms for both were present, only the dependence diagnosis was made while the abuse diagnosis required the absence of a prior history of dependence [92]. The dependence diagnosis was thus inclusive of abuse. In DSM-5, that inclusion was simplified into a unitary diagnosis of SUD, with both groups of symptoms combined, plus "craving" and minus "legal problems."

It is noteworthy that withdrawal and tolerance, included among the diagnostic criteria, are physiological manifestations rather than behavioral pattern symptoms. In DSM-IV, these two symptoms were among the criteria for the more severe form of the disorder, "dependence." Although from the clinical viewpoint the physiological symptoms are part of the disorder syndrome, they present problems from the biological and statistical perspectives. Biologically, tolerance and withdrawal are part of normal physiological responses to long-term exposure to psychoactive substances. These responses do not per se *determine* or constitute human behavior—even if they make repeated consumption and the addiction diagnosis more likely, incentivizing use when present. As emphasized by the National Institute on Drug Abuse, "[u]nlike tolerance and physical dependence, addiction develops more slowly than these physiological responses" [93]. The distinction of the disorder, which is persistent drug-seeking *behavior*, from the physiological response [34] that may contribute to this behavior as a mechanism, militates against the use of this response as a diagnostic criterion. An unwelcome corollary to the diagnostical use of physiological symptoms including craving, another part of the physiological syndrome that has become a diagnostic criterion in DSM-5, is that clinicians "assume that this means addiction" and "patients requiring additional pain medication are made to suffer" and "may forgo proper treatment because of the fear of dependence" [34]. A physiological symptom is similarly misapplied when it is proposed to be used for "[p]redicting optimal dose [of an opioid medication] for each individual" for the "clinician to provide carefully the dose to each individual patient's needs" [94]. Indicators of physiological dependence (craving in the latter study) have nothing to do with the patient's needs for which the medication is used, likely pain treatment, and can be dealt with separately.

The objectively identified and measured biological characteristics are often applied to reify the psychiatric nomenclature by reducing behavior to its biological correlates, shifting the plane of consideration to lower levels of biological organization. Reification is assured: since diagnoses dichotomize, however imprecisely, the dimensions underlying the symptoms, any lower-level processes correlated with these dimensions are guaranteed to evince differences between the "norm" and the "pathology" given a large enough sample size, thus "confirming" the diagnostic classification. This is an unfailing way to label any sufficiently high range of values on a behavioral dimension a "brain disease": inasmuch as the behavior is a brain product, there will inevitably be brain biology-level differences between that high end and an appropriate control. It is thereupon concluded that "[a]dvances in neuroscience identified addiction as a chronic brain disease" [95]. It is quite possible that the correlations between the biological and behavioral phenomena are of a mechanistically causal nature, even though that is hard to prove due to limitations in experiments on human brain (with the exception of genetic associations where the directionality of the relationships is certain). Even if proven, however, that would not change the continuous distribution of the behavioral trait and does not turn addiction into a neurological disease.

We will consider the statistical perspective on the physiological symptoms in further discussion, including their analysis as indicators of SUD presented in the last part of this chapter. Here, it should be noted that the diagnostic symptoms are indicators of a valid continuous trait, a construct that can be modeled as a source of the high correlations among them. Therefore, they provide no true foundation for a binary diagnosis.

An additional complexity is imposed by the societal rules. Not only are different substances, with their specific metabolic pathways, routes of administration, and pharmacologic effects often (ab)used concurrently, a natural barrier between legal and illegal drugs is absent. The legal barriers, an environmental factor that depends on time and location, induce genetic distinctions between sources of individual variation in liabilities to specific addictions. In particular, as noted, genetic correlations among liabilities related to licit substances and among those related to illicit substances are higher than liability correlations between these two groups, thus accounted for by two correlated but distinct genetic factors [47]. While useful in clinical practice, the diagnosis, therefore, bears numerous shortcomings as a variable.

Dimensional Approaches

Research Domain Criteria (RDoC)

The inadequacy and arbitrariness of the categorical classification in psychiatric, particularly substance use, disorders has long been recognized (e.g., [96–103]). Recently, the National Institutes of Health (NIH) have also arrived to the conclusion that "[d]iagnostic categories based on clinical consensus fail to align with findings emerging from clinical neuroscience and genetics" [104]. To remedy that, a putative alternative, the Research Domain Criteria (RDoC), was conceived of by the National Institute of Mental Health (NIMH) "as a dimensional system… spanning the range from normal to abnormal" [105]. This system is said to be "agnostic about current disorder categories." Instead, it aims to "generate classifications stemming from basic behavioral neuroscience" by subdividing human psychological functioning into five "domains" or "systems" (positive valence, negative valence, cognitive, social processes, and arousal/regulatory processes), each containing "constructs" that summarize a "functional dimension of behavior," to be studied according to a matrix of "different classes of variables (or units of analysis)," including "genes, molecules, cells, neural circuits, physiology (e.g., cortisol, heart rate, startle reflex), behaviors, and self-reports." Circuits are the "core" aspect "both because they are central to the various biological and behavioral levels of analysis, and because they are used to constrain the number of constructs that are defined."

As can be seen, apart from the question whether these domains and constructs exhaustively account for human behavior, the RDoC approach indeed distances research from the medical aspect, allowing a greater freedom for biopsychological studies while retaining them within the funding purview of the NIH—particularly, the NIMH that generated the RDoC. There is little doubt that this approach better than the diagnostic system reflects the complexity of human behavior, its determination, and the sources of its variation. As a general descriptor of the organismic function, it is scientifically more adequate than the Procrustean bed of psychiatric diagnoses within the categorical confines of a DSM/ICD nomenclature.

Nevertheless, the same recasting of human behavior away from the psychiatric diagnostic scheme conflicts with the NIH mission of research in "understanding of mental, addictive and physical disorders" [106]: obviously, disorders cannot be studied without referring to the diagnosis. To serve that mission, the diagnosis would need to be incorporated into the RDoC research paradigm rather than detached from it entirely. This detachment is implied by RDoC stated diagnostic agnosticism, which in turn also contradicts the reference to the "range from normal to abnormal." Whereas the symptom *combinations* that correspond to a diagnosis, and the minimal number of symptoms that serves as a diagnostic classifier, are a matter of medical/social consensus rather than based on an objective criterion, the *symptoms* themselves are more objective, especially when assessed directly rather than self-reported. Highly correlated, they reflect a latent behavioral dimension, which, in the case of substance use disorder symptoms, is also shared across various drugs [75, 107–109], in addition to substance-specific variance components [75]. This dimension is by design unaccounted for in the RDoC. The measurement that is provided by the RDoC hierarchy matrix does not map, by design, to the behavior indicated by symptoms. Instead, this hierarchy organizes variables representing potential mechanisms, leaving out what those mechanisms are hypothesized to underlie or cause, or to whose variation they are supposed to contribute. The same pertains to all psychiatric conditions.

The RDoC is not an adequate replacement of the diagnosis also because a domain or construct cannot be treated or prevented, in contrast to symptoms. While it is debated whether substance use disorders, which largely result from the voluntary consumption of knowingly habit-forming and toxic substances, are *diseases* on a par with other chronic conditions [110–113], it is the disorders that remain the main target of intervention. Although an alternative to the diagnostic disorder classification and symptoms is needed, the RDoC is not such an alternative but a different set of variables, many pertaining to basic science, which may or may not be applied by researchers to a mental health problem. For that application, and for the resulting knowledge to be used in clinical practice, prevention, medication development, etc., the problem, under current conditions, is still going to be diagnosed categorically, using symptoms.

Liability as a Trait

There is, however, an alternative to the categorical medical classification that does allow research to remain aligned with the dimension indicated by the symptoms, while avoiding the shortcomings of the diagnostic dichotomization, and to account for the various conceptualizations of addiction as well as related findings. In principle, consistent adoption of this alternative would allow discontinuation of development of the versions of the diagnostic manuals and schemes and could place the behavioral spectrum pertaining to substances on a common scale. This alternative is provided by the concept of *liability* [52], developed in human genetics.

Liability to a disorder is a continuous latent (unobserved directly) trait underlying individual variation in the probability of the disorder's development. Liability is determined by all factors influencing this probability—genetic, epigenetic, as well as environmental and interactions thereof. A point on the liability scale termed the threshold, which divides the affected and unaffected areas of the distribution—e.g., addiction phenotypes from the nonaddicted ones,—is defined by a set of diagnostic symptoms. For complex (non-Mendelian) disorders such as addiction, with continuous liability distributions, the threshold as a point is a statistical abstraction, summarizing a range of liability values, as there are hundreds of symptom combinations qualifying as a positive diagnosis, which nonetheless is mappable onto the liability scale. The diagnostic symptoms of substance use disorder, mostly characterizing behavior in response to the presence of psychoactive substances in the environment, are themselves dichotomous representations of continuous variation in the severity of each of these respective behaviors, with a zero-inflated distribution in the general population, and with drug users and those deemed affected comprising the truncated tail of the liability distribution above the respective thresholds. The concept of a continuous trait with a loosely defined threshold obviates the need to classify the suprathreshold addiction phenotype as a disease, which is a matter of substantial argument (e.g., [80]). The search for mechanisms influencing variation in liability is unbiased by such ideological assumptions.

More precisely defined than similarly used "vulnerability," "susceptibility," and "diathesis," liability is a trait (variable) that is measurable. The liability concept can be extended to any identifiable outcome phenotype (e.g., liability to substance use initiation, to using a particular substance, to developing a particular characteristic such as withdrawal, etc.). If liability is quantified on a numerical scale of an index (e.g., as intelligence, another latent trait, is measured by using IQ), a threshold value or a range of liability index values could replace the categorical diagnosis for medical needs. That index would also enable quantitative assessment of subdiagnostic phenotypes and of severity of the disorder.

For non-Mendelian disorders (i.e., those where *variation of liability in the population* is not due to mutations in a single gene but rather results from multiple factors, genetic and non-genetic), the liability distribution is likely normal—according to the central limit theorem of statistics, considering the large number of variables contributing to liability variation. It is for these disorders, termed polygenic, multifactorial, or complex, that the liability concept was originally developed. In principle, it is applicable to Mendelian disorders as well, with the difference that the distributions of liabilities to those conditions are (more or less) discrete rather than continuous, as the norm and pathology classes correspond to genotypes for a single gene, with a natural gap(s) between them. In reality, the number of factors involved in liability variation, genetic or otherwise, is seldom if ever limited to one. In addition to genocopies (similar strong phenotypic effects of variants of different genes/loci) and phenocopies (non-genetic effects similar to strong genetic ones), variants of different factors with smaller effects, genetic or non-genetic, may combine to produce the same/similar phenotype.

As supported by theoretical considerations and empirical data, regardless of the order of initiation, the entire process of drug use development—from the first exposure to psychoactive substances to the development of addiction or its absence—is driven by the mechanisms subsumed under liability [32, 101]. Although there is certainly specificity in the organismic response to specific drugs, due to the differences in their administration, biotransformation, and neurobiological response, the mechanisms comprising general (common) liability to addiction account for a substantial part of drug action and overlap with those underlying behavior regulation, socialization, and other consummatory/appetitive behaviors. These common liability mechanisms explain high polydrug use and comorbidity as well as high genetic correlations among not only liabilities to various drug-specific addictions but also these liabilities' correlations with numerous characteristics of those general psychological domains. In contrast to the prevention corollary of the "gateway hypothesis," which calls for restricting access specifically to nicotine and alcohol as the beginning stage of the "gateway" substance use initiation sequence, "prevention within the CLA framework emphasizes deployment of interventions beginning in early childhood that could potentiate normative socialization" [114]. The reoccurring "epidemics" related to specific substances, such as the current opioid one, are manifestations of CLA, the background to substance-specific physiological and behavioral adaptations.

For the complex disorders such as addiction, it is assumed and has been proven that liability variation is contributed by numerous polymorphisms in the genes encoding structural and functional components of the nervous system as well as by diverse environmental factors capable of modulating behavior and its development. Like other latent traits, liability can potentially be measured using its observable indicators. To measure, e.g., the latent trait of intelligence, certain tasks of different difficulty and quality, a priori related to intellectual abilities, are used to enable coverage of the trait's distribution. Liability, however, is more difficult to estimate. Measurement employing the symptoms cannot be applied to the asymptomatic *majority* population regardless of how close the individual is to the threshold. There are no face-valid indicators of liability in the asymptomatic area of the liability distribution. Absent the symptoms, which are indicators of disorder severity that can be scaled into an interval variable (or levels of severity as specified for addiction in DSM-5, i.e., "mild," "moderate," and "severe"), the "norm," the larger portion of the distribution, is undifferentiated, collapsed into one phenotypic class.

Despite having been for quite a long time the prevailing conceptualization of complex psychiatric disorders including addiction [97, 115–117], the liability framework has still not been consistently implemented in most psychiatric and addiction research—neither in conducting it nor in its interpretation. This particularly concerns using it in analyzing putatively etiologic mechanisms. Virtually none among the multiple studies performing genetic association analysis, including large scale GWASs, employs continuous indices of liability. Instead, the crude diagnostic definitions, incomparably less precise than genotyping methods, are most often used. The interpretation of research findings, due to either the lack of insight into their biological meaning or the use of scientific lingo, is also frequently misleading. For instance, an association of a biological variable (e.g., a genetic polymorphism or enzyme activity) with a binary diagnosis is reported as a proof of a role of the respective gene or the enzyme in the disorder—instead of that variable's accounting for some portion of variance in (dichotomized) liability. Indeed, as noted in the Introduction and explained in more detail below, the absence of such an association does not mean that the gene/enzyme does not play a role in the disorder, nor does the association prove an etiological role.

Consistently applying the liability concept to etiological, including genetic, research would incur benefits from not only a greater phenotyping precision, afforded by methods of latent variable analysis, but also from using continuous rather than arbitrarily dichotomized variables. Nevertheless, while at some point considered by the National Institute on Drug Abuse in the form of applying "a framework of functional domains, similar to the NIMH RDoC framework" [118], and the arguments for implementing the dimensional perspective on substance use behavior (e.g., [102, 103], it remains largely unutilized.

Most of substance use-related research treats specific-substance use disorders as separate entities, in accordance with the clinical nomenclature (e.g., opioid use disorder, cocaine use disorder, cannabis use disorder, etc.). To characterize the use behavior/disorder severity, it is possible to use dimensional indices, such as the number of cigarettes smoked or frequency-quantity of alcohol consumption, instead of categorical diagnoses, which, in turn, may increase the probability of detecting the usually very small effects of genetic polymorphisms on substance-specific liability variation. Indeed, one of the few consistent findings in genetic studies of addiction, that of the *CHRNA5/A3/B4* gene cluster, was first obtained in relation to the number of cigarettes smoked and smoking behavior as summarized by the Fagerstrom Test for Nicotine Dependence (FTND) rather than, as stated in the publications, risk for nicotine dependence once exposed to smoking [119, 120]. This type of phenotype quantification, however, is complicated when, as is common, several substances are used concurrently.

One of the problems with genetic studies of substance-specific addictions, exemplified by these latter reports, is that not only the definition of the affected phenotype is by necessity arbitrary and wide, but the controls are often selected largely by referring to the target substance only. Ignoring other substances in defining a control group may substantially decrease the power of analysis. This is because the focus on a specific substance class, whether alcohol, cocaine, opiates, or nicotine, downplays an important phenotypic component of all substance abuse: the mechanisms of common (general; non-substance-specific) liability to addiction (CLA; GLA) [32, 79, 100, 101, 121–123]. Obviously, the liability concept can be applied to disorder related to a particular drug, or to substance use regardless of whether it is classified as pathological. Nonetheless, several lines of evidence indicate that in addition to drug-specific liabilities, there is a set of common sources of variance [32, 101, 121], expressed in high correlations among behaviors related to various substances (concurrent or consecutive use) and their consequences. Not only the symptoms pertaining to the use of a variety of specific substances demonstrate their alignment on a unidimensional trait scale [124], but research supports the existence of nonspecific, general or common liability to addiction beyond statistical abstraction.

Common liability to addiction is reflected in the shared genetic variance in liabilities to drug-specific addictions: biometric genetic studies, particularly, twin research, indicate that there is little if any substance-specific genetic variation in the variance of addiction risk [46, 77, 125]. Importantly, virtually all genetic findings in addiction so far, with a possible rule-proving exception of alcohol-specific ethanol-metabolizing enzymes, are not substance-specific either [18, 19, 126, 127], which is understandable considering that they pertain to general mechanisms of nervous system functioning. The underappreciation of common liability not only results in ensuring the reemergence of the "drug epidemic" with another substance from the endlessly growing variety of abusable chemistry but may also lead to misdirection of research, resources, and effort.

Liability Mechanisms and Biomedical Research

Illegal substances obviously call for legal measures and law enforcement. Nonetheless, although interdiction of illegal drugs is important, as is addressing any law violation, it cannot affect the main source of the problem, its behavioral component, and the motivations for it. As discussed above, recreational substance use is voluntary, in conflict with the attempts to reduce behavior to the biological mechanisms that contribute to but are not synonymous with it. Moreover, after having long used the language of *war*, with real military generals appointed to wage it as "drug czars" and the involvement of armed forces and military expeditions abroad, there is a striking inconsistency of legal drug policies and of the policy makers' positions. Just as inconsistency in parental discipline may lead to a "reinforcement trap" resulting in maintaining the child's difficult behavior [128–130], the negative measures fail under these conditions. Senators' and former presidents' statements about acceptability of illegal drugs, and states' legalizing them, are likely to be perceived by the social consciousness as defeat and surrender in that war.

Indeed, one component of the reciprocal influence between personal and social constraints is via positions taken by public figures who are widely considered role models. Such individuals may follow the risk perception trends (e.g., to gain sympathy among their constituencies/audiences) as well as contribute to their development, thus forming de facto behavioral rules. As positive role models, they give their weighty imprimatur to defying social norms they themselves defy, but promoting thereby norm violation in general, not only a specific opposite behavior, inasmuch as certain behaviors are correlated (e.g., antisocial behavior with substance use). In effect, a formerly societally disapproved behavior then may, in reverse, become part of what is termed "promotion goals" [131, 132], pursuit of positive outcome, or at least be downplayed as an obstacle to that outcome. A similar influence of positive role models, lowering motivation to avoid a negative outcome and dampening the effect of negative role models, is possible on the other, "prevention" aspect of role modeling, pertaining to success or failure in that avoidance. This influence is thus relevant regardless of personal regulatory focus, to both "promotion-" and "prevention-focused" individuals (unlikely as they are to constitute a true dichotomy), combining the effects of changes in both descriptive (inferred from typical behavior) and injunctive (inferred from typical approval/disapproval) [133] social norms. As a facet of behavior self-regulation, the regulatory focus effect is compounded by the other component of self-regulation, hedonic, sought by users and satisfied by drugs. Secular changes in role models' behavior may thus both directly and indirectly contribute to the evolution of societal and individual norms regarding drugs.

Such changes have indeed been exemplified by public figures. The former President Obama, a recognized role model [134], has endorsed use of marijuana, cocaine, and heroin by referring to the former as no more harmful than alcohol and by informing the public that he had used cocaine and would use heroin too but did not like the pusher [135]. Obama's unsolicited voluntary disclosure preceded his presidential campaign but, as a politician, likely targeted a certain constituency. It was also a giant leap beyond the reluctant campaign time admission just 3 years earlier by another future president, Clinton, that he had "experimented with marijuana a time or two" but "did not inhale" [136]. President G. W. Bush refused to answer drug use-related questions and secretly instructed an aide to avoid "the marijuana question" because, as it was later leaked, he did not "want some little kid doing what [he had] tried" [137]. President Obama, in turn, asserted that inhaling "was the point" allowing one to cope with the surrounding world's "cheap moralism" [135], thereby correctly extending its significance beyond merely violation of a then still predominant and legally codified drug-specific moral/behavioral norm. In line with the societal lack of consistency or as reflection of conflicting interests in handling the problem, he also did recognize that our continuing "to see elevated rates of marijuana use among young people [is] likely driven by declines in perceptions of risk" [138]. That is a plausible cause, and those rates have indeed risen, as shown by the comparison of frequent cannabis use (six times or more in the past month) in 16–18-year-old cohorts by decade group, from 1991–2000 to 2011–2018 [139]. Moreover, the effect of age period within the cohort, from 13 to 18 years of age, was 60% greater in 2018 compared to 2005 (having climbed from the prior drop after its peak in 1995), suggesting faster development of cannabis involvement.

Clinton's "did not inhale" excuse, widely ridiculed as disingenuous, was at the same time a tribute to a soon-to-be antiquated behavioral/social norm. As noted by a reporter, "[t]here was a time when what Clinton said today would have ended a political career. Now, he apparently feels that time has passed" [136]. Indeed, on the background of marijuana decriminalization and legalization by states, a public figure of a lawmaker's stature and now US vice-president, Kamala Harris, has emphatically declared that she did smoke marijuana—and inhaled [140], while the majority of the 2020 presidential candidates who competed for nomination were for its legalization. This has happened as a very fast change from H. Clinton's 2016 position of merely reclassifying marijuana from Schedule I to Schedule II and allowing states to decriminalize it. To be sure, the point of providing these examples is not to characterize or compare the politicians but to demonstrate temporal changes in the societal attitude to drugs, which public figures well reflect.

As extensively discussed previously [32] and addressed in some detail below, marijuana as a substance has no specific "gateway" role, nor does any substance—even though research in that area still continues [141]. Initiation of use of any drug makes further involvement with drugs likelier. A role model's *endorsement* of its use can, however, play such a role—or, rather, lower the internalized societal barriers to drug use, a behavior formerly shunned, "stigmatized." Moreover, the drug use confessions by the politicians are also admissions to felony offenses, thus normalizing in public perception the *legally* proscribed norm violations that commonly entail fines, incarceration, and criminal records. Marijuana remains illegal under federal law as a Schedule I drug like heroin or peyote, i.e., classified as having "no currently accepted medical use and a high potential for abuse" [60].

At the same time, despite that classification, three cannabinoid medications are approved by the FDA, a tetrahydrocannabinol (THC) preparation, a THC synthetic analog, and a cannabidiol (CBD) medication, used for the same medical purposes for which natural marijuana has been traditionally used: treatment of nausea, loss of appetite, and epilepsy and severe childhood seizure syndromes (CBD from hemp oil). The US Patent and Trademark Office grants patents for cannabis breeding and cannabinoid production [142]. Moreover, in conflict with federal law, medical use of marijuana is by now legal in 40 states and territories, and its recreational use has been decriminalized or legalized in half of the states. Unsurprisingly, in contrast to some earlier reports [143], legalization and thus increase in cannabis availability do lead to increase in marijuana use, cannabis use disorder, and cannabis potency [144, 145]. Opioid use, although not as ostensibly normative, is *legally* in a way more normative than marijuana: DEA recognizes medical use of opioids, which are commonly prescribed for pain treatment. Tied to the legalization of cannabis use, however, even heroin, also a Schedule I drug, has been proposed to be rescheduled [146], which would inevitably result in its appearance on the illegal market via its additional supply source as a prescription drug, with a likely price drop.

Focus on drug supply is one side of misplacing agency from the user to the drug, part of the general tendency of ascribing agency to inanimate objects and phenomena, especially where problems of high social impact are concerned. Whereas substance use is a behavior for which the individual is ultimately responsible, legalization is a potent environmental factor directly influencing that behavior by facilitating access to a psychoactive substance and, indirectly, resulting in changes in societal attitudes and lowering barriers to substance use in general.

Yet another, subtler way of shifting agency from the user elsewhere is, paradoxically, the most common form of biomedical research. As indicated by Winick [87] and discussed in detail elsewhere [72, 147–149], this research, with few exceptions like vaccine development, has historically been confined mainly to "*risk* factors," associated with *disease* rather than absence thereof. In addictions, adopting the same approach along with the language of "epidemics" means not only focusing on the apparent pathogen but also searching for biological factors, such as genes and neurobiological processes, that are associated with and presumably drive the pathological behavior. The individual is not responsible for the biological factors but also is relieved of responsibility for the presence of drugs in the environment, which ignores the individual's choice of the environment and what is consumed from it. The identification of the high-risk individuals is viewed as not only the means of discovery of those factors but also a step to what has lately been described as "personalized medicine."

Nevertheless, unfortunate though it may be and thus hardly ever discussed, this risk factor search is arguably largely futile from the *practical* standpoint. Moreover, the elimination of the presumed "risk" factors is often in principle impossible (e.g., one of such factors is male sex [150]). It is true that the removal of drugs could prevent all addictions. As experience shows, however, that is infeasible despite all costly drug warfare (which is, again, not an argument for legalization). There is no other necessary (or, for that matter, sufficient) singular condition for drug use, unless we view as such the organismic component of addiction liability, virtually the entire system of reinforcement and behavior regulation.

That system's mechanisms, however, do not exist to react specifically to drugs, to produce the effects abusable substances are sought for. It is difficult to preventively turn it down to preclude addictions—at least, not without producing anhedonia if not a greater functional disruption. In fact, drug use serves to raise the hedonic amplitude, with drugs then exhausting the hedonic mechanisms' capacity due to their overloading the system. This leads to anhedonia as one of the drug effects manifest particularly in withdrawal and calling for further drug use. An example of the disruption is disabling just a single component of the cannabis response system, the cannabinoid CB1 receptor, by its inverse agonist rimonabant. Applied in attempting to control obesity by its action on peripheral receptors, rimonabant was once considered promising in restoring insulin sensitivity, normalizing fat cell size and distribution, and decreasing body mass. It has failed therapeutically, however, due to its adverse CNS/behavioral effects, suicidal ideation and depression [151], which are consistent with anhedonia.

Another drug effect is blunted affect. Notably, blunted affect may also be a factor that predates drug use and predisposes a person to seek ways, including drug use, to augment the amplitude of affective states (AAS [32]), a more general view on the hedonic motivation. This is a concept close to hedonic responsiveness or tone that is defined as the ability to feel pleasure [152]. A broader concept, the AAS refers to the individual range of magnitudes of positive affect changes (narrow if blunted), which in evolutionary terms are indicative of events' providing a fitness gain/loss. Drug use is thus hypothesized to be instrumental in counteracting the general decrease of the AAS that results from the relatively increased everyday life stability as compared to that under the environment of human evolutionary adaptedness (EEA [153]), "red in tooth and claw," an evolutionary mismatch. This is consistent with the strong relationship of anhedonia with drug craving and with its sharing the dopaminergic circuitry with the neural substrate of drug action [154]. Fittingly, naltrexone, an opioid antagonist, particularly its extended-release form, does not appear to induce anhedonia in opiate addicts, but it does so, as expected, in non-addicted individuals.

A shift of hedonic set point that results from drug use, termed "allostasis" [155], in line with the AAS's diminishing after its initial increase under drug influence, is one of hypothesized mechanisms of addiction development. This shift, however, can be subsumed under the long-standing concept of stress, applied to the limits of the organism's adaptation to the addictive substances. Considering that many addicts return to normative behavior, the physiological changes thus either do not determine addictive behavior and/or are not stable enough to maintain it into the permanence of a *new* set point that would be necessary for allostasis as a non-redundant concept.

Discrete biological "risk" factors are numerous, each of small effect on liability variation, such as that of genetic polymorphisms. The latter attract special attention, due to the rapid analytic technology development and the view on the genes as virtually unequivocally located in the top upstream position in the biological causal chains. This view has somewhat changed relatively recently, with the discovery of epigenetic mechanisms influencing gene expression in response/adjustment to environmental influences. Moreover, there is an often-neglected difference between tracing such chains when dealing with type 1 mechanistic causes of individual development and function, as in finding genes responsible for the structure and function of a protein or an organ, and with the type 2 causes of trait variation. As noted above, it is those latter causes that are the actual targets of genetic association studies in biomedical research.

This distinction between the causes is critical because the statistical associations, even when true, do not necessarily point at a direct cause of a disorder such as SUD or are etiological at all. Despite that, the misleading truisms like "[g] enetic factors contribute to the risk for developing alcohol use disorder" are commonplace [156]. It is a truism because there are no traits of the organism to which genetic factors do not contribute mechanistically. It is misleading, because it is an inaccurate conclusion from the legitimate results of biometric genetic analyses of phenotypic differences between individuals in the population. These analyses are based mostly on the differences in intrapair similarity of monozygotic (MZ) and dizygotic (DZ) twins for that trait. MZ twins in a pair share all their genes in common, whereas DZ twins, like regular siblings, share, on average, only half of their segregating genes (i.e., those where allelic variation exists). Relating differences in the genetic intrapair similarity of MZ and DZ twins to the differences in the phenotypic similarity affords estimation of how much the former accounts for the latter and, therefore, what proportion of phenotypic variance, e.g., in the risk for the disorder, in a particular population at a specific point in time, is accounted for by genetic variance. This proportion is termed "heritability." As can be seen, heritability has little to do with traits' genetic mechanisms as such.

Whereas low heritability of a trait means that on the background of currently existing environmental/non-genetic causes of variation in a trait in a population the contribution of genetic causes is comparatively low, high heritability also does not translate into the chances of detecting genetic associations with specific polymorphisms [157]. Much fewer genetic associations have been discovered than even the number of genes that are long known to be involved mechanistically in the outcome of the human-drug interaction. Statistical associations depend on the frequencies and thus detectability of variants, if any, and on liability variances. As mentioned above [12], genetic studies are able to discover an etiologically causal mechanism only when a genetic polymorphism detectably contributes to variation in disorder liabilities on the background of all other natural sources of phenotypic variation (i.e., the phenotypic difference between respective genotypes is significant).

Notably, the "unnatural" (pharmacological) action on a gene's expression, when applied to a mechanism, may be utilized regardless of existence of any genetic association with that gene. For instance, the disulfiram effect's serendipitous discovery history in Caucasians [158], which started with a plant physician's observation of "inability to drink" in workers who dealt with its production at a rubber factory [159], was unrelated to the genetic association findings for AlDH in Japanese [2, 4]. In Caucasians, that association would not be found at all, even though the AlDH activity is functionally among the *etiologic* mechanisms of alcoholism regardless of the population.

Many of the genetic association findings are not of the polymorphisms contributing to the risk variation (i.e., not in the regions variably coding for a relevant structural/functional gene product or a regulatory element), but rather of those in *linkage disequilibrium* (non-random co-occurrence of alleles of different polymorphisms) with such "causal" polymorphisms. Due to the smallness of the latter's contribution to liability variation, many of them may be below the radar of the current mainstream approach, genome-wide association scan (GWAS), even with very large samples employed to enable statistically significant detection of small effects. On the other hand, despite the stringent significance thresholds, the association may still be spurious.

The assumption guiding the GWAS approach is that the risk-elevating alleles of single nucleotide polymorphisms (SNPs) contributing to risk variation (i.e., the risk related to one allele is greater than with the other allele) are common, with ensuing large attributable risks in the population [160]. However, the polygenic character of the genetic component of phenotypic variation entails high genetic heterogeneity of the affected population, thus lessening possibility of high attributable risks for particular alleles. To illustrate, imagine a disorder that is mechanistically caused by mutations in numerous genes, each sufficient to result in the same phenotypic defect, i.e., the multiple genocopies (which may happen, e.g., when the phenotypic defect results from a product at the end of a long metabolic chain). It would be very difficult to discover those genes by purely genetic association approaches because of their small attributable risk despite their very large etiologic effect, especially considering that a gene's function can be changed by mutations in numerous loci in a gene's coding sequence and outside of it, as well as by epigenetic events, variation in which has its own mechanisms of determination, genetic as well as environmental. Moreover, in addition to the ~20,000 protein-coding sequences in human genome, there are an order of magnitude more intergenic transcription start sites related to generation of noncoding RNAs (e.g., micro-RNAs, long noncoding RNAs, circular RNAs, and micropeptide-coding RNAs), which are affected by psychoactive substances (up- or downregulated) and likely influence nervous system development and teratogenesis [161]. Now consider that none of those mutations nor even all of them together are sufficient to result in the disorder phenotype (small effects), while the attributable risks are still small because of those alleles' relative rarity. Moreover, hard-to-specify environmental variables are no less important contributors to phenotypic variation, directly and indirectly, as well as likely interacting with the genotype. Statistical effects, which are averages over the individual ones, may be unable to detect mechanistic effects in part because those may be individually ambiguous: e.g., parental or a sibling's substance abuse may in the offspring/sibling cause aversion to it or serve to facilitate drug use [162]. Behavioral phenotypic development, including exposure to drugs, is superimposed on the physiological development and age changes, adding enormous complexity.

Suppose, however, a truly risk-elevating ("causal") allele is discovered and there is a way to counteract its mechanistic effect—e.g., inhibit an enzyme encoded by that gene. Since the allele's statistical effect is averaged across the population (sample), the individual mechanistic effect of such counteraction may vary from negligible to large, i.e., from useless to potentially harmful (the latter will be prone to affect natural reward mechanisms as well—see above), or may have a relatively low range of variation around the mean and hence be simply small, not only statistically but etiologically. It is also not necessarily generalizable across populations, as is also illustrated by the disulfiram-like effect of the AlDH deficiency that exists among East Asians but not Caucasians. Moreover, as discussed above, even such strong effects are far from absolute.

The most important genetic result would perhaps be a newly detected polymorphism effect pointing to a gene directly contributing to the etiological mechanisms of the disorder and previously unknown (so-called novel) from biochemical, neurobiological, and physiological mechanistic research. An example is the discovery of the role of the *BRCA1* ("breast cancer 1") gene in breast cancer. Various mutations in this gene encoding a component of RNA polymerase II [163], which were traced by linkage analysis in different families, result in a defective gene product. Only a small proportion, about 2% [164], of breast cancer cases in the US non-Ashkenazi population are related to those mutations. The presence of those mutations has, however, a strong effect, with ~50% of carriers becoming affected by age 80 [165]. Another example is the relationship of apolipoprotein E (APOE) with the risk for Alzheimer disease. Although it has been over 20 years since that relationship was discovered [166], the practical implementation of the findings is still under discussion as holding "a great deal of promise" in the future [167].

For drug addiction, however, virtually no strong effect mechanistic genes have been or are likely to be found, barring the possible exceptions of the AlDH kind. Considering that liability to addiction is a complex behavioral trait, the lack of strong genetic associations with it is what is expected. A strong association would correspond to the virtually single-gene (or oligo- rather than polygenic) determination of behavioral variation in relation to psychoactive drugs, an unlikely scenario because of the number of variable organismic processes and environmental variables involved in addiction development. Considering that drug-related behavior in its mechanisms piggybacks on natural consummatory behaviors in pursuit of targets pertaining to Darwinian fitness (food; sex), such strong associations would also be expected in regard to those targets, but they are not observed. The lack of a strong genetic determinism of behavior variation enables immense flexibility of behavioral response to environmental changes. By the same token, changing, for prevention or treatment purposes, gene expression beyond the magnitude observed under natural conditions would likely result in pleiotropic behavioral changes, going beyond anything pertaining to addiction as such and being tantamount to behavior control if not otherwise noxious.

As noted above, whereas a singular cause of substance use disorders and associated conditions, such as a gene let alone a specific allele of a gene, is unlikely, a substantial amount of liability variance is shared among numerous behavioral/psychiatric traits, forming general (common) liability. Unsurprisingly, while most genetic research is focused on drug-specific addictions, most drug-related genetic association findings are with the loci that are not specific—not only to any drug but to drugs in general [127, 168–171]. For instance, an "opioid overdose risk locus" detected in a GWAS in opioid users is "close to" *MCOLN1* [172], the gene encoding mucolipin-1, a lysosome and endosome membrane protein participating in cellular lipid and protein transport and mechanistically important in many processes, including brain development. While the cited report is introduced with a paragraph on the "opioid use and overdose crisis," it is unclear what role the *MCOLN1* or any such finding can potentially play in that crisis. Similarly, a SNP in *DNMT3B*, the gene encoding a DNA methyltransferase that is part of general epigenetic mechanisms, has been found in a GWAS to "contribute to nicotine dependence" [173] (i.e., it is putatively associated with variation in smoking severity among those who have smoked at least 100 cigarettes lifetime). The study is introduced with an accurate description of harm from smoking, but nothing in the discussion portends any potential use of the finding to lessen that harm. Clearly, that is not for the lack of the researchers' desire to see their results translated into practice, even though some consider translational research as "detracting from an equivalent appreciation of fundamental research of broad applicability, without obvious connections to medicine" [174]. While the choice between the two broad kinds of research is a red herring argument (both are necessary), translation, limited as it has been, is definitely no threat to fundamental research in terms of resources and effort.

Accordingly, few if any practical approaches have been suggested based on either previously known or newly *genetically discovered* mechanisms of addiction development. The same pertains to "novel" physiological processes. Indeed, the alcohol aversion effect of AlDH2 inhibition had been known long before the enzyme-inactivating mutation was found. Significantly, the mutant (i.e., less common) allele increases not the *risk* for but *resistance* to drinking and thereby resistance to alcoholism (see the discussion of resistance below). Another well-confirmed addiction-related genetic finding, of the associations between characteristics of tobacco-smoking and the acetylcholine nicotinic receptor subunit *CHRNA5/A3/B4* gene cluster, is also not novel from the mechanistic standpoint. Appositely, it was detected not only in a hypothesis-free GWAS [175] but also in a parallel candidate gene study [120] guided by hypotheses based on prior mechanistic knowledge. This finding has not resulted in practical applications either. The development of effective anti-nicotine-craving compounds, such as varenicline used for assisting smoking cessation, is unrelated to genetic findings. While it does pertain to the nicotinic receptors (neuronal nicotinic acetylcholine receptors, nAChRs), of which varenicline is an agonist, those are a different group, $\alpha4\beta2$ [176] and $\alpha7$ [177]. In general, pharmacotherapy in drug addiction, when a medication's mechanism of action is known, targets neurotransmitters, their receptors, or enzymes, etc., that are known to be involved in physiological drug response (e.g., [178, 179])—regardless of any observed natural variation in their function.

Deriving benefits from the current mainstream biomedical research is also problematic. Let us again consider genes, a frequent target of that research. The firmware of the organism, the genes code for the entire gamut of its components as well as delimit their potential changes, including gene expression reactions to any possible changes in the environment. While the genes' physiologically upstream location makes the interpretation of phenotypic associations with the genes free from doubts about directionality, this location also makes their detection difficult. If/when detected, those associations may also be unusable or no longer relevant even when they are relevant to etiology. As a comparison, the match that started a forest fire would be difficult to find in the fire; it would also be useless in dealing with the fire even if found against all odds.

Nevertheless, starting with the model applied to monogenic disorders, search for "disease" genes continues, meaning a "disease" allele, a mutation of a normal gene that results in a disorder. Driven by technology development, updates to the genetic firmware, e.g., via gene editing, will inevitably be considered and attempts will be likely made. A recent report on the human genome editing "supports crossing what has been a bright red line by recommending that clinical trials of heritable human genome editing be allowed" to prevent "a serious disease or condition" [180]. Without doubt, psychiatric disorders, including addiction, are "serious" despite their fuzzy diagnostic thresholds. It is doubtful, however, if intervention in the genome is a reasonable strategy for those disorders. Notably, the rate of *discordance* in MZ twins is high even for ostensibly more endogenous disorders like schizophrenia (reaching 60%) [181], with unknown environmental triggers, one of which could be the preventable prenatal vitamin D deficiency [182]. Moreover, there is no clear boundary between psychosis and the "norm" [183]. It is even more important to draw distinctions between those diseases that have no conscious volitional component, such as PKU or schizophrenia, and behavioral conditions such as addiction. The dystopian genetic manipulations of human behavior are hardly within ethical limits. Considering that voluntary exposure to drugs is a recent factor in human evolutionary history (animals must avoid poisons and intoxicants lest their Darwinian fitness declines), likely afforded by the increased lenience of natural selection and/or becoming a form of Zahavi's handicap [32, 184], specific addiction liability-increasing genetic variants may be beneficial in other settings.

The same pertains to the possible intermediate traits like personality characteristics that have been proposed as "endophenotypes" for studying genetic associations in SUD [185]. In contrast to the original concept of endophenotype in psychiatry [186], personality traits do not underlie liability to addiction (like an enzyme deficiency underlies mental manifestations of PKU). Far from being, by definition, "biochemical test or microscopic examination," they are also not relatively elementary physiological or biochemical units but manifest at the same high level of organization, behavioral, as liability to addiction. The same pertains to liabilities to other psychiatric disorders. Accordingly, the genetics of these multifactorial traits is much more complex than would correspond to the concept of endophenotype, their heritability is no higher than the traits' for which they are supposed to be "endophenotypes," and the chances to discover actionable genetic variation are similar as well. It is thus not surprising that "endophenotypes have not lived up to their promise in facilitating gene discovery for disease risk" [187], and unlikely will.

It has also been noted that heritability does not predict discoverability [157], and that is true even for structural neuroimaging measures, the traits that are closer to the gene products and more objectively defined than behavioral traits like addiction liability, manifest far downstream from gene expression. The hypothesis-based genetic association ("candidate gene") studies in complex traits have long been criticized for their irreproducibility, including a recent prominent publication pertaining to the widely publicized and studied 5-HTTLPR variable number tandem repeat polymorphism in the promoter region of the serotonin transporter *SLC6A4* gene [188]. Technology development has afforded GWAS, initially turning every gene in the genome into a candidate one with no hypotheses posed. It is noteworthy, however, that GWAS, usually viewed as a preferred alternative to candidate gene studies, whether using increasingly dense genome coverage by tagging SNPs or full genome sequencing, is in fact an alternative means of selection of candidate genes—based on the detection of their statistical associations with liability rather than by their known or likely mechanistic involvement. Upon detection of an association, the locus must be made sense of by explaining its mechanistic involvement (in so-called post-GWAS functional studies [189]). Those studies are currently greatly behind.

Balancing between the difficulty of detecting expectedly small true association effects and thus high type II error (not rejecting wrong null hypothesis) on the one hand and, on the other hand, false positives due to the millions of explicit tests (type I error, rejecting correct null hypothesis), increasingly large samples in GWAS are employed, growing into millions (e.g., [190]). The effects detected by GWAS due to high statistical power achieved by very large samples are usually small and thus more congruent with expectations for complex trait associations than the relatively large effects that historically have been observed for "candidate genes" in smaller samples. These effects, however, are not replicated well either (e.g., [191]). Even if they are, however, they are expectedly trivial. Moreover, as large samples are unlikely to be accrued in one particular population, the possibility grows that unaccounted-for heterogeneity will efface the power gains, similar to what has been noted as a potential problem for large-scale analyses of MRI data [192].

GWAS cannot take into account the complexity of the genetic architecture of liability variation. As previously noted [72], the genes in genome-wide studies are largely treated as independent of each other, while their products frequently comprise intersecting cascades, with each subsequent reaction/process dependent on the outcome of the previous one(s), thus forming complex functional gene-gene as well as genotype-environment interactions. In addition to the large number of polymorphic genes that may contribute to addiction liability's heritability, even a functional association (due to the relevant gene product's changes) is mediated by numerous variables at different levels of biological organization between the gene and the behavior. The association is thus prone to erode to statistical nonsignificance/nondetection even if strong between the adjacent links. While pathway analysis, combining the existing knowledge of the biochemical pathways with GWAS data, may allow avoiding such type II errors, it seems to negate the goal of genetic research: instead of discovering a previously unknown pathway by a genetic association, the association gets confirmed by a known mechanistic pathway.

Moreover, the likelihood is low that the "novel targets" [193] would be any more useful for prevention and treatment than the processes and myriad of their components already known to mechanistically contribute to the development of addiction. Replacing with a "normal" allele the one associated with risk elevation, even when it becomes possible with gene editing, or changing the activity of a gene or its product in the "needed" direction, is not justified by the small "natural" effect sizes. More generally, it is not justified without a proof that a polymorphism's contribution to mechanisms of variation reflects its contribution to biological etiological mechanisms. If, on the contrary, a pharmacologic application results in a substantial effect (e.g., compensating for the supposed deficiency), it is likely to be associated with adverse CNS/mood consequences, as in the above-cited case with rimonabant. That is a corollary to the nonspecificity of such an effect to drugs.

For the same reasons, it is uncertain if genetic variation findings will benefit substance use/addiction prevention. As a potential practical target, personalized medicine pertaining to drug addiction can hardly be derived from the genetic "risk" discoveries. A strong deleterious genetic effect, while usually incurable (with rare partial success exceptions as that with the low phenylalanine diet for phenylketonuria), could be used for predicting and evaluating personal risk—in genetic testing for drug use generally or, particularly, for using opioids in pain treatment. There is, for instance, a large functional effect of *CYP2D6*, a gene encoding an enzyme catalyzing biotransformation of opioids such as codeine into an active derivative, morphine. That effect can be expressed in low metabolizing with no analgesic benefit or in very fast metabolizing with a possibility of poisoning. Guidelines based on the genetic testing data have been developed [194] to prevent either possibility when used therapeutically. While as few as 7% of the population fall into both categories, with a potential benefit, genotyping even for this purpose is difficult, however, because there are over 70 known single nucleotide and copy number variation polymorphisms (SNP and CNV) in this locus.

In the absence of strong effects for complex disorders including addictions, other methods of utilization of genetic data consisting of risk-associated genetic polymorphisms have been proposed—more recently, polygenic risk score (PRS), a sum of (elevated-) "risk" alleles derived from GWAS, including those below the "genome-wide" significance level, weighted by the respective polymorphisms' association coefficients (e.g., [195]). The goal is largely "to ascertain who among an at-risk population have the highest likelihood of developing a condition or of progressing to a more severe state" [196], which "depends on [PRS's] ability to stratify a population into categories with sufficiently distinct risks to substantially affect the risk–benefit balance of public health or clinical interventions" [195]. The utility of this method as applied to addictions or, for that matter, to other psychiatric conditions [197] is yet to be proven. For instance, a recent high-profile study of smoking and alcohol use, involving samples up to 1.2 million individuals, determined that PRS accounted for only trivial proportions of variance in characteristics of these behaviors, one to four percent [190]. A commercially developed test for prescribing opioids, based on 11 SNPs associated with addiction liability in general, has a low accuracy as well, so that "the majority of the small percentage of patients recommended not to take opioids would actually not be at high risk of addiction" [196], thus needlessly denied treatment benefit. Considering the low frequency of overdosing among the patients legally receiving opioid prescriptions, it may be easier among them to predict low rather than high risk. In principle, PRS cannot account for more variance than the proportion of heritability that is due to SNPs used for tagging genetic variation in GWAS or, ultimately, from full genome sequencing [198]. In general, not only reliable predictors but even disease biomarkers in psychiatry hardly exist. That is consistent with the lack of qualitative physiological differences between the "norm" and mental disorders. A rare exception is a rather accurate prediction of transition to psychosis based on proteomic analysis—but that prediction, among other limitations, was made for a group that already had prodromal symptoms [199].

Drug use reflects some humans' willingness to take a chemical shortcut to the core mechanisms of reward that is more naturally derived from regular consummatory behaviors. Purely medical and law enforcement measures cannot prevent this "pursuit of happiness," positive affect, which *falsely* signifies a Darwinian fitness benefit (e.g., [200]). It is the means of that pursuit, as well as the understanding of what happiness is, that differentiate between health and disorder, if not between law-abiding and crime. Psychoactive substances acting as agonists of receptors like opioids or mitragynine (kratom), or as neurotransmitter reuptake inhibitors like cocaine, provide a relatively effortless if noxious way to reach a variant of "happiness."

When unbounded by social, including legal, rules that derive from moral and/or health considerations, hedonic pursuit in humans may and frequently does become comparable to that of rats pressing a pedal to obtain cocaine to the point of starvation, in its ability of self-inflicting morbid or even lethal harm. Unless those rules are internalized, even the cruelest persecution may fail to stop and prevent it. In the 1656 book by a Turkish scholar Kâtip Çelebi [201], the history of tobacco use under the Sultan Murad IV (1623–1640) provides a compelling example. The sultan banned tobacco smoking on pain of death, either convinced that it was an innovation, forbidden in Islam, or due to fires caused by smokers. Nevertheless, some people "found the opportunity to smoke even during the executions… with severest torture" of those caught smoking. The author's conclusion is that "the best course is not to interfere with anyone in this respect"; "if the rulers interfere, they will be taking upon themselves more than they should." In the totalitarian Soviet Union, where alcoholism treatment was often coercive, placed under the purview of the harsh police system, alcoholism remained rampant. Alcoholics were not deterred by the prospects of a month or more of compulsory "labor therapy," managing to sneak alcohol even into the locked-down semi-prison hospital. These examples, including the repressive measures against substance users that have been sanctioned by the US justice and political system, illustrate the general inefficacy of attempts at direct external social control of behavior. As discussed above, however, whereas it may have been wrong to criminalize substance use, this does not mean that the reversal of existing legal drug use restrictions is epidemiologically neutral or beneficial. Behavioral changes, facilitated by restrictions, that resulted in the fall of prevalence of smoking appear to be an example of a more reasonable alternative.

Finally, it should be noted that drug abuse exerts a powerful systemic attack on the same human brain that produces it. In its effects, this attack, especially poisoning ("overdose"), could be compared with another self-destructive behavioral act, a suicide attempt with consequent brain damage or death. It is likely that numerous biochemical brain changes can be found in such an assault as well, some probably preceding it and even related to genetic variation. Regardless of those differences at the deep phenotypic and even genetic levels, it is the behavioral act that needs to be prevented. Just because the effect of drugs may take longer to unfold does not mean that the biological factors related to the act as such have necessarily any relevance to it, or are usable in its primary, secondary, or tertiary prevention.

To summarize, the main approaches in dealing with drug problems, including recurrent drug "epidemics," have been largely oriented to causes external to the individual. When considering the individual, the focus has been on the sources of *variation in the risk* that are not necessarily the same as actual etiological mechanisms and may even erroneously lead to discarding the latter when related research results are negative. The consequences of these perspectives in policy and research may be thus ineffective, uncoupled from the actionable factors.

The Resistance Aspect of Liability

It has been noted that when analyzing disease-related data, "[g]eneticists generally report composite measures of sensitivity and specificity…, which only measure how good a test is at identifying *affected* individuals" [202] (emphasis added). In fact, this statement reflects the general state of biomedical research. The studies conducted under the aegis of the National Institutes of *Health* in their overwhelming majority pertain to *Disease*. This is understandable: it is diseases that are the problems to be solved. Despite the repeated calls for greater attention to prevention, medicine remains a field focused on treating and, hopefully, curing diseases, rather than maintaining health. Prophylactic dental procedures, which are substantially related to behavior (from abstaining from sweets to regular visits to a dentist), are relatively common likely because of their high efficiency and facility as well as the immediate impact of tooth decay on the quality of life. Yet, even in dentistry, prevention is still considered a desirable but incomplete "paradigm shift" [203]. Along with many other disorders, dental problems in their preventability take a place in the range between (as yet) unpreventable conditions like schizophrenia and entirely preventable if often not prevented drug addictions.

In considering drug-related behaviors (addiction and its prodrome, drug use), the requirement of prevention of the *illegal behavior* is also inevitably involved. As more readily conceived of from the society's standpoint, substance use therefore tends to be reduced to its illegality aspect, with no qualitative differences from any other criminal behavior. Thus, while dealing with a problem classified as medical, prevention of drug use is in a large part placed outside of medical domain, in the hands of law enforcement. Nevertheless, drug use is not a public safety issue like crime or warfare and becomes so only when crime is involved. Consumption is an individual's action upon himself, voluntary, strictly speaking, even when prescribed. Relegation of at least some responsibility for it to the government deprives the individual of agency even in consumption, before drug response makes the choice more difficult. Interdiction and punitive measures, which is all the government can do, do not result in lasting success.

Such contradictions are likely to hinder the problem's solution. They also illustrate that categorical institutional distinctions between various human activities and conditions (legal vs. medical), made exactly to facilitate solutions, may be formal and nonexistent in reality, which is the continuous variation of multidimensional human behavior. This also points to the need in a shift from the disease-oriented (or crime-oriented) and thus artificially dichotomous medical (or law-enforcement) outlook to the realistic consideration of the *entire phenotypic distribution* pertaining to relevant individual differences.

This distribution of liability to addiction covers the full range of phenotypes varying in their degree of "normality" and, if affected, of disorder severity [52]. Absent an objective boundary, the threshold between them is defined by the changing and numerous combinations of diagnostic criteria, providing for a heterogeneous and variably arbitrary description of the disease phenotype. Thus, recall that the current US classification of SUD (DSM-5) is based on 11 symptoms. The number of those symptoms present determines gradations of severity, also a part of the classification. This classification is common to all substances. Corresponding to the degree of manifestation, however, psychometric properties of the symptoms are different for each abused substance.

Moreover, as noted above, despite the prevailing designation of addiction as a "brain disease" [204], most of these symptoms are descriptors of *behavior*. The few that are indicative of physiological ("brain") level changes (withdrawal, tolerance, and perhaps craving) could be causally related to the rest of the symptoms when present, i.e., to behavioral changes. The physiology-based symptoms do not fit conceptually: inasmuch as the addiction phenotype is defined as a behavioral disorder (persistent drug *use* despite negative consequences), liability to it is a behavioral rather than physiological trait, while physiological changes, as one of the emergent causes of the drug pursuit behavior, may facilitate it. Indeed, in opioid addiction, withdrawal was observed as the most frequent and earliest developing symptom [109, 205], thus corresponding counterintuitively to low severity of that disorder as measured by diagnostic criteria. At the same time, it was not observed in all addicts or in the absence of at least one other symptom, which suggests that addiction as behavior does not necessarily follow from withdrawal (physical dependence). Arguably, physiological events and changes underlie any behavior, which is not, however, reducible to them, let alone to a single mechanism—e.g., dopaminergic, as in "Reward Deficiency Syndrome" [206].

From the statistical perspective, in the analysis of the structure of the relationships among the symptoms, withdrawal and tolerance are upstream to behavioral symptoms related to them. This is a critical distinction: they belong to the determinants of the trait's variation rather than the latent trait's being the determinant of their variation and covariation. As part of physiological mechanisms of the behavioral phenotype, consistent with biological perspective, they are *causal* rather than *effect* indicators of the latent behavioral trait [207]. The differences between the two kinds of indicators as well as addiction liability as a latent trait are discussed below, but here it should be noted that causal indicators are inappropriate in latent trait measurement. Withdrawal and tolerance are also not truly categorical but, like any manifestation of a complex trait, vary in severity. Moreover, in opioid use disorder, withdrawal, having a relatively low manifestation threshold [109, 205], does not fit the role of an indicator of high severity.

Inasmuch as the focus of research remains on the disease, it is also on identifying risk factors. Such factors are approached as those that raise liability over the population average, because the mean liability of usual control groups, drawn from 90–99% of the population, is close to that average. This is commonly done with a straightforward but seldom feasible objective of the elimination or neutralization of risk factors, or a less translation-oriented goal of "understanding of the biological mechanisms" of a disorder (e.g., [208]). In the latter case, it is uncertain whether this understanding will bring about any practical benefits that are implicit in search for "risk variants." Importantly but almost never addressed, however, risk is only one of the two opposite aspects of liability: while risk pertains to growth in liability, *resistance* corresponds to liability decrease [148]. The resistance conceptualization, co-dimensional with risk, implies major differences from the notion of "resilience," which is contingent on overcoming "adversity" (e.g., [209]) and is subsumed under resistance. Similarly, "protective factors," commonly considered the alternatives to risk factors (e.g., an allele that is more common among the controls), are subsumed under resistance factors (if they indeed have liability-lowering effect) but are only a subset thereof. In other words, resistance factors are any that lower liability.

While symmetric and ostensibly only nominally different, the two liability aspects have important and asymmetric practical implications. As illustrated on Fig. 1.1, research directed at *risk* factors relies on the "high-risk" populations/samples where they aggregate, i.e., affected individuals and their relatives, comparing them with "normal" controls, i.e., individuals representing the rest of the population, its overwhelming majority. Sometimes, as in the transmission-disequilibrium test of genetic association/linkage (TDT [210]), the unaffected individuals are not even involved: "cases" and "controls" are, respectively, alleles transmitted and nontransmitted to the *affected* offspring from heterozygous parents. As disorder is the target, the genes that are looked for are termed accordingly, e.g., "genes for addiction" [211], and the average effect of "overtransmitted" alleles (those more frequent among the "cases") is related to higher than average liability. Obviously, if the power to discover high-*risk*-related variants is notoriously low, it is lower yet for a high-*resistance* variant to be discoverable in such a setup. As noted, the alleles that are alternative to the potential high-risk ones—and only those can come out of the controls used—confer on average only average risk. Accordingly, even if a TDT evaluated transmission/nontransmission of alleles to the *un*affected offspring of heterozygotes, it would not turn the perspective around

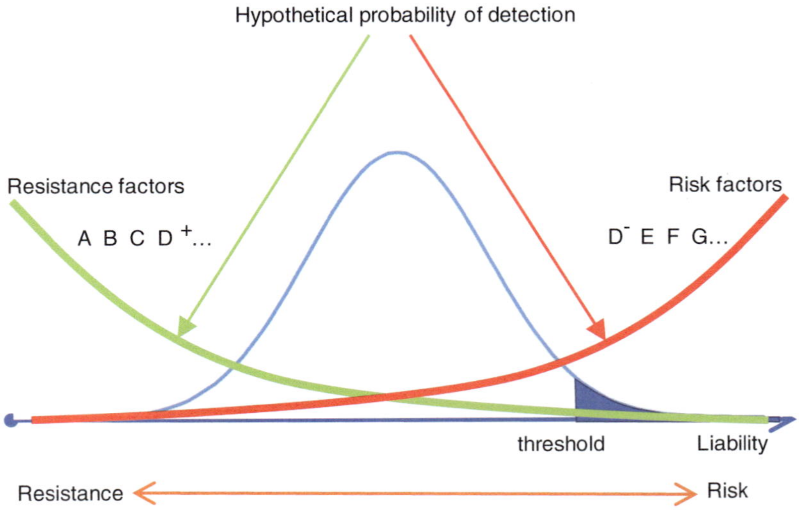

Fig. 1.1 Liability: risk and resistance aspects

from high risk to high resistance: the average effect of overtransmitted alleles would correspond to approximately average rather than low liability.

Another type of control used, in particular, in genetic studies of addictions, is the so-called exposed controls—e.g., in a study of smoking [172], those with "a significant history of smoking" (100 or more cigarettes in their lifetimes) but no "nicotine dependence" as per zero score on the six-item FTND during the period of heaviest smoking. The FTND items reflect smoking frequency, quantity, and timing and desire to smoke. As indicated by that study's authors, by comparing these controls with individuals who score four or higher allows examining "the genetic effects that are specific to nicotine dependence." Notably, however, using such controls precludes investigation of factors that are related to the *initiation of smoking* as well as *continuation of smoking without developing a heavy consumption regimen and signs of physiological dependence*, both quite important health-wise. Interestingly, the authors note ([120], p. 44) that

> [b]ecause our controls were highly selected and could even be considered 'protected' against susceptibility to nicotine dependence, interpretation of our results must consider the possibility that an association signal from our study may actually represent protective rather than risk effects. We used the allele more frequent in cases for reporting these data as a convention to facilitate comparison of the odds ratios among SNPs; this should not be viewed as a conclusion of how a particular variant influences the risk for nicotine dependence. The precise determination of the mechanism by which a variant alters risk can only come from functional studies.

This comment is relevant to critical differences between two alternative approaches to studying liability to disorders, risk/disease, and resistance/health, detailed further on. Importantly, no attempt was made to identify the protective effects, which quite possibly resulted in the ability of people to smoke without becoming dependent—however arbitrary the lines delimiting dependence may be, and regardless of the fact that tobacco harm is determined largely by the products of tobacco combustion rather than by nicotine itself. Germane to the discussion of the differences between dependence and addiction, it is not that study's target phenotype, nicotine dependence as such, that is of most health significance but the behavior of inhaling tobacco smoke—regardless of dependence (which, to be sure, does make smoking more likely but is not necessary for that). Research in factors that lead to smoking initiation and continuation would require different controls. Studying factors that preclude these behaviors would require a different sampling methodology.

Unsurprisingly, the few genetic findings related to the *non*development of the disorder, "protective" alleles, are mostly inadvertent (e.g., [127]), including those where an allele's risk/

resistance modality flip-flops depending on the substance (e.g., nicotine vs. cocaine [18]), or on the type of drug use behavior (addiction vs. less severe use [19]). It is noteworthy that these modality changes illustrate the difficulty of possible translation efforts involving behavior modification based on genetic findings. There have been studies in addiction, however, that can be categorized as resistance-related, such as pertaining to cessation of heroin use [212].

The resistance factors, both genetic and non-genetic, aggregate on the low end of the liability distribution, symmetric to risk factors. The aggregation of transmissible (e.g., heritable) resistance factors in the respective population extends to the relatives of individuals with high resistance. For instance, first-degree relatives of abstinent alcoholics (i.e., *resistant* to relapse) were three times as likely to be abstinent themselves as relatives of individuals with persistent AUD [213]. This supports an approach to the identification of a high-resistance population that mirrors a standard high-risk approach that is based on relatives of affected individuals. This is, not, however, the only possible way to identify resistance factors. The possible methodological suggestions for implementing the resistance perspective are described below.

Resistance Analysis

It follows from the above discussion that the high-risk paradigm, common in addiction and generally psychiatric research, needs to be reversed to enable the resistance perspective therein. Namely, just as a high-risk population is required for a disease-oriented study, identifying high-resistance populations is a means for detecting factors conferring/elevating resistance. An example can be drawn from the history of smallpox vaccine development (vaccinations in general are among the few examples of the practical implementation of the resistance paradigm). Its beginning was in the identification of the high-resistance population, milkmaids who had had a more benign cowpox and been long known to be resistant to smallpox, which then informed of the source of material for preventive inoculation. This was a method much preferable to another one and historically much older, variolation, also using a highly resistant population: people who were infected with but surviving smallpox. Variolation, inoculation with the material taken from a ripe pustule of such an individual, preceded vaccination by centuries [214]. Remarkably, in contrast to variolation, vaccination, which is derived from vaccinia virus, has nothing to do with the agent causing the dangerous disease, variola virus, illustrating the asymmetry of risk and resistance factors.

In other words, while resistance factors subsume "protective" ones (conceptualized as opposite ends of the same continuum as risk factors or those that moderate or buffer the effects of risk factors [215]), they can be entirely different and non-codimensional with the "risk" factors. Accordingly, as shown on Fig. 1.1, the sets of discrete risk and resistance factors overlap (e.g., factor "D" in its two opposite variants—e.g., for simplicity, exposure and non-exposure to a drug), but only partially. It is likely due to this asymmetry that even the estimates of heritability differ for the dimensions defined by the diagnosis and by the definitions of resistance: in contrast to risk for alcohol use disorder, the contribution of genetic variation to individual differences in resistance to its relapse (ability to asymptomatic remission) is very low [216].

Other examples of the asymmetry of risk and resistance approaches can be found in existing treatment methods. For instance, whereas the cause of PKU is genetic, mutations related to phenylalanine metabolism, its prevention is environmental, the phenylalanine-poor diet. Obviously, it is phenylalanine that is the agent that acts abnormally upon the defective metabolic system, but it is also an essential amino acid that the human organism must obtain from food to develop and function, and at the levels available from food causes no disorder in the absence of mutations. In psychiatric disorders, despite the long history of etiology research, successful medications have little to do with its results, and their mechanisms of action are largely either unknown (lithium) or were partially elucidated after the medication had been put into practice (chlorpromazine). The development of fluoxetine and its success in treating depression were due to targeting a specific neurochemical mechanism, serotonin reuptake, but it is uncertain if that is indeed the etiological mechanism. In effect, these medications' ability to raise organismic resistance to the disorder (its symptoms) was discovered without connection to the mechanisms that determined the high risk—those are still unclear. Nevertheless, even when it is recognized that effective interventions have yet to be identified for psychiatric disorders, the methods for it are commonly planned to be based on identifying "individuals with sufficient risk enrichment" [217].

Driven by the disease outlook, the risk perspective is defined to a large degree by the disorder diagnosis or, more seldom, another negative outcome such as a relapse or dropout from treatment. In contrast, the resistance perspective may have various end phenotypes to define the dimension studied, as illustrated by a remission study as well as research in resistance to relapse to heroin and cocaine addiction upon cessation (i.e., in prolonged abstinence from heroin and cocaine) [212, 218, 219]. This further differentiates resistance methodologies from the risk/disease paradigm. Importantly, in the latter publications, the genes found to be associated with resistance are consistent with the concept of general liability to addiction in that they resulted from a hypothesis-driven study into the genes mechanistically associated with stress, nonspecific to any drug or drugs in general.

Clearly, further research into the differences between relapse-resistant and relapsing individuals may result in determining, first and foremost, malleable factors enabling the phenotype that indeed is sought: disease-free recovery. The reason for relative confidence in obtaining that result is the fact that such individuals are well known to exist despite having had a disorder, whether they were assisted by existing methods (e.g., Alcoholics/Narcotics Anonymous) or "matured out" of addiction. Even if relatively rare in the diverse and heterogeneous recovered population, those factors may have wide applicability—similar to how the milkmaid-informed vaccination could be used for the entire population. The same principle, of course, is true for any prevention, primary (smallpox) or secondary (addiction relapse).

Compared to smallpox, for the complex disorders like addiction, however, the tables are turned: it is easy to identify a high-resistance sample to study resistance to relapse, but it is difficult to identify a high-resistance sample to ensure aggregation and discoverability of factors that could be used for *primary* prevention of addiction. As noted, resistance factors do not aggregate in the unaffected population as such. It is thus necessary to devise means to measure liability, particularly to identify individuals at the low end of its population distribution.

This problem has been approached using several designs, involving family and/or longitudinal data. First, capitalizing on the transmissibility of addiction liability (largely accounted for by its heritability), a transmissible liability index (TLI) has been developed, based on the item response theory (IRT) analysis of psychological indicators that differentiate offspring of addicted parents and normal controls before the children are exposed to drugs [220]. The TLI interval scale covers the entire liability distribution, while being more precise (lower error) in its higher portion because the items usually employed in psychological assessment tools are often indicators of behavior deviance rather than normality. The TLI is predictive of SUD in adulthood [221]. As expected, it has high heritability [220, 222, 223]. The TLI is included in the PhenX Toolkit [224], the NIH-funded collection of consensus protocols for biomedical research data collection. Another approach is to use the children's own outcome as adults, instead of parental diagnosis, to select their childhood liability indicators from among the psychological items assessed in childhood [147].

Liability measurement can also be accomplished in adults [147]. Whereas in the affected portion of the liability distribution the disorder symptoms can be scaled into a severity measure by applying, e.g., an appropriate IRT model [75], the asymptomatic population is not covered by that scale. The behavioral/psychological dimensions correlated with severity but "normal" rather than referencing a behavioral deviance should be identified, with respective non-symptom indicator items then used to scale the entire span of the liability distribution, given there is no differential item functioning in the two portions of the distribution. Obviously, the same measurement approaches can be applied to any complex disorder liability, enabling the identification of high-resistance groups as well as tracking liability development across time.

It should be kept in mind that while these tools are by design valid measures of liability, their ability to *forecast* the outcome is naturally restricted by the limited continuity of human behavior. In other words, the probability of disorder development is only a manifestation but not the synonym of liability, which is a labile and dynamic trait, in contrast to more stable traits like eye color or ridge count. Liability measurement, as exemplified by its application in sample selection, has importance besides prediction—similar to the importance of knowing a child's weight regardless of how predictive it is for the body mass in adulthood.

The application of the high-resistance approach further entails differences from the high-risk designs in that the controls in non-twin sample comparisons need to be selected from the rest of the "normal" population rather than the one that includes the symptomatic/affected individuals. As described in detail previously [147], the exclusion of symptomatic individuals is needed to minimize the impact of risk factors on comparisons. Two high-resistance groupings can be derived from measuring childhood liability: (1) pertaining to high outset resistance, i.e., *low* childhood liability *and* no SUD in adulthood, and (2) pertaining to high realized resistance, i.e., *high* childhood liability *but* no SUD in adulthood. The former would provide information about lifelong resistance factors while the latter about the factors that could potentially offset high outset liability. Respective cutoff points on the childhood liability scale can be established at a low and a high percentile for identifying low- and high-liability (high- and low-outset resistance) individuals, respectively, with grouping further indicated by their adult SUD-free phenotype.

A resistance approach unrelated to measurement and focused specifically on non-genetic factors is afforded by twins. Specifically, childhood and life span environmental resistance factors may be identifiable retroactively by using a co-twin design: differences, if any, between affected and unaffected twins in discordant MZ pairs are due to environmental factors (and possibly stochastic epigenetic differences) [225], because the effects of genetic differences are largely removed (except for possible postzygotic mutations). Such differences may be potentially drawn to effects in epigenetic mechanisms, although with obvious limitations pertaining to lack of access to the brain and the need to employ peripheral epigenetic indicators. However, the practical significance of the environmental findings derives directly from themselves, regardless of the neurobiological and gene expression mechanisms mediating their effects. DZ twins afford further extensions of this design, and discordance can also be operationalized in quantitative terms.

Specific resistance aspects may also be studied outside the quantitative framework, such as resistance to development of addiction or its particular aspects/symptoms in substance users, identifying a high-resistance group as those who have not developed these phenotypes despite long-term use, with the control group of those who have. It is difficult, however, to ensure the absence of addiction among substance users, particularly considering the variety of substances and the predominance of polysubstance use [45]). Power of such designs could be also increased by the quantification of use and abstinence duration.

Whereas resistance research, especially if supported to the degree comparable to the resources that have been expended in search of risk factors, is highly likely to result in translatable findings facilitating progress in prevention and recovery, adoption of the resistance perspective also brings about immediate benefits. Namely, it entails moving the focus of attention from the external circumstances, including the drugs, to the individual as the active agent dealing with those circumstances. In turn, this implies the need to alter the contradictory treatment of substance use as both a disease and a crime, removing both official labels and related limitations and recategorizing it into a *behavior to be prevented or recovered from*. This leaves responsibility for it with the individual—without either criminalizing or shifting it to another agent, human (e.g., physicians) or inanimate (drug).

It is unnecessary for a condition to be labeled a disease to qualify for medical help. Pregnancy is an example, as are regular checkups in the absence of any health concerns. While opioid poisonings present a public health problem, they are no different in this respect from alcohol poisonings or indeed any type of poisonings that follow voluntary substance consumption, sometimes lethal, with or without a suicidal intent. Although such intent may be absent in a particular case, such as a poisoning following recreational use of opioids, the hazard of concomitant self-destruction is common knowledge, as certain as the danger from other means of dangerous entertainment. Like in substance use, the extreme sensations produced, e.g., by skydiving (thrill), are due to neurobiological events produced by extreme circumstances, albeit via endogenous mechanisms. The main difference, however, is that responsible measures are taken, parachute and training, to offset the actual danger from skydiving. No such measures are taken to avoid the risk to become addicted, and if any concern about poisoning is present in substance use, it is clearly not sufficient in too many cases. Using clean syringes and other methods to avoid infections do deal with an aspect of potential harm, but not with the one that derives from drug consumption as such. The only responsible measure to prevent drug problems is to resist recreational drugs.

It is both logical and supported by the history of effective prevention measures that pivoting research from the risk/disease to the resistance aspect of liability or, in other words, to the health- (or behavior-adjustment)-oriented perspective promises a greater long-term success than the currently prevailing disease/risk orientation. The differences of the high-resistance populations from the controls on the key variables, empirically supported and/or hypothesized as candidates, particularly the environmental ones, have a high likelihood to be actionable and generalizable to the rest of the population. This is evidenced by their corresponding to the factors that have *in reality resulted* in the needed and predominant outcome of the disorder's nondevelopment or in successful recovery from it in the overwhelming majority of the population, in contrast to unknown and hardly ever observed neutralized risk factors.

Short term, without diminishing the medical help and social support (such as AA/NA) needed for coping with effects of substance use including addiction, the responsibility for one's behavior needs to be clearly defined as the individual's own, in contrast to unknowingly contracting an infection. The drug "epidemic" will remain, waxing and waning, now with one disabling or lethal substance, now with another, a tunnel with no light and no end, until mechanisms of behavioral resistance to the appetitive consummatory behavior of drug use gain significantly in their impact in the general population. This should be supported by understanding of personal responsibility for one's behavior and its structure inculcated in the young generation, thus creating the foundation for prevention of behavior deviations including problematic involvement with addictive/intoxicating substances. Research results may help achieving that, identifying successful resistance-raising strategies.

It would be wrong to conclude that research in biological variables such as genetic polymorphisms, or neurobiological mechanisms such as neuroimaging, is to be abandoned as unproductive from the standpoint of health significance. On the contrary, it leads to the accumulation of basic knowledge of the sources of human variation that eventually may lead, as basic knowledge often does, to as yet unforeseen advances. However, the approach to those variables also requires the reversal of common risk factor designs to the resistance perspective, if such research is intended for maximal health impact. Arguably, this reversal would facilitate the establishment of the *culture of prevention* [226] that still has not been fully embraced for substance use/addiction.

Dimensionality of the SUD Symptoms and Physiological Indicators: A Case Analysis

As noted above, the physiological symptoms (withdrawal, tolerance, and—added in DSM-5—craving) do not conceptually fit the liability/severity measurement model. Most of the symptoms denote persistent *use* of substances, a behavioral trait. Physiological symptoms are *causal* in relation to the trait indicated by the rest of the symptoms, since the physiological consequences of use elevate the probability of its continuation. In turn, substance use increases the probability of development, exacerbation, and maintenance of physiological dependence and its manifestations, withdrawal and tolerance, in a feedback loop. Inasmuch as the latent trait under study is concerned, i.e., the severity of substance use/addiction, this mechanistic process is captured by the labile *liability trait itself* that is reflected in the *behavioral* indicators. There is thus no need to model that loop in measuring the trait. For the model that would include the physiological indicators to be equivalent to the unidimensional one, a reverse indicator rule could be applied if there were one physiological symptom only, with an arrow pointing either directly from that symptom to the latent trait or in a reciprocal relationship [227], but there are at least two such symptoms (or three if the DSM-5 craving is included). A recursive model, i.e., the one that defines the physiological symptoms as the same kind of indicators of the latent trait as the behavioral symptoms, is not equivalent to the model that includes the feedback loop for the physiological symptoms and thus would be misspecified.

To statistically evaluate the diagnostic conceptualization of SUD liability, this study tested three bi-factor models (Fig. 1.2): (i) Model 1, all DSM-IV SUD symptoms are indicators of the common and substance-specific latent factors; (ii) Model 2, all SUD symptoms with the exception of tolerance and withdrawal as indicators of the latent factors; and (iii) Model 3 where tolerance and withdrawal were not indicators of the common and substance-specific factors, but these latent factors were regressed on these two symptoms.

The data used were from participants in a longitudinal family study of SUD etiology, the Center for Education and Drug Abuse Research (CEDAR) funded by NIDA. The sample consisted of families of adult men who qualified for DSM-IV SUD related to an illicit substance (abuse or dependence) (n = 349) and women (n = 173), their spouses/mates, as well as families of adult men and women who did not qualify for a SUD diagnosis (men, n = 190; women, n = 133). To be included in the study, at least one SUD symptom had to be present. The family was excluded from study if the father had a history of neurological disorders, schizophrenia, or uncorrectable sensory incapacity, or the participant child had a history of neurological injury requiring hospitalization, an IQ below 70, a chronic physical disability, uncorrectable sensory incapacity, or psychosis.

The mean age of the men was 40 years. European- and African-Americans comprised 77% and 22% of the sample. Mean family socioeconomic status according to Hollingshead criteria was 40, indicating that this sample was primarily middle class [228]. The mean age of the women was 38 years. Table 1.1 presents the lifetime SUD diagnoses in men and women. The most common SUD diagnoses are related to alcohol, cannabis, and cocaine in both men and women.

In this study, lifetime DSM-IV abuse and dependence symptoms related to use of alcohol, cannabis, cocaine, opioids, sedatives, and stimulants were used in the analyses. The abuse symptoms are (1) failure to fulfill major role obligations at work, school, or home, (2) hazardous use, (3) legal problems, and (4) continued substance use despite having persistent or recurrent social or interpersonal problems. The dependence symptoms are (1) tolerance; (2) withdrawal; (3) con-

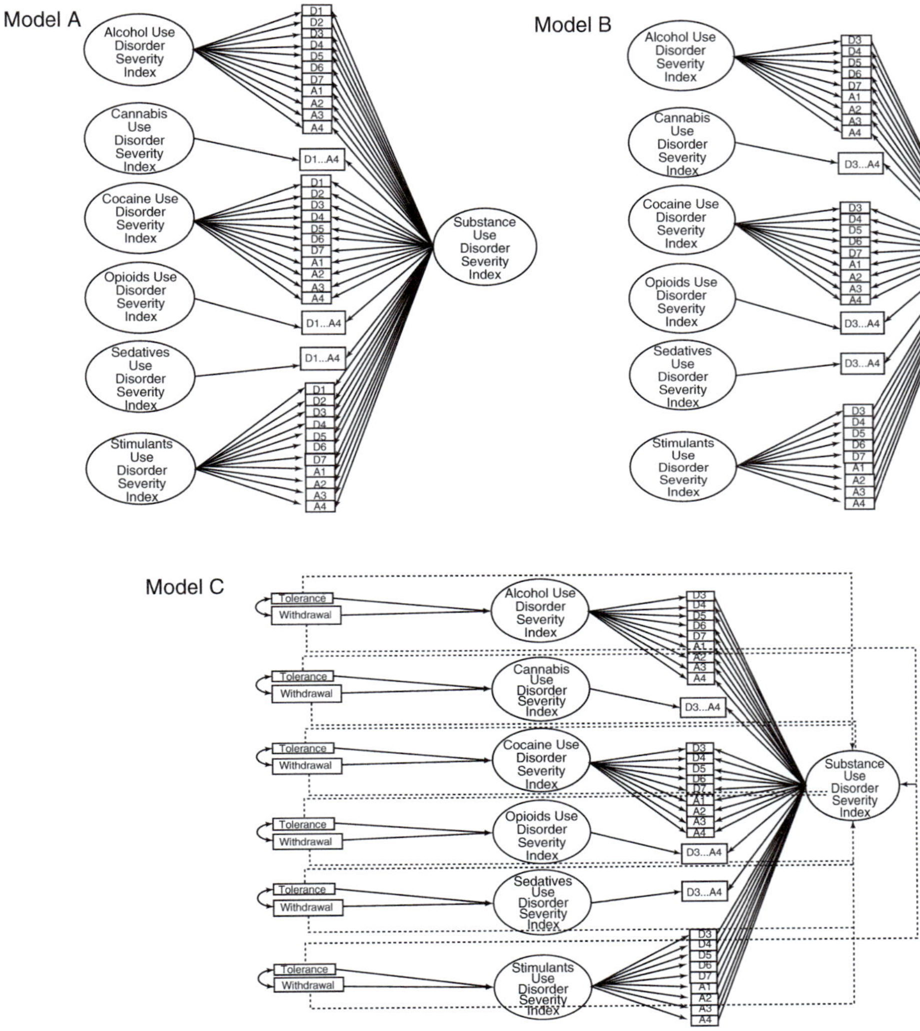

Fig. 1.2 Modeling substance use disorder symptoms

Table 1.1 Lifetime SUD diagnosis in men and women

	Men ($N = 539$)	Women ($N = 306$)
Alcohol	52%	43%
Cannabis	41%	21%
Cocaine	30%	16%
Opioids	15%	12%
Sedative	5%	5%
Stimulants	8%	19%

sumption of larger amounts or over a longer period than intended; (4) unsuccessful efforts to cut down; and (5) a great deal of time spent taking/using the substance; (6) reduced social, occupational, and recreational activities; and (7) persisting consumption despite physical or psychological problems. An expanded version of the Structured Clinical Interview for DSM-IV (SCID) [229] was administered to characterize lifetime and current substance use disorders. Diagnoses were formulated during a clinical conference chaired by a psychiatrist certified in addiction psychiatry and attended by another psychiatrist or a psychologist, along with the clinical associates who conducted the interviews. The best estimate procedure was used to formulate the diagnoses [230]. In this procedure, the results of the diagnostic interview, along with medical, legal, and social history information obtained from other facets of the research protocol and official records, were considered in aggregate when formulating the diagnoses.

Written informed consent was obtained from the participants prior to administering the protocols. All the study participants were additionally informed that the findings from this research were protected by a Certificate of Confidentiality issued to CEDAR by NIDA.

First, exploratory factor analysis was conducted to estimate the percent of variance accounted for by the first, second, and the rest of the sizable factors, using Mplus [231] to show the existence of the unidimensional general (global) factor. Mplus was also used to document the psychometric properties of the SUD symptoms: the item discrimination and item threshold parameters that characterized the symptom.

Mplus utilizes the maximum likelihood parameter estimates with standard errors and a chi-square test statistic (when applicable) that are robust to non-normality and non-independence of observations. A good fit is suggested by root mean square error of approximation (RMSEA) less than 0.05, comparative fit index (CFI) greater than 0.95, and/or Tucker-Lewis Index (TLI) greater than 0.95 [231]. In addition, −2log likelihood (−2logL), Akaike Information Criterion (AIC) [232], Bayesian Information Criterion (BIC), and sample size adjusted nBIC [233] are computed to determine the best fitting model. For the AIC, BIC, and nBIC, a lower value indicates a better model-data fit [234].

Model testing was followed by item response theory (IRT) analysis. The advantages of using IRT for psychometric trait measurement compared to traditional (or classical) psychometric approaches are well documented [235]. In particular, classical psychometric theory, although widely used in constructing and evaluating scales for measuring alcohol and drug use, is limited because subject characteristics and scale characteristics are correlated and cannot be separated. Item threshold and item discrimination parameters as well as reliability and validity of a scale must also be interpreted in the context of a particular sample. Hence, scale and item parameters vary across samples. This limitation of classical measurement theory is referred to as group dependency. In addition, in classical measurement theory, reliability is quantified as the correlation between test scores on parallel scales, which is constant across the continuum of the trait. In contrast, IRT provides a reliability score for each trait level.

Moreover, in IRT, item response function (IRF) informs on the relationship between responses to sets of items (e.g., endorsement/nonendorsement of SUD symptoms) and the person's latent trait value (e.g., SUD severity phenotype). Therefore, contingent on satisfactory model-data fit, the information obtained from IRT analyses enables documenting SUD severity across the gradient of latent trait severity while taking into account the difference between items' capacity to be discriminative across the spectrum of trait level.

In this study, a two-parameter (intercept and discrimination) IRT bi-factor logistic model, used to model global SUD severity and drug-specific dimensions, is described as

$$P_i(\theta_j) = 1 \Big/ \left(1 + \exp\left(-D\left(\sum a_{ik}\theta_{jk} + d_i\right)\right)\right); j = 1,\ldots,n; k = 1,\ldots,p$$

where θ_j is a number of unobserved continuous latent variables (such as global SUD severity, θ_1, and drug-specific dimensions, $\theta_2,\ldots, \theta_p$), to model a subject's response to an item; $P_i(\theta_j)$ is the probability the subject endorses an SUD symptom; a_i is the item discrimination parameter (slope), indicating the probability of endorsement of a symptom associated with changes in a subject's standing along the p-dimensions; d_i is the item intercept or scalar parameter that replaces item threshold parameter of the unidimensional two-parameter logistic model and is not interpreted as the threshold (or difficulty); n is the number of subjects; p is the number of dimensions ($\theta_1,\ldots,\theta_p$) such as global SUD severity and drug-specific dimensions; and $D = 1.7$ is the scaling constant used to approximate the logistic model to the normal ogive model in computing $P_i(\theta_j)$. The exponent in this model is a linear combination of a_i, θ_j values written as $a_{i1}\theta_{j1} + a_{i2}\theta_{j2} + \cdots + a_{i2}\theta_{jp} + d_i$, in which a_{i1} is the slope, or discrimination, parameter for symptom i for subject j's standing on the first dimension, $\theta_{1,p}$ is for the pth dimension, and d_i is the intercept. The higher the value of the sum, the higher the probability of endorsement of a symptom. The more discriminative item, with a higher a_i, on a particular dimension has a stronger effect on the probability of endorsing a symptom. In the bi-factor model, the probability of endorsing a SUD symptom item is related to the global SUD severity and drug-specific dimensions as a monotonically increasing S-shaped item response surface (IRS). In this study we focus mostly on the association between SUD symptoms and the global SUD severity. The item discrimination parameter has the same interpretation as the a parameter for univariate IRT models, proportional to the slope of the item response function (IRF) at the global SUD severity (θ_1); that is, the rate at which the probability of endorsement of a symptom changes as the latent trait score increases at the point of inflection. Higher item discrimination values are associated with steeper IRFs. In other words, higher discrimination parameters indicate a stronger relationship between SUD severity and observed symptom. A symptom with a low value of the item discrimination parameter would result in an IRF that increases gradually as a function of SUD severity.

The item threshold parameter (or item difficulty), which is defined as $b_i = \frac{-d_i}{\sqrt{\sum a_{ik}^2}}$, has the same interpretation as the b parameter for univariate IRT models and determines the position of the curve relative to the latent trait, which corresponds to the severity of the symptom. It is usually called summary difficulty (MDIFF or b) for an item. A higher threshold parameter indicates that fewer subjects endorse a particular symptom. In other words, a higher trait value (higher score on the continuum of the SUD severity scale) is required for the person to endorse the particular symptom; hence, individuals whose scores fall on the right of the scale are more severe cases compared to individuals whose scores are on the left of the scale.

The assumptions underlying the multidimensional IRT are very similar to those of unidimensional IRT. Two assumptions are crucial to apply IRT models to a SUD severity scale. (i) Unidimensionality implies that only one latent trait is measured by the symptoms used in developing the scale, i.e., the probability of endorsing a diagnosis is a function of only one latent trait. This corresponds to the situation where the latent trait is the only (or the main) source of covariance among the item (symptom) responses. If the residual covariances among symptoms are small (rather than zero) at a given trait level, there may exist a dominant factor, even though other factors may be present, corresponding to essential unidimensionality [236]. (ii) The second assumption is local independence, that is, for any group of subjects that are characterized by the $\theta_1,\ldots,\theta_p$, no relationship is present among the subject's responses to different symptoms after taking into account the subject's latent trait level [237]. Essentially, endorsement of a symptom is independent of endorsement of other symptoms, given all of the subject's exhibited scores on dimensions. Unidimensionality is a sufficient condition for satisfying the local independence assumption.

Furthermore, we used the following formula [238] to estimate IRT-based reliability of the global SUD severity index of the bi-factor model: $\rho = \left(\sigma_\theta^2 + \sigma_e^2\right) / \sigma_\theta^2$, where σ_θ^2 is the observed scale score variance and σ_e^2 is the average measurement error of variance across the levels of the latent trait of SUD severity. In addition, an average IRT-based reliability for the entire trait is provided.

The most frequently endorsed dependence symptoms were "tolerance" for alcohol, "a great deal time spent taking and using it" for cannabis, and "need for larger amounts or over a longer period than intended" for cocaine in both men and women (see Table 1.2). The most frequently

Table 1.2 Percent of endorsement and corrected item-total test correlations (r) of lifetime DSM-IV SUD dependence and abuse symptoms in men and women

	Men (N = 539)						Women (N = 306)					
Symptoms	Alcohol %, r	Cannabis %, r	Cocaine %, r	Opioids %, r	Sedative %, r	Stimulants %, r	Alcohol %, r	Cannabis %, r	Cocaine %, r	Opioids %, r	Sedative %, r	Stimulants %, r
D1	36, 0.62	15, 0.31	20, 0.52	10, 0.40	3, 0.29	4, 0.16	32, 0.57	6, 0.25	14, 0.73	5, 0.33	4, 0.23	15, 0.72
D2	15, 0.47	10, 0.30	11, 0.47	12, 0.40	3, 0.30	5, 0.24	12, 0.34	10, 0.18	10, 0.63	6, 0.37	4, 0.22	17, 0.75
D3	34, 0.64	19, 0.34	25, 0.56	11, 0.40	3, 0.31	5, 0.17	29, 0.49	10, 0.27	17, 0.75	5, 0.37	3, 0.26	18, 0.76
D4	26, 0.56	11, 0.32	22, 0.55	11, 0.37	2, 0.26	3, 0.19	20, 0.53	8, 0.20	17, 0.75	4, 0.38	3, 0.20	18, 0.76
D5	31, 0.62	22, 0.38	23, 0.57	12, 0.43	3, 0.37	5, 0.19	24, 0.53	11, 0.30	16, 0.77	6, 0.38	1, 0.19	17, 0.78
D6	20, 0.59	10, 0.36	19, 0.55	8, 0.44	2, 0.32	2, 0.16	18, 0.60	9, 0.25	13, 0.73	3, 0.32	2, 0.19	13, 0.74
D7	25, 0.60	10, 0.22	14, 0.55	6, 0.34	3, 0.32	5, 0.18	30, 0.43	8, 0.11	13, 0.70	3, 0.30	4, 0.25	16, 0.60
A1	27, 0.59	20, 0.36	17, 0.55	7, 0.34	2, 0.31	3, 0.19	25, 0.50	12, 0.18	14, 0.72	3, 0.21	3, 0.22	11, 0.64
A2	46, 0.54	32, 0.26	18, 0.50	7, 0.34	4, 0.32	7, 0.20	32, 0.34	10, 0.14	7, 0.64	3, 0.26	2, 0.17	8, 0.66
A3	20, 0.51	16, 0.37	8, 0.35	11, 0.40	3, 0.34	3, 0.20	8, 0.42	3, 0.05	6, 0.48	4, 0.28	2, 0.10	12, 0.65
A4	39, 0.64	17, 0.43	25, 0.62	11, 0.45	3, 0.35	4, 0.22	34, 0.48	9, 0.17	17, 0.76	5, 0.29	2, 0.18	17, 0.76

Note: Dependence symptoms. D1, tolerance; D2, withdrawal; D3, need for larger amounts or over a longer period than intended; D4, unsuccessful efforts to cut down; D5, a great deal of time spent taking/using it; D6, reduced social, occupational, and recreational activities; D7, substance use is continued despite physical or psychological problems. Abuse symptoms. A1, failure to fulfill major role obligations at work, school, or home; A2, hazardous use; A3, substance use-related legal problems; A4, continued substance use despite having persistent or recurrent social or interpersonal problems endorsed abuse items were "hazardous use" for alcohol and cannabis and "social and interpersonal problems" for cocaine in men, whereas "social and interpersonal problems" related to alcohol and cocaine use, and "failure to fulfill major role obligations" related to cannabis use, were most frequent in women. Most of the abuse and dependence symptoms have item-test correlations exceeding the 0.2 threshold, indicating a significant item relationship with the severity scale.

The principal component analysis showed that the first six factors accounted for 20%, 12%, 10%, 8%, 6%, 4%, and 2% of the variance in men and 27%, 15%, 8%, 7%, 5%, and 2% in women. The first factor's accounting for 20% or higher of the variance in males and females suggests a unidimensional factor structure of SUD abuse and dependence symptoms in both sexes [239]. The factor loadings of the symptoms on the global factor in the bi-factor model are all higher than 0.4 in males and, with few exceptions, in females.

We observed significant correlations among all six substance-specific classes (males, mean correlation = 0.33, SD = 0.17; females, mean correlation = 0.29, SD = 0.21), reflecting the common variance among them, suggesting the possibility of a global factor [240], and corresponding to general (common; non-drug-specific) liability to addiction. The bi-factor results also suggest that substance class-specific factors account for residual symptom covariation that is independent of the covariation due to the global factor.

Model fit statistics are presented in Table 1.3. Model C (the bi-factor model where tolerance and withdrawal are predictors rather than indicators of global and drug-specific factors) had the best fit statistics in both sexes; Model C had the smallest AIC, BIC, and sample-size-corrected BIC indices in men and women. Model B (bi-factor model without tolerance and withdrawal as indicators of general and drug-specific factors) had the second best fit indices.

The item discrimination and item intercept parameters of Model C of the bi-factor model for the global factor and substance-specific factors are presented in Tables 1.4 and 1.5 and also the estimates of regression coefficients of tolerance and withdrawal symptoms on the global and drug-specific factors in Table 1.6 for men and women, respectively. All symptoms indicating the global factor have high ability to discriminate between trait values (severity) in both males and females. The probability of endorsing any symptom is higher in men than in women, with the exception of stimulants. Alcohol use disorder symptoms are more likely to be endorsed than any other symptoms in both males and females.

Table 1.3 Comparison of three bi-factor models in men and women

	Men			Women		
	Model A	Model B	Model C	Model A	Model B	Model C
Sample size	539	539	539	306	306	306
−2logL	14138.47	12497.98	11042.64	6643.08	6188.40	5438.14
Number of parameters	193	157	209	193	157	209
χ^2	2233.01	1635.26	N/A	2271.80	1677.15	N/A
Df	2014	1328	N/A	2014	1328	N/A
P	<0.001	<0.001	N/A	<0.001	<0.001	N/A
RMSEA	0.014	0.021	N/A	0.020	0.029	N/A
CFI	0.99	0.99	N/A	0.99	0.99	N/A
TLI	0.99	0.99	N/A	0.99	0.99	N/A
AIC	14532.84	12811.61	11460.63	7029.08	6502.40	5856.14
BIC	15377.91	13485.09	12357.19	7749.61	7088.53	6634.37
nBIC	14752.56	12986.71	11693.75	7186.55	6590.59	5971.52

Note: Model fit indices: −2logL, −2log of likelihood
RMSEA root mean square error of approximation, *CFI* comparative fit index, *TLI* Tucker-Lewis Index, *AIC* Akaike Information Criterion, *BIC* Bayesian Information Criterion, *nBIC* sample size adjusted BIC

Table 1.4 Item parameter estimates of the bi-factor model for men, logit: aθ + *d*, *where a = item discrimination and d = item intercept parameters*

		Global factor	Alcohol factor	Cannabis factor	Cocaine factor	Opioids factor	Sedatives factor	Stimulants factor	
Item	Symptom	*A*	*a*	*a*	*a*	*a*	*a*	*a*	*d*
1	Alcohol D3	5.1890	3.8210						−0.6731
2	Alcohol D4	3.1566	1.8617						−1.1550
3	Alcohol D5	5.0306	3.4290						−0.9415
4	Alcohol D6	4.7742	2.8892						−2.4596
5	Alcohol D7	3.5825	1.0653						−1.0460
6	Alcohol A1	3.7816	1.2855						−0.9125
7	Alcohol A2	3.0746	0.9501						0.8796
8	Alcohol A3	2.7608	0.7035						−1.4075
9	Alcohol A4	5.1302	1.4778						0.5618
10	Cannabis D3	2.4483		3.4388					−2.9891
11	Cannabis D4	2.1473		2.7595					−3.6738
12	Cannabis D5	2.8354		3.1339					−2.3501
13	Cannabis D6	2.7925		2.5524					−3.6640
14	Cannabis D7	1.5522		0.9006					−2.3835
15	Cannabis A1	2.7299		1.3019					−1.5422
16	Cannabis A2	1.5433		1.5281					−0.6170
17	Cannabis A3	2.2953		1.4269					−2.0447
18	Cannabis A4	3.5711		1.8629					−2.2982
19	Cocaine D3	6.9531			9.3351				−5.6762
20	Cocaine D4	3.9849			4.7796				−3.5085
21	Cocaine D5	8.6178			9.7372				−6.6388
22	Cocaine D6	4.0451			4.3290				−3.7097
23	Cocaine D7	4.8442			3.7140				−4.2599
24	Cocaine A1	4.4464			5.1047				−4.6904
25	Cocaine A2	2.5232			2.2857				−2.2522
26	Cocaine A3	1.8580			1.9411				−3.5001
27	Cocaine A4	12.510			10.7859				−6.4879
28	Opioids D3	3.4692				9.6248			−11.6245
29	Opioids D4	3.1892				8.6993			−10.8771
30	Opioids D5	6.6732				14.1440			−16.8593
31	Opioids D6	6.2847				10.8388			−14.9663
32	Opioids D7	3.0958				4.5377			−7.4898
33	Opioids A1	3.2383				6.8373			−10.2099
34	Opioids A2	2.8708				4.5729			−6.9477
35	Opioids A3	3.7886				7.9019			−9.6273
36	Opioids A4	6.2008				9.3367			−11.5669
37	Sedatives D3	19.4254					22.8374		−11.4551
38	Sedatives D4	59.5169					72.5322		−36.6304
39	Sedatives D5	91.2321					92.1939		−45.4395
40	Sedatives D6	90.5012					92.9407		−47.0887
41	Sedatives D7	12.4736					12.7963		−6.7274
42	Sedatives A1	10.9197					9.2654		−6.0927
43	Sedatives A2	16.1057					15.3038		−7.2949
44	Sedatives A3	15.9028					13.6971		−7.8459

(continued)

Table 1.4 (continued)

		Global factor	Alcohol factor	Cannabis factor	Cocaine factor	Opioids factor	Sedatives factor	Stimulants factor	
45	Sedatives A4	99.5307					94.9702		−47.9854
46	Stimulants D3	4.5628						13.1244	−21.8357
47	Stimulants D4	2.5209						4.9435	−9.5823
48	Stimulants D5	3.1659						7.8877	−13.0054
49	Stimulants D6	2.1620						4.5102	−9.8447
50	Stimulants D7	2.2852						3.5685	−6.5313
51	Stimulants A1	2.8218						3.0109	−6.4650
52	Stimulants A2	2.9839						3.9371	−6.0988
53	Stimulants A3	2.6705						3.4554	−7.2486
54	Stimulants A4	5.8302						6.8019	−12.5011

Table 1.5 Item parameter estimates of the bi-factor model for women, logit: aθ + *d*, *where a = item discrimination and d = item intercept parameters*

		Global factor	Alcohol factor	Cannabis factor	Cocaine factor	Opioids factor	Sedatives factor	Stimulants factor	
Item	Symptom	*A*	*a*	*a*	*a*	*a*	*a*	*a*	*d*
1	Alcohol D3	2.4148	3.1209						0.2320
2	Alcohol D4	2.6973	3.4894						−0.9891
3	Alcohol D5	2.7374	3.4366						−0.3323
4	Alcohol D6	3.8816	3.5446						−0.5108
5	Alcohol D7	1.4955	2.1014						−0.0687
6	Alcohol A1	2.1459	2.0928						0.0480
7	Alcohol A2	0.7610	1.3420						−0.2883
8	Alcohol A3	2.2385	1.7928						−2.0533
9	Alcohol A4	2.2104	2.3261						0.8453
10	Cannabis D3	1.9647		3.0885					42.5550
11	Cannabis D4	1.5029		3.7546					3.8243
12	Cannabis D5	5.3757		8.4001					41.7198
13	Cannabis D6	2.1596		3.6755					35.3997
14	Cannabis D7	0.5509		1.3287					1.1023
15	Cannabis A1	1.4166		2.0385					1.7060
16	Cannabis A2	0.3980		1.9036					33.6530
17	Cannabis A3	0.0218		2.4572					−1.3232
18	Cannabis A4	0.5529		2.0231					3.4715
19	Cocaine D3	136.5690			59.9136				−2.9084
20	Cocaine D4	12.8233			5.2076				−4.4674
21	Cocaine D5	125.3270			32.9560				−6.6597
22	Cocaine D6	202.0310			101.4330				−3.6430
23	Cocaine D7	7.0961			1.8275				−2.5728
24	Cocaine A1	7.9998			2.1366				−2.0296
25	Cocaine A2	1196.1400			91.9805				−2.8969
26	Cocaine A3	4.0332			1.6714				−5.6267
27	Cocaine A4	10.9397			3.7173				−3.0291
28	Opioids D3	5.1084				8.3511			−9.1463
29	Opioids D4	7.6216				11.8728			−13.8876

(continued)

Table 1.5 (continued)

		Global factor	Alcohol factor	Cannabis factor	Cocaine factor	Opioids factor	Sedatives factor	Stimulants factor	
30	Opioids D5	6.7509				9.0243			−8.5047
31	Opioids D6	54.5872				79.2701			−50.6007
32	Opioids D7	4.4095				7.6919			−10.4394
33	Opioids A1	1.0769				6.2055			−10.4031
34	Opioids A2	5.0061				14.0121			−19.7629
35	Opioids A3	2.8710				4.2328			−5.5682
36	Opioids A4	3.3283				8.2137			−10.0123
37	Sedatives D3	111.4950					125.8260		−48.3544
38	Sedatives D4	4.7484					6.6705		−4.6341
39	Sedatives D5	79.2672					83.9005		−46.5090
40	Sedatives D6	72.5946					76.2034		−39.5875
41	Sedatives D7	9.5490					11.1498		−5.0510
42	Sedatives A1	25.2635					33.8960		−17.1996
43	Sedatives A2	28.3772					60.3116		−46.7688
44	Sedatives A3	2.7433					5.6832		−6.0071
45	Sedatives A4	61.2161					87.7921		−48.9526
46	Stimulants D3	133.6840						58.7764	41.8151
47	Stimulants D4	12.0984						4.9348	3.7398
48	Stimulants D5	120.1690						26.8082	42.2636
49	Stimulants D6	260.8590						137.9160	39.0613
50	Stimulants D7	4.1725						1.0993	0.6916
51	Stimulants A1	5.6390						1.7200	0.1777
52	Stimulants A2	1597.0800						89.3574	33.3187
53	Stimulants A3	4.9554						1.0370	0.4232
54	Stimulants A4	10.3168						3.6575	2.9636

Table 1.6 presents the estimates of regression coefficients of tolerance and withdrawal for males and females. The global factor is predicted significantly by the tolerance and withdrawal symptoms of alcohol use disorder in men and the withdrawal symptom of the stimulants in women. The tolerance and withdrawal symptoms, with the exception of the withdrawal symptom for alcohol in men, predict all substance-specific factors. Both withdrawal and tolerance predict the alcohol-specific factor, and withdrawal predicts marijuana and opioid use disorder factors.

The standard error of measurement of the global SUD severity factor is presented in Fig. 1.3. The global SUD severity factor in men has better precision and is more discriminating at low to moderate (−2 to −0.9) and moderate to high (−0.4 to 2.0) levels of SUD severity, whereas measurements in women are more precise than in men at moderate levels below the mean (−0.8 to −0.3). The measurement in women is also more precise than in men at the extreme values of the global SUD severity factor (−3 to −2.3 and 2.3 to 3). Concomitantly, the IRT-based reliability coefficient is in the good range for both men ($\rho = 0.95$) and women ($\rho = 0.87$).

To summarize, this research complements and extends previous studies showing that the SUD symptoms are scalable as indicators of a single common factor [107, 241], corresponding to general (non-drug-specific, common) liability to addiction, combined with drug-specific liabilities [99, 101, 220–222]. This study shows that (i) bi-factor model provides the most optimal representation of the factor structure of SUD symptoms in males and females and (ii) tolerance and withdrawal symptoms are not indicators of the global factor and drug-specific factors, but instead they are significant predictors of global factor and drug-specific factors.

Table 1.6 Regression coefficients from tolerance and withdrawal to global factor and drug-specific factors in men and women

	Men		Women	
	Tolerance	Withdrawal	Tolerance	Withdrawal
	b	b	b	b
Global factor				
Alcohol	0.31c	0.23c	−0.04	−0.01
Marijuana	0.06	0.09	−0.02	−0.05
Cocaine	0.18b	0.02	0.14	−0.01
Opioids	−0.01	0.11	−0.02	0.01
Sedative	0.07	−0.03	−0.07	0.01
Stimulants	−0.04	0.07	0.13	0.33c
Drug-specific factors				
Alcohol	0.72c	0.10	0.39c	0.32c
Marijuana	0.35c	0.32c	0.15	0.39a
Cocaine	0.64c	0.14b	−0.34	0.19
Opioids	0.10a	0.57c	0.20a	0.24a
Sedative	0.20b	0.19b	0.31	0.08
Stimulants	0.24c	0.32c	−0.14	0.39

a: $p < 0.05$, b: $p < 0.01$, c: $p < 0.001$

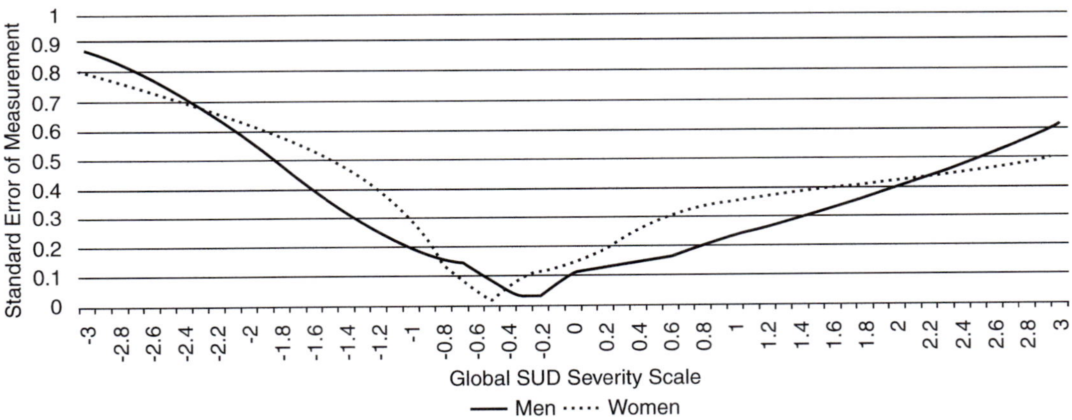

Fig. 1.3 Substance use disorder severity scale

The study has its limitations. The pattern and rate of SUD observed in women may be, in part, due to the influence of homogamy, including the possibility of contagion (direct influence of the mate's phenotype) [242]. The sample of women was also relatively small. Nonetheless, the results support the definition of addiction liability as a behavioral trait with a substantial non-substance-specific, common component termed common/general liability to addiction, as well as demonstrate the lack of support for using physiological symptoms for addiction severity/liability measurement, consistent with these symptoms' contribution to the emergence of behavioral symptoms. This trait can be quantified using latent variable approaches such as IRT, enabling individual liability measurement along the entire distribution of the trait in the population.

References

1. Dobzhansky T. Genetics and the origin of species. 3d ed. New York: Columbia University Press; 1951.

2. Goedde HW, Agarwal DP, Harada S, Meier-Tackmann D, Ruofu D, Bienzle U, et al. Population genetic studies on aldehyde dehydrogenase isozyme deficiency and alcohol sensitivity. Am J Hum Genet. 1983;35(4):769–72.
3. Harada S, Agarwal DP, Goedde HW. Aldehyde dehydrogenase polymorphism and alcohol metabolism in alcoholics. Alcohol. 1985;2(3):391–2.
4. Harada S, Agarwal DP, Goedde HW, Tagaki S, Ishikawa B. Possible protective role against alcoholism for aldehyde dehydrogenase isozyme deficiency in Japan. Lancet. 1982;2(8302):827.
5. American Psychiatric Association DSM-5 Task Force. Diagnostic and statistical manual of mental disorders : DSM-5, vol. xliv. 5th ed. Washington, D.C.: American Psychiatric Association; 2013. p. 947.
6. Macgregor S, Lind PA, Bucholz KK, Hansell NK, Madden PA, Richter MM, et al. Associations of ADH and ALDH2 gene variation with self report alcohol reactions, consumption and dependence: an integrated analysis. Hum Mol Genet. 2009;18(3):580–93.
7. Blum K. Allelic association of human dopamine D2 receptor gene in alcoholism. JAMA. 1990;263(15):2055.
8. Dick DM, Wang JC, Plunkett J, Aliev F, Hinrichs A, Bertelsen S, et al. Family-based association analyses of alcohol dependence phenotypes across DRD2 and neighboring gene ANKK1. Alcohol Clin Exp Res. 2007;31(10):1645–53.
9. Neville MJ, Johnstone EC, Walton RT. Identification and characterization of ANKK1: A novel kinase gene closely linked to DRD2 on chromosome band 11q23.1. Hum Mutat. 2004;23(6):540–5.
10. Jung Y, Montel RA, Shen P-H, Mash DC, Goldman D. Assessment of the association of D2 dopamine receptor gene and reported allele frequencies with alcohol use disorders. JAMA Netw Open. 2019;2(11):e1914940.
11. Terwilliger JD. Gene mapping and human disease. In: Vanyukov MM, editor. Genetics of substance use. Switzerland: Springer Nature.
12. Thoday JM, Thompson JN. The number of segregating genes implied by continuous variation. Genetica. 1976;4:335–44.
13. Munafo MR, Zammit S, Flint J. Practitioner review: a critical perspective on gene-environment interaction models--what impact should they have on clinical perceptions and practice? J Child Psychol Psychiatry. 2014;55(10):1092–101.
14. Terwilliger JD, Weiss KM. Confounding, ascertainment bias, and the blind quest for a genetic 'fountain of youth'. Ann Med. 2003;35(7):532–44.
15. Maher B. Personal genomes: the case of the missing heritability. Nature. 2008;456(7218):18–21.
16. Blum K, Sheridan PJ, Wood RC, Braverman ER, Chen TJ, Cull JG, et al. The D2 dopamine receptor gene as a determinant of reward deficiency syndrome. J R Soc Med. 1996;89(7):396–400.
17. Wei X, Nielsen R. CCR5-32 is deleterious in the homozygous state in humans. Nat Med. 2019;25(6):909–10.
18. Grucza RA, Wang JC, Stitzel JA, Hinrichs AL, Saccone SF, Saccone NL, et al. A risk allele for nicotine dependence in CHRNA5 is a protective allele for cocaine dependence. Biol Psychiatry. 2008;64(11):922–9.
19. Maher BS, Vladimirov VI, Latendresse SJ, Thiselton DL, McNamee R, Kang M, et al. The AVPR1A gene and substance use disorders: association, replication, and functional evidence. Biol Psychiatry. 2011;70(6):519–27.
20. Watanabe K, Stringer S, Frei O, Umićević Mirkov M, De Leeuw C, Polderman TJC, et al. A global overview of pleiotropy and genetic architecture in complex traits. Nat Genet. 2019;51(9):1339–48.
21. Darwin C. The descent of man, and selection in relation to sex. London: John Murray; 1871.
22. Wilson EO. Sociobiology : the new synthesis. 25th anniversary ed. Cambridge, MA: Belknap Press of Harvard University Press; 2000. xiii. p. 697.
23. Kandel D. Stages in adolescent involvement in drug use. Science. 1975;190(4217):912–4.
24. Kandel D, Faust R. Sequence and stages in patterns of adolescent drug use. Arch Gen Psychiatry. 1975;32(7):923–32.
25. Kandel D, Jessor R. The gateway hypothesis revisited. In: Kandel DB, editor. Stages and pathways of drug involvement: examining the gateway hypothesis. Cambridge, MA: Cambridge University Press; 2002. p. 365–72.
26. Kandel DB. Does marijuana use cause the use of other drugs? JAMA. 2003;289(4):482–3.
27. Kandel DB. Stages and pathways of drug involvement: examining the gateway hypothesis. Cambridge, UK ; New York: Cambridge University Press; 2002. xvi. p. 384.
28. Kandel DB, Kandel ER. A molecular basis for nicotine as a gateway drug. N Engl J Med. 2014;371(21):2038–9.
29. Kandel DB, Yamaguchi K, Klein LC. Testing the gateway hypothesis. Addiction. 2006;101(4):470–2. discussion 4-6
30. Levine A, Huang Y, Drisaldi B, Griffin EA, Pollak DD, Xu S, et al. Molecular mechanism for a gateway drug: epigenetic changes initiated by nicotine prime gene expression by cocaine. Science Translat Med. 2011;3(107):107ra109.
31. Cook T, Davenport S, Trusler J. The Works of William Hogarth; containing one hundred and fifty-nine engravings, by Mr. Cooke, and Mr. Davenport, with descriptions, in which are pointed out many beauties that have hitherto escaped notice, with a comment on their moral tendency by the Rev. John Trusler. In two volumes. London: J. Sharpe, King Street, Covent-Garden; R. Griffin and Co. Glasgow; 1821.
32. Vanyukov MM, Tarter RE, Kirillova GP, Kirisci L, Reynolds MD, Kreek MJ, et al. Common liability

to addiction and "gateway hypothesis": theoretical, empirical and evolutionary perspective. Drug Alcohol Depend. 2012;123(Suppl 1):S3–17.
33. Kandel D. Setting the record straight on the phrase 'gateway drug'. In: Rath A, editor. NPR: All Things Considered. https://www.npr.org/2015/04/18/400658693/setting-the-record-straight-on-the-phrase-gateway-drug: NPR; 2015.
34. O'Brien CP, Volkow N, Li TK. What's in a word? Addiction versus dependence in DSM-V. Am J Psychiatry. 2006;163(5):764–5.
35. Golub A, Johnson B. Substance use progression and hard drug use in inner city New York. In: Kandel DB, editor. Stages and pathways of drug involvement: examining the gateway hypothesis. Cambridge: Cambridge University Press; 2002. p. 90–112.
36. Mackesy-Amiti ME, Fendrich M, Goldstein PJ. Sequence of drug use among serious drug users: typical vs atypical progression. Drug Alcohol Depend. 1997;45(3):185–96.
37. Tarter RE, Vanyukov M, Kirisci L, Reynolds M, Clark DB. Predictors of marijuana use in adolescents before and after licit drug use: examination of the gateway hypothesis. Am J Psychiatry. 2006;163(12):2134–40.
38. Irons DE, McGue M, Iacono WG, Oetting WS. Mendelian randomization: a novel test of the gateway hypothesis and models of gene-environment interplay. Dev Psychopathol. 2007;19(4):1181–95.
39. Furr-Holden CD, Ialongo NS, Anthony JC, Petras H, Kellam SG. Developmentally inspired drug prevention: middle school outcomes in a school-based randomized prevention trial. Drug Alcohol Depend. 2004;73(2):149–58.
40. Morral AR, McCaffrey DF, Paddock SM. Reassessing the marijuana gateway effect. Addiction. 2002;97(12):1493–504.
41. Morral AR, McCafrey DF, Paddock SM. Evidence does not favor marijuana gateway effects over a common-factor interpretation of drug use initiation: responses to Anthony, Kenkel & Mathios and Lynskey. Addiction. 2002;97(12):1509–10.
42. Kandel DB. Examining the gateway hypothesis: stages and pathways of drug involvement. In: Kandel DB, editor. Stages and pathways of drug involvement: examining the gateway hypothesis. Cambridge: Cambridge University Press; 2002. p. 3–16.
43. Degenhardt L, Dierker L, Chiu WT, Medina-Mora ME, Neumark Y, Sampson N, et al. Evaluating the drug use "gateway" theory using cross-national data: consistency and associations of the order of initiation of drug use among participants in the WHO world mental health surveys. Drug Alcohol Depend. 2010;108(1-2):84–97.
44. Anthony JC. Death of the 'stepping-stone' hypothesis and the 'gateway' model? Comments on Morral et al. Addiction. 2002;97(12):1505–7.
45. Darke S, Hall W. Levels and correlates of polydrug use among heroin users and regular amphetamine users. Drug Alcohol Depend. 1995;39(3):231–5.
46. Tsuang MT, Lyons MJ, Meyer JM, Doyle T, Eisen SA, Goldberg J, et al. Co-occurrence of abuse of different drugs in men: the role of drug-specific and shared vulnerabilities. Arch Gen Psychiatry. 1998;55(11):967–72.
47. Kendler KS, Myers J, Prescott CA. Specificity of genetic and environmental risk factors for symptoms of cannabis, cocaine, alcohol, caffeine, and nicotine dependence. Arch Gen Psychiatry. 2007;64(11):1313–20.
48. Whitehead PC, Smart RG, Laforest L. Multiple drug use among marijuana smokers in eastern Canada. Int J Addict. 1972;7(1):179–90.
49. Johnston L. University of Michigan. Survey research center. Drugs and American youth. A report from the youth in transition project, vol. xiii. Ann Arbor: Institute for Social Research; 1973. p. 273.
50. Jessor R, Jessor SL. Problem behavior and psychosocial development : a longitudinal study of youth, vol. xv. New York: Academic Press; 1977. p. 281.
51. Kandel DB, Yamaguchi K. Developmental stages of involvement in substance use. Sourcebook on substance abuse: etiology, epidemiology, assessment, and treatment. Needham Heights: Allyn & Bacon; 1999. p. 50–74.
52. Falconer DS. The inheritance of liability to certain diseases, estimated from the incidence among relatives. Ann Hum Genet. 1965;29:51–76.
53. Scherma M, Qvist JS, Asok A, Huang S-SC, Masia P, Deidda M, et al. Cannabinoid exposure in rat adolescence reprograms the initial behavioral, molecular, and epigenetic response to cocaine. Proc Natl Acad Sci. 2020:201920866.
54. Vanyukov MM. A gateway that never was. Behav Genet. 2022;52(1):65–8.
55. Young SE, Stallings MC, Corley RP, Krauter KS, Hewitt JK. Genetic and environmental influences on behavioral disinhibition. Am J Med Genet. 2000;96(5):684–95.
56. Iacono WG, Carlson SR, Taylor J, Elkins IJ, McGue M. Behavioral disinhibition and the development of substance-use disorders: findings from the Minnesota twin family study. Dev Psychopathol. 1999;11(4):869–900.
57. Tarter R, Vanyukov M, Giancola P, Dawes M, Blackson T, Mezzich A, et al. Etiology of early age onset substance use disorder: a maturational perspective. Dev Psychopathol. 1999;11(4):657–83.
58. Windle M. Psychopathy and antisocial personality disorder among alcoholic inpatients. J Stud Alcohol. 1999;60(3):330–6.
59. Tarter RE, Kirisci L, Habeych M, Reynolds M, Vanyukov M. Neurobehavior disinhibition in childhood predisposes boys to substance use disorder by

young adulthood: direct and mediated etiologic pathways. Drug Alcohol Depend. 2004;73(2):121–32.
60. DEA. DEA, United States Drug Enforcement Administration: Drug Scheduling. undated. Available from: https://www.dea.gov/drug-scheduling.
61. Roditis ML, Delucchi K, Chang A, Halpern-Felsher B. Perceptions of social norms and exposure to pro-marijuana messages are associated with adolescent marijuana use. Prev Med. 2016;93:171–6.
62. Talati A, Wickramaratne PJ, Keyes KM, Hasin DS, Levin FR, Weissman MM. Smoking and psychopathology increasingly associated in recent birth cohorts. Drug Alcohol Depend. 2013;133(2):724–32.
63. Kaye AD, Granier AL, Garcia AJ, Carlson SF, Fuller MC, Haroldson AR, et al. Non-opioid perioperative pain strategies for the clinician: a narrative review. Pain Ther. 2020.
64. Lieber CS. Perspectives: do alcohol calories count? Am J Clin Nutr. 1991;54(6):976–82.
65. Richard EL, Kritz-Silverstein D, Laughlin GA, Fung TT, Barrett-Connor E, McEvoy LK. Alcohol intake and cognitively healthy longevity in community-dwelling adults: the rancho Bernardo study. J Alzheimers Dis. 2017;59(3):803–14.
66. Zhang R, Shen L, Miles T, Shen Y, Cordero J, Qi Y, et al. Association of low to moderate alcohol drinking with cognitive functions from middle to older age among US adults. JAMA Netw Open. 2020;3(6):e207922.
67. Enculescu C, Kerr ED, Yeo KYB, Schenk G, Fortes MRS, Schulz BL. Proteomics reveals profound metabolic changes in the alcohol use disorder brain. ACS Chem Neurosci. 2019;10(5):2364–73.
68. Shwayder ME. Marijuana advocate. Harvard Magazine. May-June 2011. ed2011.
69. Courtwright DT. Commentary on Hall (2010): the difference a word makes - a short history of 'prohibition'. Addiction. 2010;105(7):1174–5.
70. Blocker JS Jr. Did prohibition really work? Alcohol prohibition as a public health innovation. Am J Public Health. 2006;96(2):233–43.
71. Schoenaker D, Brennan E, Wakefield MA, Durkin SJ. Anti-smoking social norms are associated with increased cessation behaviours among lower and higher socioeconomic status smokers: a population-based cohort study. PLoS One. 2018;13(12):e0208950.
72. Vanyukov MM, Tarter RE. Genetics and epigenetics of substance use. In: Sloboda Z, Petras H, Robertson EB, Hingson R, editors. Prevention of substance use. New York: Springer Publishers; 2019. p. 57–73.
73. Mill J. Editorial note. In: Mill JS, editor. Analysis of the phenomena of the human mind, A New Edition, with notes illustrative and critical by Alexander Bain, Andrew Findlater and George Grote, edited with additional notes by John Stuart Mill, in two volumes. London: Longmans Green Reader and Dyer; 1869. Volume II, p. 5.
74. WHO. ICD-11 Reference Guide. https://icd.who.int/icd11refguide/en/index.html. World Health Organization; 2019.
75. Kirisci L, Tarter RE, Reynolds M, Vanyukov MM. Item response theory analysis to assess dimensionality of substance use disorder abuse and dependence symptoms. Int J Pers Cent Med. 2016;6(4):260–73.
76. MacCoun RJ. The puzzling unidimensionality of DSM-5 substance use disorder diagnoses. Front Psych. 2013;4:153.
77. Kendler KS, Jacobson KC, Prescott CA, Neale MC. Specificity of genetic and environmental risk factors for use and abuse/dependence of cannabis, cocaine, hallucinogens, sedatives, stimulants, and opiates in male twins. Am J Psychiatry. 2003;160(4):687–95.
78. Haberstick BC, Zeiger JS, Corley RP, Hopfer CJ, Stallings MC, Rhee SH, et al. Common and drug-specific genetic influences on subjective effects to alcohol, tobacco and marijuana use. Addiction. 2011;106(1):215–24.
79. Palmer RH, Button TM, Rhee SH, Corley RP, Young SE, Stallings MC, et al. Genetic etiology of the common liability to drug dependence: evidence of common and specific mechanisms for DSM-IV dependence symptoms. Drug Alcohol Depend. 2012;123(Suppl 1):S24–32.
80. Pickard S, Ahmed SH, Foddy B, editors. Alternative models of addiction. Front Psychiatry. 2015;6.
81. American Psychiatric Association. Task Force on DSM-IV. Diagnostic and statistical manual of mental disorders: DSM-IV. 4th ed. Washington, DC: American Psychiatric Association; 1994;xxvii. p. 886.
82. Stein DJ, Phillips KA, Bolton D, Fulford KWM, Sadler JZ, Kendler KS. What is a mental/psychiatric disorder? From DSM-IV to DSM-V. Psychol Med. 2010;40(11):1759–65.
83. Leshner AI. Foreword. In: Kandel DB, editor. Stages and pathways of drug involvement: examining the gateway hypothesis. Cambridge: Cambridge University Press; 2002. p. xiii.
84. NIDA. Dr. Nora Volkow on addiction: a disease of free will. National Institute on Drug Abuse Director, Dr. Nora Volkow, delivers the William C. Menninger Memorial Convocation Lecture during the 168th Annual Meeting of the American Psychiatric Association in Toronto, Canada: NIDA; 2015. Available from: https://www.drugabuse.gov/videos/dr-nora-volkow-addiction-disease-free-will.
85. Robins LN, Helzer JE, Hesselbrock M, Wish E. Vietnam veterans three years after Vietnam: how our study changed our view of heroin. Am J Addict. 2010;19(3):203–11.
86. Robins LN, Slobodyan S. Post-Vietnam heroin use and injection by returning US veterans:

clues to preventing injection today. Addiction. 2003;98(8):1053–60.
87. Winick C. Maturing out of narcotic addiction: United Nations Office on Drugs and Crime; 1962 [updated 1/1/1962]. Available from: https://www.unodc.org/unodc/en/data-and-analysis/bulletin/bulletin_1962-01-01_1_page002.html.
88. Lindell M. What are the odds? From crack addict to CEO. Lindell Publishing; 2019.
89. Prince D, McGuiness K. Aiming high: how a prominent sports and celebrity agent hit bottom at the top. Los Angeles: Light Hustler; 2018.
90. Cohen P. The clinician's illusion. Arch Gen Psychiatry. 1984;41(12):1178.
91. Lopez-Quintero C, Hasin DS, De Los Cobos JP, Pines A, Wang S, Grant BF, et al. Probability and predictors of remission from life-time nicotine, alcohol, cannabis or cocaine dependence: results from the National Epidemiologic Survey on alcohol and related conditions. Addiction. 2011;106(3):657–69.
92. SAMHSA. Impact of the DSM-IV to DSM-5 changes on the national survey on drug use and health [Internet 2016 4/15/2020]. Available from: https://www.ncbi.nlm.nih.gov/books/NBK519697/.
93. Volkow ND, McLellan AT. Opioid abuse in chronic pain--misconceptions and mitigation strategies. N Engl J Med. 2016;374(13):1253–63.
94. Chang H-W, Ho W-C, Huang C-L, Wang R-Y. Precision therapeutic opioid dosing implications from genetic biomarkers and craving score. Medicine. 2020;99(22):e20429.
95. Volkow ND, Morales M. The brain on drugs: from reward to addiction. Cell. 2015;162(4):712–25.
96. Tarter R, Vanyukov M. Re-visiting the validity of the construct of resilience. In: Glantz MD, Johnson JL, editors. Resilience and Development: Positive Life Adaptations. New York: Plenum Press; 1999. p. 85–100.
97. Tarter RE, Moss HB, Arria A, Mezzich AC, Vanyukov MM. The psychiatric diagnosis of alcoholism: critique and proposed reformulation. Alcohol Clin Exp Res. 1992;16(1):106–16.
98. Tarter RE, Vanyukov M. Alcoholism: a developmental disorder. J Consult Clin Psychol. 1994;62(6):1096–107.
99. Vanyukov MM, Kirisci L, Tarter RE, Simkevitz HF, Kirillova GP, Maher BS, et al. Liability to substance use disorders: 2. A measurement approach. Neurosci Biobehav Rev. 2003;27(6):517–26.
100. Vanyukov MM, Tarter RE. Genetic studies of substance abuse. Drug Alcohol Depend. 2000;59(2):101–23.
101. Vanyukov MM, Tarter RE, Kirisci L, Kirillova GP, Maher BS, Clark DB. Liability to substance use disorders: 1. Common mechanisms and manifestations. Neurosci Biobehav Rev. 2003;27(6):507–15.
102. Conway KP, Levy J, Vanyukov M, Chandler R, Rutter J, Swan GE, et al. Measuring addiction propensity and severity: the need for a new instrument. Drug Alcohol Depend. 2010;111(1-2):4–12.
103. Vanyukov MM, Moss HB, Plail JA, Blackson T, Mezzich AC, Tarter RE. Antisocial symptoms in preadolescent boys and in their parents: associations with cortisol. Psychiatry Res. 1993;46(1):9–17.
104. Insel T, Cuthbert B, Garvey M, Heinssen R, Pine DS, Quinn K, et al. Research domain criteria (RDoC): toward a new classification framework for research on mental disorders. Am J Psychiatr. 2010;167(7):748–51.
105. NIMH. NIMH Research Domain Criteria (RDoC): National Institute of Mental Health; 2011. Available from: http://www.nimh.nih.gov/research-priorities/rdoc/nimh-research-domain-criteria-rdoc.shtml; currently archived at https://web.archive.org/web/20140330070232/http://www.nimh.nih.gov/research-priorities/rdoc/nimh-research-domain-criteria-rdoc.shtml.
106. NIH. Missions and Goals, undated [updated July 27, 2017]. Available from: https://www.nih.gov/about-nih/what-we-do/mission-goals.
107. Kirisci L, Tarter RE, Vanyukov M, Martin C, Mezzich A, Brown S. Application of item response theory to quantify substance use disorder severity. Addict Behav. 2006;31(6):1035–49.
108. Kirisci L, Vanyukov M, Dunn M, Tarter R. Item response theory modeling of substance use: an index based on 10 drug categories. Psychol Addict Behav. 2002;16(4):290–8.
109. Wu LT, Pan JJ, Blazer DG, Tai B, Brooner RK, Stitzer ML, et al. The construct and measurement equivalence of cocaine and opioid dependences: a National Drug Abuse Treatment Clinical Trials Network (CTN) study. Drug Alcohol Depend. 2009;103(3):114–23.
110. Heyman GM. Addiction and choice: theory and new data. Front Psych. 2013;4:7–11.
111. Satel S, Lilienfeld SO. Addiction and the brain-disease fallacy. Front Psych. 2013;4:17–27.
112. Vanyukov MM. Evolution, genes, and environment - Neurobiological outcomes. In: Fishbein DH, editor. The Science, Treatment, and Prevention of Antisocial Behaviors: Application to the Criminal Justice System. Chapter 4. Kingston: Civic Research Institute; 2004. p. 4-1–4-29.
113. Vanyukov MM. An Eternal Epidemic: 1. Why substance use problems persist. PsyArXiv, 14 July 2021. https://doi.org/10.31234/osf.io/tkm5u.
114. Tarter RE, Kirisci L, Mezzich A, Ridenour T, Fishbein D, Horner M, et al. Does the "gateway" sequence increase prediction of cannabis use disorder development beyond deviant socialization? Implications for prevention practice and policy. Drug Alcohol Depend. 2012;123(Suppl 1):S72–8.
115. Cloninger RC, Reich T, Guze SB. The multifactorial model of disease transmission: II. Sex differences in the familial transmission of sociopathy (antisocial personality). Br J Psychiatry. 1975;127:11–22.
116. Reich R, Cloninger CR, Guze SB. The multifactorial model of disease transmission: I. Description of

the model and its use in psychiatry. Br J Psychiatry. 1975;127:1–10.

117. Bucholz KK, Heath AC, Reich T, Hesselbrock VM, Kramer JR, Nurnberger JI Jr, et al. Can we subtype alcoholism? A latent class analysis of data from relatives of alcoholics in a multicenter family study of alcoholism. Alcohol Clin Exp Res. 1996;20(8):1462–71.
118. NIDA. Strategic planning workgroup on the complexity of substance use disorders and the continuum of substance use problems: workgroup proposal: National Institute on Drug Abuse; 2015. Available from: https://www.drugabuse.gov/about-nida/strategic-plan/strategic-plan-workgroup-reports-past-plans/strategic-planning-workgroup-complexity-substance-use-disorders-continuum-substance.
119. Saccone NL, Wang JC, Breslau N, Johnson EO, Hatsukami D, Saccone SF, et al. The CHRNA5-CHRNA3-CHRNB4 nicotinic receptor subunit gene cluster affects risk for nicotine dependence in African-Americans and in European-Americans. Cancer Res. 2009;69(17):6848–56.
120. Saccone SF, Hinrichs AL, Saccone NL, Chase GA, Konvicka K, Madden PA, et al. Cholinergic nicotinic receptor genes implicated in a nicotine dependence association study targeting 348 candidate genes with 3713 SNPs. Hum Mol Genet. 2007;16(1):36–49.
121. Vanyukov MM. Substance-specific symptoms and general liability to addiction. Am J Psychiatry. 2012;169(10):1016–8.
122. Vanyukov MM, Ridenour TA. Common liability to drug addictions: theory, research, practice. Drug Alcohol Depend. 2012;123(Suppl 1):S1–2.
123. Iacono WG, Malone SM, McGue M. Behavioral disinhibition and the development of early-onset addiction: common and specific influences. Annu Rev Clin Psychol. 2008;4:325–48.
124. Kirisci L, Tarter RE, Reynolds M, Vanyukov MM. Item response theory analysis to assess dimensionality of substance use disorder abuse and dependence symptoms. Int J Pers Cent Med. 2016;6(4):260–73.
125. Karkowski LM, Prescott CA, Kendler KS. Multivariate assessment of factors influencing illicit substance use in twins from female-female pairs. Am J Med Genet. 2000;96(5):665–70.
126. Munn-Chernoff MA, Johnson EC, Chou Y-L, Coleman JRI, Thornton LM, Walters RK, et al. Shared genetic risk between eating disorder- and substance-use-related phenotypes: Evidence from genome-wide association studies. Addiction Biology. 2020:e12880.
127. Schwantes-An TH, Zhang J, Chen LS, Hartz SM, Culverhouse RC, Chen X, et al. Association of the OPRM1 variant rs1799971 (A118G) with non-specific liability to substance dependence in a collaborative de novo meta-analysis of European-ancestry cohorts. Behav Genet. 2016;46(2):151–69.
128. Gardner FE. Inconsistent parenting: is there evidence for a link with children's conduct problems? J Abnorm Child Psychol. 1989;17(2):223–33.
129. Patterson GR. A performance theory for coercive family interaction. In: Cairns RB, editor. The analysis of social interactions: Methods, issues and illustrations. Hillsdale: Erlbaum; 1979. p. 119–63.
130. Patterson GR. Coercive family process. Eugene: Castalia; 1982.
131. Higgins ET. Promotion and prevention: regulatory focus as a motivational principle. Adv Exp Soc Psychol. 1998;30:1–46.
132. Lockwood P, Jordan CH, Kunda Z. Motivation by positive or negative role models: regulatory focus determines who will best inspire us. J Pers Soc Psychol. 2002;83(4):854–64.
133. Cialdini RB, Kallgren CA, Reno RR. A focus theory of normative conduct: a theoretical refinement and reevaluation of the role of norms in human behavior. In: Zanna MP, editor. Advances in experimental social psychology. 24. London: Academic Press; 1991. p. 201–34.
134. Marx DM, Ko SJ, Friedman RA. The "Obama effect": how a salient role model reduces race-based performance differences. J Exp Soc Psychol. 2009;45(4):953–6.
135. Obama B. Dreams from my father: a story of race and inheritance. New York: Times Books; 1995.
136. CNN.com transcripts. Morning News CNN 20: 'I Didn't Inhale,' March 29, 1992, Aired March 29, 2000 - 10:49 a.m. ET 2000. Available from: http://transcripts.cnn.com/TRANSCRIPTS/0003/29/mn.12.html.
137. BBC News. Bush hinted at use of marijuana 2005. updated 21 February, 2005, 11:44 GMT. Available from: http://news.bbc.co.uk/2/hi/americas/4282799.stm.
138. Obama B. To the Congress of the United States. National Drug Control Strategy: Executive Office of the President of the United States; 2013. Available from: https://obamawhitehouse.archives.gov/sites/default/files/ondcp/policy-and-research/ndcs_2013.pdf.
139. Hamilton AD, Jang JB, Patrick ME, Schulenberg JE, Keyes KM. Age, period and cohort effects in frequent cannabis use among US students: 1991-2018. Addiction. 2019;14:1763–72.
140. Zhao C. Kamala Harris's father slams her for 'fraudulently stereotyping' Jamaicans with pot comments, accuses her of pursuing 'identity politics': Report. Newsweek [Internet]. 2019 4/16/2019. Available from: https://www.newsweek.com/kamala-harris-father-slams-her-fraudulently-stereotyping-jamaicans-pro-pot-1338092.
141. Miller ML, Hurd YL. Testing the gateway hypothesis. Neuropsychopharmacology. 2017;42(5):985–6.
142. Dolgin E. The bioengineering of cannabis. Nature. 2019;572(7771):S5–7.

143. Hall W, Weier M. Assessing the public health impacts of legalizing recreational cannabis use in the USA. Clin Pharmacol Ther. 2015;97(6):607–15.
144. Cerdá M, Mauro C, Hamilton A, Levy NS, Santaella-Tenorio J, Hasin D, et al. Association between recreational marijuana legalization in the United States and changes in marijuana use and cannabis use disorder from 2008 to 2016. JAMA Psychiat. 2020;77(2):165–71.
145. Hall W, Lynskey M. Assessing the public health impacts of legalizing recreational cannabis use: the US experience. World Psychiatry. 2020;19(2):179–86.
146. Kleinman RA, Morris NP. Is it time to reschedule heroin? JAMA Psychiat. 2020;77(8):781–2.
147. Vanyukov MM, Cornelius MD, De Genna NM, Reynolds MD, Kirillova GP, Maher BS, et al. Measurement of liability to addiction: dimensional approaches. Int J Pers Cent Med. 2016;6:250–9.
148. Vanyukov MM, Tarter RE, Conway KP, Kirillova GP, Chandler RK, Daley DC. Risk and resistance perspectives in translation-oriented etiology research. Transl Behav Med. 2016;6(1):44–54.
149. Maher BS, Latendresse S, Vanyukov MM. Informing prevention and intervention policy using genetic studies of resistance. Prev Sci. 2018;19:49–57.
150. Gilbertson R, Prather R, Nixon SJ. The role of selected factors in the development and consequences of alcohol dependence. Alcohol Res Health. 2008;31(4):389–99.
151. Richey JM, Woolcott O. Re-visiting the endocannabinoid system and its therapeutic potential in obesity and associated diseases. Curr Diab Rep. 2017;17(10):99.
152. Sternat T, Katzman MA. Neurobiology of hedonic tone: the relationship between treatment-resistant depression, attention-deficit hyperactivity disorder, and substance abuse. Neuropsychiatr Dis Treat. 2016;12:2149–64.
153. Bowlby J. Attachment and loss. New York: Basic Books; 1969.
154. Hatzigiakoumis DS, Martinotti G, Giannantonio MD, Janiri L. Anhedonia and substance dependence: clinical correlates and treatment options. Front Psych. 2011;2:10.
155. Koob GF, Le Moal M. Drug addiction, dysregulation of reward, and allostasis. Neuropsychopharmacology. 2001;24(2):97–129.
156. Sanchez-Roige S, Fontanillas P, Elson SL, Gray JC, De Wit H, Davis LK, et al. Genome-wide association study of alcohol use disorder identification test (AUDIT) scores in 20 328 research participants of European ancestry. Addict Biol. 2019;24(1):121–31.
157. Fan CC, Smeland OB, Schork AJ, Chen CH, Holland D, Lo MT, et al. Beyond heritability: improving discoverability in imaging genetics. Hum Mol Genet. 2018;27(R1):R22–R8.
158. Kragh H. From disulfiram to antabuse: the invention of a drug. Bull Hist Chem. 2008;33(2):82–8.
159. Williams EE. Effects of alcohol on workers with carbon disulfide. JAMA. 1937;109:1472–3.
160. Risch N, Merikangas K. The future of genetic studies of complex human diseases. Science. 1996;273(5281):1516–7.
161. Pinson MR, Miranda RC. Noncoding RNAs in development and teratology, with focus on effects of cannabis, cocaine, nicotine, and ethanol. Birth Defects Res. 2019;111(17):1308–19.
162. Goodwin DW. Drinking problems in adopted and nonadopted sons of alcoholics. Arch Gen Psychiatry. 1974;31(2):164–9.
163. Scully R, Anderson SF, Chao DM, Wei W, Ye L, Young RA, et al. BRCA1 is a component of the RNA polymerase II holoenzyme. Proc Natl Acad Sci U S A. 1997;94(11):5605–10.
164. Malone KE, Daling JR, Doody DR, Hsu L, Bernstein L, Coates RJ, et al. Prevalence and predictors of BRCA1 and BRCA2 mutations in a population-based study of breast cancer in white and black American women ages 35 to 64 years. Cancer Res. 2006;66(16):8297–308.
165. Anglian Breast Cancer Study Group. Prevalence and penetrance of BRCA1 and BRCA2 mutations in a population-based series of breast cancer cases. Anglian Breast Cancer Study Group. Br J Cancer. 2000;83(10):1301–8.
166. Farrer LA, Cupples LA, Haines JL, Hyman B, Kukull WA, Mayeux R, et al. Effects of age, sex, and ethnicity on the association between apolipoprotein E genotype and Alzheimer disease. A meta-analysis. APOE and Alzheimer disease meta analysis consortium. JAMA. 1997;278(16):1349–56.
167. Berkowitz CL, Mosconi L, Rahman A, Scheyer O, Hristov H, Isaacson RS. Clinical application of APOE in Alzheimer's prevention: a precision medicine approach. J Prev Alzheimers Dis. 2018;5(4):245–52.
168. Pasman JA, Verweij KJH, Gerring Z, Stringer S, Sanchez-Roige S, Treur JL, et al. GWAS of lifetime cannabis use reveals new risk loci, genetic overlap with psychiatric traits, and a causal influence of schizophrenia. Nat Neurosci. 2018;21(9):1161–70.
169. Munn-Chernoff MA, Grant JD, Agrawal A, Sartor CE, Werner KB, Bucholz KK, et al. Genetic overlap between alcohol use disorder and bulimic behaviors in European American and African American women. Drug Alcohol Depend. 2015;153:335–40.
170. Munn-Chernoff MA, Johnson EC, Chou Y-L, Coleman JRI, Thornton LM, Walters RK, et al. Shared genetic risk between eating disorder- and substance-use-related phenotypes: evidence from genome-wide association studies. Addict Biol. in press.
171. Iob E, Schoeler T, Cecil CM, Walton E, McQuillin A, Pingault J-B. Identifying risk factors involved in the common versus specific liabilities to substance

use: A genetically informed approach. Addict Biol. 2020:e12944.
172. Cheng Z, Yang BZ, Zhou H, Nunez Y, Kranzler HR, Gelernter J. Genome-wide scan identifies opioid overdose risk locus close to MCOLN1. Addict Biol. 2019:e12811.
173. Hancock DB, Guo Y, Reginsson GW, Gaddis NC, Lutz SM, Sherva R, et al. Genome-wide association study across European and African American ancestries identifies a SNP in DNMT3B contributing to nicotine dependence. Mol Psychiatry. 2018;23(9):1911–9.
174. Alberts B, Kirschner MW, Tilghman S, Varmus H. Rescuing US biomedical research from its systemic flaws. Proc Natl Acad Sci U S A. 2014;111(16):5773–7.
175. Bierut LJ, Madden PA, Breslau N, Johnson EO, Hatsukami D, Pomerleau OF, et al. Novel genes identified in a high-density genome wide association study for nicotine dependence. Hum Mol Genet. 2007;16(1):24–35.
176. Coe JW, Brooks PR, Vetelino MG, Wirtz MC, Arnold EP, Huang J, et al. Varenicline: an alpha4beta2 nicotinic receptor partial agonist for smoking cessation. J Med Chem. 2005;48(10):3474–7.
177. Mihalak KB, Carroll FI, Luetje CW. Varenicline is a partial agonist at alpha4beta2 and a full agonist at alpha7 neuronal nicotinic receptors. Mol Pharmacol. 2006;70(3):801–5.
178. Butelman ER, Kreek MJ. Medications for substance use disorders (SUD): emerging approaches. Expert Opin Emerg Drugs. 2017;22(4):301–15.
179. Kreek MJ, Laforge KS, Butelman E. Pharmacotherapy of addictions. Nat Rev Drug Discov. 2002;1(9):710–26.
180. Coller BS. Ethics of human genome editing. Annu Rev Med. 2019;70:289–305.
181. Petronis A, Gottesman II, Kan P, Kennedy JL, Basile VS, Paterson AD, et al. Monozygotic twins exhibit numerous epigenetic differences: clues to twin discordance? Schizophr Bull. 2003;29(1):169–78.
182. Eyles DW, Trzaskowski M, Vinkhuyzen AAE, Mattheisen M, Meier S, Gooch H, et al. The association between neonatal vitamin D status and risk of schizophrenia. Sci Rep. 2018;8(1):17692.
183. Johns LC, van Os J. The continuity of psychotic experiences in the general population. Clin Psychol Rev. 2001;21(8):1125–41.
184. Zahavi A. Mate selection - a selection for a handicap. J Theor Biol. 1975;53(1):205–14.
185. Belcher AM, Volkow ND, Moeller FG, Ferre S. Personality traits and vulnerability or resilience to substance use disorders. Trends Cogn Sci. 2014;18(4):211–7.
186. Gottesman II, Gould TD. The endophenotype concept in psychiatry: etymology and strategic intentions. Am J Psychiatry. 2003;160(4):636–45.
187. Iacono WG. Endophenotypes in psychiatric disease: prospects and challenges. Genome Med. 2018;10(1):1–3.
188. Border R, Johnson EC, Evans LM, Smolen A, Berley N, Sullivan PF, et al. No support for historical candidate gene or candidate gene-by-interaction hypotheses for major depression across multiple large samples. Am J Psychiatry. 2019;176(5):376–87.
189. Gallagher MD, Chen-Plotkin AS. The post-GWAS era: from association to function. Am J Hum Genet. 2018;102(5):717–30.
190. Liu M, Jiang Y, Wedow R, Li Y, Brazel DM, Chen F, et al. Association studies of up to 1.2 million individuals yield new insights into the genetic etiology of tobacco and alcohol use. Nat Genet. 2019;51(2):237–44.
191. Mullins N, Bigdeli TB, Borglum AD, Coleman JRI, Demontis D, Mehta D, et al. GWAS of suicide attempt in psychiatric disorders and association with major depression polygenic risk scores. Am J Psychiatry. 2019;176(8):651–60.
192. Vita A, De Peri L. New meta- and mega-analyses of magnetic resonance imaging findings in schizophrenia: do they really increase our knowledge about the nature of the disease process? Biol Psychiatry. 2019;85(7):e33.
193. Lassi G, Taylor AE, Timpson NJ, Kenny PJ, Mather RJ, Eisen T, et al. The CHRNA5-A3-B4 gene cluster and smoking: from discovery to therapeutics. Trends Neurosci. 2016;39(12):851–61.
194. Crews KR, Gaedigk A, Dunnenberger HM, Leeder JS, Klein TE, Caudle KE, et al. Clinical pharmacogenetics implementation consortium guidelines for cytochrome P450 2D6 genotype and codeine therapy: 2014 update. Clin Pharmacol Ther. 2014;95(4):376–82.
195. Chatterjee N, Shi J, Garcia-Closas M. Developing and evaluating polygenic risk prediction models for stratified disease prevention. Nat Rev Genet. 2016;17(7):392–406.
196. Gibson G. On the utilization of polygenic risk scores for therapeutic targeting. PLoS Genet. 2019;15(4):e1008060.
197. Murray GK, Lin T, Austin J, McGrath JJ, Hickie IB, Wray NR. Could polygenic risk scores be useful in psychiatry? JAMA psychiatry. 2020.
198. Wray NR, Lin T, Austin J, McGrath JJ, Hickie IB, Murray GK, et al. From basic science to clinical application of polygenic risk scores. JAMA Psychiat. 2021;78(1):101–9.
199. Mongan D, Föcking M, Healy C, Susai SR, Heurich M, Wynne K, et al. Development of proteomic prediction models for transition to psychotic disorder in the clinical high-risk state and psychotic experiences in adolescence. JAMA Psychiat. 2021;78(1):77–90.

200. Panksepp J, Knutson B, Burgdorf J. The role of brain emotional systems in addictions: a neuro-evolutionary perspective and new 'self-report' animal model. Addiction. 2002;97(4):459–69.
201. Çelebi K. The balance of truth. Transl. by G.L. Lewis. London: George Allen and Unwin Ltd.; 1957. Available from: https://archive.org/details/MN40230ucmf_5/mode/2up.
202. Gibson G. Going to the negative: genomics for optimized medical prescription. Nat Rev Genet. 2019;20(1):1–2.
203. Garcia RI, Sohn W. The paradigm shift to prevention and its relationship to dental education. J Dent Educ. 2012;76(1):36–45.
204. Leshner AI. Addiction is a brain disease, and it matters. Science. 1997;278(5335):45–7.
205. Kirisci L, Tarter RE, Reynolds M, Hayes KN, Cochran G, Vanyukov M. Derivation and assessment of the opioid use disorder severity scale: prediction of health and behavioral adjustment problems. Am J Drug Alcohol Abuse. 2020;46(6):699–707.
206. Blum K, Oscar-Berman M, Demetrovics Z, Barh D, Gold MS. Genetic addiction risk score (GARS): molecular neurogenetic evidence for predisposition to reward deficiency syndrome (RDS). Mol Neurobiol. 2014;50(3):765–96.
207. Bollen K, Lennox R. Conventional wisdom on measurement: a structural equation perspective. Psychol Bull. 1991;110:305–14.
208. Zhou H, Rentsch CT, Cheng Z, Kember RL, Nunez YZ, Sherva RM, et al. Association of OPRM1 functional coding variant with opioid use disorder. JAMA Psychiat. 2020;77(10):1072–80.
209. Masten AS, Best KM, Garmezy N. Resilience and development: contributions from the study of children who overcome adversity. Dev Psychopathol. 1990;2:425–44.
210. Spielman RS, McGinnis RE, Ewens WJ. Transmission test for linkage disequilibrium: the insulin gene region and insulin-dependent diabetes mellitus (IDDM). Am J Hum Genet. 1993;52(3):506–16.
211. Agrawal A, Verweij KJ, Gillespie NA, Heath AC, Lessov-Schlaggar CN, Martin NG, et al. The genetics of addiction-a translational perspective. Transl Psychiatry. 2012;2:e140.
212. Peles E, Levran O, Randesi M, Ott J, Kreek MJ, Adelson M. Genetic variant in the CRH-binding protein gene (CRHBP) is associated with cessation of cocaine use in methadone maintenance patients with opioid addiction. J Addict Med. 2019;13(6):430–5.
213. McCutcheon VV, Schuckit MA, Kramer JR, Chan G, Edenberg HJ, Smith TL, et al. Familial association of abstinent remission from alcohol use disorder in first-degree relatives of alcohol-dependent treatment-seeking probands. Addiction. 2017;112(11):1909–17.
214. Riedel S. Edward Jenner and the history of smallpox and vaccination. Proc (Baylor Univ Med Center). 2005;18(1):21–5.
215. Schulenberg JE, Maggs JL. A developmental perspective on alcohol use and heavy drinking during adolescence and the transition to young adulthood. J Stud Alcohol Suppl. 2002;14:54–70.
216. McCutcheon VV, Grant JD, Heath AC, Bucholz KK, Sartor CE, Nelson EC, et al. Environmental influences predominate in remission from alcohol use disorder in young adult twins. Psychol Med. 2012;42(11):2421–31.
217. Fusar-Poli P. Salazar De Pablo G, Correll CU, Meyer-Lindenberg a, Millan MJ, Borgwardt S, et al. prevention of psychosis: advances in detection, prognosis, and intervention. JAMA Psychiat. 2020;77(7):755–65.
218. Levran O, Peles E, Randesi M, Correa da Rosa J, Shen PH, Rotrosen J, et al. Genetic variations in genes of the stress response pathway are associated with prolonged abstinence from heroin. Pharmacogenomics. 2018;19(4):333–41.
219. Levran O, Peles E, Randesi M, da Rosa JC, Adelson M, Kreek MJ. The mu-opioid receptor nonsynonymous variant 118A>G is associated with prolonged abstinence from heroin without agonist treatment. Pharmacogenomics. 2017;18(15):1387–91.
220. Vanyukov MM, Kirisci L, Moss L, Tarter RE, Reynolds MD, Maher BS, et al. Measurement of the risk for substance use disorders: phenotypic and genetic analysis of an index of common liability. Behav Genet. 2009;39(3):233–44.
221. Kirisci L, Tarter R, Mezzich A, Ridenour T, Reynolds M, Vanyukov M. Prediction of cannabis use disorder between boyhood and young adulthood: clarifying the phenotype and environtype. Am J Addict. 2009;18(1):36–47.
222. Vanyukov M, Kim K, Irons D, Kirisci L, Neale M, Ridenour T, et al. Genetic relationship between the addiction diagnosis in adults and their childhood measure of addiction liability. Behav Genet. 2015;45(1):1–11.
223. Hicks BM, Iacono WG, McGue M. Index of the transmissible common liability to addiction: heritability and prospective associations with substance abuse and related outcomes. Drug Alcohol Depend. 2012;123(Suppl 1):S18–23.
224. PhenX. Addiction Vulnerability - Child. RTI International. https://www.phenxtoolkit.org/toolkit_content/supplemental_info/saa_intermediate_phenotypes/measures/Addiction_Vulnerability_Child.doc: PhenX; 2016.
225. Castillo-Fernandez JE, Spector TD, Bell JT. Epigenetics of discordant monozygotic twins: implications for disease. Genome Med. 2014;6(7):60.
226. Sloboda Z, David SB. Commentary on the culture of prevention. Prev Sci. 2021;22(1):84–90.
227. Hershberger SL. The specification of equivalent models before the collection of data. In: von Eye A, Clogg C, editors. The analysis of latent variables in

developmental research. Beverly Hills: CA Sage; 1994. p. 68–108.
228. Hollingshead AB. Four-factor index of social status. New Haven, CT: Department of Sociology, Yale University; 1975.
229. Spitzer RL, Williams JB, Rieder R. Another perspective on "putting DSM-IV in perspective". Am J Psychiatry. 1999;156(3):499. author reply 500
230. Leckman JF, Sholomskas D, Thompson WD, Belanger A, Weissman MM. Best estimate of lifetime psychiatric diagnosis: a methodological study. Arch Gen Psychiatry. 1982;39(8):879–83.
231. Muthen L, Muthen BO. Mplus user's manual, version 7, computer program. Los Angeles: Muthen & Muthen; 2015.
232. Akaike H. Factor analysis and AIC. Psychometrika. 1987;52:317–32.
233. Schwarz G. Estimating the dimension of a model. Ann Stat. 1978;6:461–4.
234. Nylund K, Asparouhov T, Muthen B. Deciding on the number of classes in latent class analysis and growth mixture modeling, a Monte Carlo simulation study. Struct Equ Model. 2007;14:535–69.
235. Embretson SE, Reise SP. Item response theory for psychologists. Mahwah, NJ: Lawrence Erlbaum Associates; 2000.
236. Stout W, Habing B, Dougles J, Kim HR, Rousses L, Zhang J. Conditional covariance-based nonparametric multidimensionality assessment. Appl Psychol Meas. 1996;20:331–54.
237. Lord F. Application of item response theory to practical problems. Hillsdale: Lawrence Erlbaum; 1980.
238. Samejima F. A use of the information function in tailored testing. Appl Psychol Meas. 1977;1:233–47.
239. Reckase M. Unifactor latent trait models applied to multifactor tests: results and implications. J Educ Stat. 1979;4:207–30.
240. Reise SP, Morizot J, Hays RD. The role of the bifactor model in resolving dimensionality issues in health outcomes measures. Qual Life Res. 2007;16(Suppl 1):19–31.
241. Kirisci L, Tarter RE, Reynolds M, Vanyukov MM. Item response theory analysis to assess dimensionality of substance use disorder abuse and dependence symptoms. Int J Pers Cent Med. 2016;6(4):260–73.
242. Vanyukov MM, Moss HB, Tarter R. Mating assortment and the liability to substance abuse. Drug Alcohol Depend. 1996;42:1–10.

2 Neurobiological Mechanisms in Substance Use

Eduardo R. Butelman and Mary Jeanne Kreek

Abbreviations

Cannabis	*Cannabis sativa*
CB1-r	Cannabinoid receptor type 1
CNS	Central nervous system
CRF	Corticotrophin-releasing factor
DAT	Dopamine transporter
GPCR	G-protein-coupled receptors
KOP-r	Kappa opioid receptor (encoded by the *OPRK1* gene)
MOP-r	Mu-opioid receptor (encoded by the *OPRM1* gene)
SUD	Substance use disorders
Δ9-THC	Δ9-tetrahydrocannabinol

Introduction

Substance use disorders (SUD) are due to self-exposure to substances including mu-opioid receptor (MOP-r) agonists, cocaine and amphetamines, alcohol, or cannabis. Other than for alcohol, the primary site(s) of action of the aforementioned substances are fairly well understood [1–4]. The neuroanatomical distribution of these primary sites of action has been examined in humans and experimental animals, including rodents and non-human primates [5–8].

SUD are currently diagnosed based on the presence of several major clinical and behavioral criteria [9]. The major criteria focus on increasing self-exposure ("escalation"), persistent desire for the substance, substance use resulting in major health or social consequences, tolerance, and dependence (that is, presence of a withdrawal syndrome upon sudden discontinuation of drug use). Clearly, these different criteria can be subserved by different neuroanatomical pathways, which can vary across drugs of abuse, and also as a factor of the stage in disease trajectory or drug exposure (i.e., acute effects of the drug, dependence, withdrawal, or abstinence) [10–13]. Several studies have also examined specific SUD dimensionally (e.g., in terms of differential exposure or age trajectory), rather than as categorical diagnoses [14–16], and such approaches may also be fruitful for mechanistic, translational, and genetic association studies [17].

Developmental Aspects of the Neurobiological Effects of Drugs of Abuse

Initiation and escalation of use of specific drugs can follow an age trajectory in human populations with diagnosed SUD. For example, exposure to cannabis, nicotine, and alcohol is more

E. R. Butelman (✉) · M. J. Kreek
Laboratory on the Biology of Addictive Diseases, The Rockefeller University, New York, NY, USA
e-mail: butelme@rockefeller.edu

M. M. Vanyukov (ed.), *Genetics of Substance Use*, https://doi.org/10.1007/978-3-030-95350-8_2

often initiated in adolescence [18, 19], whereas exposure to heroin or cocaine is more typically (but not always) initiated in the transition from late adolescence to early adulthood [15, 20, 21]. There are also more recently reported changes in age trends in initiation of exposure to non-medical prescription opioids [22]. Several studies have shown that adolescent rodents exposed to short-acting MOP-r agonists display exaggerated neurobiological responses, for example, on dopamine dialysate levels [23, 24], and also more robust long-term neurobiological changes [25, 26], compared to adults. Likewise, adolescent rodents exhibit enhanced dopaminergic responses to cocaine, compared to adults [24].

Sex Influences on the Neurobiological Effects of Drugs of Abuse

While the primary site(s) of action of abused substances are likely to be similar in males and females, sexual dimorphism in neurobiological and behavioral effects of drugs have been observed in some specific situations, especially in rodents [27, 28], but not in others [29, 30]. The clinical trajectory of some SUD (for example, times of escalation) may also show some sex dimorphism in humans [31, 32]. However, it is critical to examine sex differences under a diverse set of clinical conditions, in order to determine how generalizable these findings are [15, 33]. It is also known that some of these differences, for example, for alcohol, can change across birth cohorts [34] and also depend on ages of initial exposure [35]. Furthermore, methodological factors can also affect the robustness of observed sex differences in experimental models [36, 37].

Importance of Animal Research in the Neurobiology of SUD and Considerations for Translational Research

It is likely that no single experimental animal assay can be used to examine all the major biological features of a SUD. Therefore, animal protocols can be designed to model specific phenomena (e.g., escalation of intake, withdrawal, relapse), and data need to be interpreted after integration across studies [38–41]. Of importance to genetic association studies of SUD and their translational examination in animal models, there can be substantial interspecies differences in regulatory regions of genes of interest [42–44]. There are also interspecies differences in neuroanatomical and functional organization of some gene products, including opioid and monoamine systems [45]. Furthermore, differences in the cognitive, affective, and ethological repertoire of experimental animals versus humans also require consideration when designing and interpreting studies.

Translational considerations should also guide the specific behavioral assay conditions used in animals and their relative homologies to human SUD [46, 47]. These assay conditions may include types and extent of operant or classical conditioning [48], amount of drug exposure [38, 39], use of experimental extinction [49, 50], or priming in reinstatement techniques [51]. Overall, animal research will continue to be indispensable to study different aspects of the neurobiological and behavioral changes associated with SUD. This is especially due to the opportunity to systematically interrogate neurobiological status at specific stages in addiction-like trajectory, mentioned above. For a variety of practical and ethical reasons, such data are very difficult to obtain in humans. Animal models of specific human polymorphisms may also be used to interrogate the mechanistic basis of genetic variations in SUD [52–54].

Stages in the Trajectory of Substance Use Disorders

As mentioned above, SUD are due to initial exposure to a substance (e.g., mu-opioid receptor [MOP-r] agonists, cocaine, or alcohol), which in a subset of persons is followed by escalating exposure and eventually regular or compulsive-like drug taking. It has been hypothesized that different parts of the brain may be involved at different stages in addiction trajectory. For example, several studies discuss a transition of mediation from ventral to dorsal striatal areas as drug self-administration becomes more habit-like or compulsive-like [12, 55]. Studies also show that other brain regions are involved at specific stages in drug-taking trajectory, including prefrontal cortical areas and limbic areas [56]. In many cases, these mechanisms have been elucidated from studies in experimental animals [57–59] and have also been examined in some neuroimaging or functional experiments in humans [60–62].

For some drugs, especially MOP-r agonists, severe SUD is associated with a daily high-dose self-exposure, in part due to tolerance and also to alleviate withdrawal symptoms [1, 63]. For other drugs (such as cocaine), severe SUD can occur with periodic moderate or high-dose "binges." These differences across types of drugs may be due in part to different patterns of neurobiological and behavioral adaptations, occurring after chronic exposure [64].

SUD are considered to be chronic relapsing disorders; attempts at abstinence and relapse may alternate. Some SUD have particularly high rates of relapse unless there is effective medication treatment. This is the case for severe OUD, which usually requires long-term maintenance with methadone or buprenorphine-naloxone, as standards of care [1, 65]. There are approved medications for the treatment of alcohol use disorders (nalmefene and naltrexone, in different countries), and these tend to target primarily MOP-r and KOP-r receptor systems [66, 67]. There are no approved medications for cocaine or amphetamine use disorders, although some recent clinical studies have been carried out [68, 69]. The disease trajectory for specific SUD has been conceptualized and modeled by various groups, including ours [1, 70–72].

Neurobiological Systems Involved in Use of Specific Substances

Opioids (Mu-Opioid Receptor Agonists, MOPr)

As mentioned above, OUD are due to self-exposure to MOP-r agonists, such as morphine and structural analogs, including heroin and prescription opioids (e.g., oxycodone), as well as fentanyl and its analogs. MOP-r are G-protein-coupled receptors (coupled primarily to Gi/Go proteins) and are encoded by the *OPRM1* gene [73]. MOP-r are distributed in several areas of the brain and spinal cord and also in the peripheral nervous system [74], and the mesolimbic dopaminergic pathway from the VTA to the nucleus accumbens in the ventral striatum has received much attention as a site mediating rewarding effects of MOP-r agonists [75]. However, other areas are also likely involved, especially at different stages in addiction trajectory. For example, the nigrostriatal dopaminergic pathway, from the substantia nigra pars compacta to dorsal striatal regions (Caudate-Putamen), is also modulated by acute and chronic MOP-r agonist exposure [76, 77]. Dorsal striatal areas may be more involved in advanced stages of OUD, possibly mediating more compulsive or habit-like drug-taking behaviors. Studies in experimental animals also show that the reinforcing effects of MOP-r agonists are not solely due to the aforementioned dopaminergic systems [78].

Other brain areas, including the prefrontal cortex and amygdala, are involved [79], and stress-related responsivity of the hypothalamic-pituitary-adrenal (HPA) axis is also affected in OUD [80]. Furthermore, brainstem areas, including the locus coeruleus, are involved in the mediation of dependence and withdrawal to MOP-r agonists, of considerable importance after chronic self-exposure to MOP-r agonists [81]. Thus, withdrawal can enhance the reinforcing effects of short-acting MOP-r agonists [82, 83] and can also underlie neurobiological changes that may be involved in relapse [84].

Acute mortality in OUD is due primarily to MOP-r agonist-induced respiratory depression, and this is thought to be mediated by specific brainstem centers which modulate sensitivity to CO_2 levels [85, 86]. Some studies also show that fentanyl analogs may have further overdose potential, due to their propensity to cause other respiratory dysfunctions, including chest wall rigidity [85].

Several groups including ours have documented complex transcriptomic changes due to repeated exposure to short-acting MOP-r agonists, such as oxycodone [77, 87, 88], including neurotransmitter and neuroinflammatory gene targets. Other studies also show that repeated self-administration of a short-acting MOP-r agonist causes changes in the transcription of gene systems involved in neuroplasticity and axon guidance, suggesting that chronic OUD may also involve neuronal remodeling [87].

It has also been shown that some of these transcriptional changes (and related neurobiological and behavioral changes) may emerge a considerable time after the end of repeated MOP-r agonist exposure, and may potentially underlie the relapsing nature of OUD [89, 90]. Overall, these studies clearly suggest variations in the level of expression at diverse gene targets (in addition to those of the MOP-r itself) may affect sensitivity to OUD, at specific stages in its trajectory [91].

We and others have shown that repeated exposure to short-acting MOP-r agonists can result in diverse changes in specific neuropeptide and neurotransmitter systems [77], which may mediate some of the neurobiological and behavioral changes that are observed in OUD models. For example, repeated exposure to short-acting MOP-r agonists such as heroin results in changes in the level of expression of kappa opioid receptor (KOP-r)/dynorphin system [92, 93]. Activation of this system may underlie in part prolonged dysphoria and anhedonia after repeated exposure to short-acting MOP-r agonists [94].

Cocaine and Amphetamines

Cocaine's rewarding effects are thought to be primarily due to blockade of the membrane dopamine reuptake transporter (DAT), resulting in increased extracellular neurotransmitter concentrations [75, 95, 96]. However, cocaine also has similar effects at serotonin and norepinephrine reuptake transporters (SERT and NET) [95, 97]. Another widely abused psychostimulant, methamphetamine, causes an increase in synaptic levels of monoamines, likely by stimulating neurotransmitter release through both vesicular and membrane transporters [3]. Other amphetamine-derived compounds, including methylenedioxymethamphetamine (MDMA, "Ecstasy"), are also self-administered by humans, and their effects are more prominently mediated by the serotonergic system [98].

Increased synaptic dopamine levels both in ventral and dorsal striatum (i.e., both mesolimbic and nigrostriatal pathways) have been examined as important mechanisms for the rewarding effects of cocaine and amphetamines and also of other drugs of abuse [76, 96]. More recent studies have examined dopaminergic tone more specifically as indicating reward prediction error, rather than reward per se [99, 100].

Other monoaminergic systems targeted by cocaine and amphetamines (i.e., via the serotonin and norepinephrine transporters) also mediate diverse behavioral functions, including arousal, dysphoria, and anhedonia, as well as responses to stress. These functions can also be relevant at specific stages in drug-taking and SUD trajectory. Repeated exposure to cocaine also causes functional changes to its direct targets (DAT, SERT, and NET) [13, 101–103]. Furthermore, repeated exposure to cocaine and selected amphetamines also results in changes in expression of other gene systems, including KOP-r/dynorphin [10, 104–106], as well as other targets including glutamate [107]. As a major example, we and others have shown that increased activity of the KOP-r/dynorphin system can underlie behavioral effects consistent with dysphoria and anhedonia [108, 109], which may be involved in the long-term relapsing course of some substance use disorders. We have also recently found that relapse-like behavior observed after chronic extended access cocaine self-administration can be reduced by a short-acting KOP-r antagonist, in rats [110]. However, the behavioral changes observed after cocaine exposure are affected by KOP-r antagonism under some, but not all, conditions [82, 108, 111].

Ethanol

Despite millennia of use, the direct pharmacodynamic target(s) of alcohol (ethanol) remain elusive. However, it has been shown that ethanol administration results in several neurobiological changes to major systems involved in the effects of other abused substances.

For example, ethanol administration or self-administration in rodents results in increases in dopamine dialysates from the terminal fields of both the mesolimbic [75, 112] and nigrostriatal systems [75], an effect also observed with mu-opioid agonists and cocaine. Furthermore, PET studies in humans also show that ethanol results in increased occupancy at D2-like receptors [113, 114].

The rewarding effects of ethanol also appear to be mediated in part by downstream mu-opioid receptor systems. For example, mu-opioid receptor (*Oprm1*) gene knockout mice show decreased ethanol-induced reward [115]. Mu-opioid receptor populations are also affected in the brains of persons with alcohol use disorders, as shown by PET radiotracer studies [116, 117].

Other studies also show that the inhibitory neurotransmitter GABA is also involved in ethanol's rewarding effects. For example, the GABA-B agonist baclofen prevents the acquisition of ethanol self-administration in rodents [118] and also ethanol-reinforced responding in ethanol-dependent rodents [119]. Other components of the GABA system, including benzodiazepine receptors, appear to be affected in limbic areas of persons with alcohol use disorders [120].

The functional status of glutamate receptor systems affects ethanol intake and also other stages including intoxication and withdrawal [121, 122]. Given the diverse roles of the excitatory neurotransmitter glutamate at its various receptor subtypes and their wide distribution in the CNS, it is useful to examine different major mechanisms.

For example, an agonist at metabotropic II glutamate receptors (given in the nucleus accumbens core) decreased oral ethanol self-administration [123]. By contrast, agonism at the ionotropic AMPA receptor appears to promote ethanol intake, possibly through actions in the amygdala [124, 125]. Early in vitro studies show that ethanol affects the function of ionotropic NMDA receptors, including a decrease in long-term potentiation [126, 127]. Ionotropic NMDA receptors are also affected at different stages of ethanol use, intoxication, and withdrawal [122].

Similarly to other abused substances, repeated exposure to ethanol results in diverse changes to several neuropeptide systems [128–131]. These neurobiological changes could underlie in part aspects of ethanol use and abuse, including escalation and relapse.

Tobacco/Nicotine

Nicotine is the main active component of tobacco and acts as an agonist at the nicotinic family of acetylcholinergic receptors. Nicotine is a chiral molecule, and (S)-nicotine is the main form active at nicotinic receptors [132]. Nicotinic receptors are pentameric; the receptor is ionotropic and when activated allows cations, especially sodium and potassium, into the cytosol. The five units are divided into alpha and beta families (each with different types, e.g., alpha 2–10). The combination of subunits varies by location in the periphery and specific areas of the CNS. The alpha-4/beta-2 forms are thought to be prominent in areas of the brain that mediate reinforcing effects of nicotine, including in the ventral tegmental area [133–135]. Other subunits may also be present in the pentamer (e.g., beta-4) and may modulate nicotine-induced reward [136]. The reinforcing actions of nicotine are thought to be mediated primarily by presynaptic receptors causing release of neurotransmitters, including dopamine, GABA, and glutamate [137–139].

Similarly to other self-administered drugs, repeated exposure to nicotine results in long-term changes in other neurobiological systems, and some of these may underlie specific stages in the disease trajectory. For example, cessation of chronic nicotine exposure results in an aversive withdrawal state, and this may be mediated by upregulation of kappa receptor/dynorphin systems [140]. Changes in the functional status of other neuropeptide systems, including CRF, have also been implicated in nicotine withdrawal [141, 142].

Cannabis and Cannabinoid Compounds

Different formulations derived from the plant *Cannabis sativa* (cannabis) have been self-administered across many centuries, ethnicities, and societies. The main active component of cannabis is Δ9-tetrahydrocannabinol (Δ9-THC), which acts as a partial agonist at CB-1 receptors, similarly to an endogenous agonist, anandamide [143]. CB-1 receptors are GPCR, primarily coupled to inhibitory G-proteins ($G_{i/o}$) [144, 145]; CB-1 receptors are present in many areas of the CNS and thus can mediate diverse neurobiological functions [8].

Δ9-THC can elevate striatal dopamine dialysates in experimental animals [146]. Reinforcing effects of THC can be observed under specific conditions in experimental animals but are less robust than those of other types of abused drugs [147, 148]. Furthermore, in contextual conditioning assays in rodents, Δ9-THC can be aversive; this aversive effect may be mediated by downstream activation of kappa receptor/dynorphin systems [149, 150]. Intriguingly, some humans report aversive subjective effects after cannabis exposure (anxiety-like and paranoia-like) [151], and it is unclear if some of these aversive effects are mediated by downstream activation of the kappa-dynorphin or other neuropeptide systems.

Cannabidiol is another component of the cannabis plant that has received much attention [152]; it is not thought to have abuse potential *per se*. The pharmacological effects of cannabidiol may be mediated by different mechanisms, including serotonergic systems and modulation of fatty acid amide hydrolase (FAAH, one of the main metabolic enzymes for the lipid anandamide, an endogenous cannabinoid agonist) [153]. Much of the interest on cannabidiol in the drug abuse field is based on its potential to modulate undesirable and rewarding effects of Δ9-THC, which has been observed under some, but not all, conditions [154].

More recently, synthetic CB1-r agonists have been self-administered by humans, under a variety of non-medical preparations and names (e.g., "spice") [155]. These synthetic CB1 agonists appear to have greater toxicity than Δ9-THC itself, due to either absolute doses self-administered, pharmacokinetic, or pharmacodynamic factors [151].

Relevance to Genetic Association Studies of Substance Use Disorders

The neuroanatomical distribution of the primary targets of the abused compounds mentioned above (e.g., MOP-r, monoamine transporters, nicotinic receptors, CB1-r) has partial overlap in the CNS. There is also partial overlap in downstream targets (including dopaminergic, neuropeptide, and glutamatergic systems) which are affected by exposure to abused drugs [10, 64, 92]. Overall, it is important to define clear phenotypes for genetic association studies, using, for example, persons who have only one severe SUD [156, 157].

However, polydrug use occurs commonly in persons with SUD, especially early in the disease trajectory (e.g., adolescence and early adulthood). For example, persons with opioid and cocaine use disorders can also present with earlier onset of exposure to cannabis and alcohol [15, 158]. Therefore, patterns of polydrug use may be of relevance to the design and interpretation of genetic association studies of specific SUD [159]. Overall, the neurobiological changes observed in SUD may include transcriptional changes in neurotransmitter and neuropeptide systems, as well as in targets commonly associated with neuroinflammation, glial function, as well as neuroplasticity [77, 87, 88, 160]. These changes may be affected by epigenetic marks [91, 161]. The type and persistence of transcriptional, protein, and behavioral changes are also affected by dimensional aspects of drug exposure, which could include frequency, duration, and unit doses, as well as its age trajectory [12, 38, 39, 162]. Therefore, dimensional aspects of drug exposure are receiving more attention in the design and analysis of preclinical, clinical, and genetic association studies [14, 163, 164].

Persons with SUD typically present for clinical care after long-term exposure to relatively high doses of abused drugs [63]; this is also relevant to the design and interpretation of preclinical studies. Studies also suggest that different stages in the trajectory of specific SUD (or its preclinical models) may have specific neurobiological and also genetic underpinnings [11, 12, 39, 64, 102, 108].

Acknowledgments The authors would like to gratefully acknowledge funding from the National Institutes of Health (NIDA, NIAID, and NCATS) and from the Dr. Miriam and Sheldon G. Adelson Medical Research Foundation.

References

1. Kreek MJ, Reed B, Butelman ER. Current status of opioid addiction treatment and related preclinical research. Sci Adv. 2019;5(10):eaax9140.
2. Pacher P, Kogan NM, Mechoulam R. Beyond THC and endocannabinoids. Annu Rev Pharmacol Toxicol. 2020;60:637–59.
3. Fleckenstein AE, Volz TJ, Riddle EL, Gibb JW, Hanson GR. New insights into the mechanism of action of amphetamines. Annu Rev Pharmacol Toxicol. 2007;47(1):681–98.
4. Ritz MC, Lamb RJ, Goldberg SR, Kuhar MJ. Cocaine receptors on dopamine transporters are related to self-administration of cocaine. Science (New York, NY). 1987;237(4819):1219–23.
5. Mansour A, Fox CA, Burke S, Meng F, Thompson RC, Akil H, et al. Mu, delta, and kappa opioid receptor mRNA expression in the rat CNS: an in situ hybridization study. J Comp Neurol. 1994;350(3):412–38.
6. Daunais JB, Letchworth SR, Sim-Selley LJ, Smith HR, Childers SR, Porrino LJ. Functional and anatomical localization of mu opioid receptors in the striatum, amygdala, and extended amygdala of the nonhuman primate. J Comp Neurol. 2001;433(4):471–85.
7. Kling MA, Carson RE, Borg L, Zametkin A, Matochik JA, Schluger J, et al. Opioid receptor imaging with positron emission tomography and [(18)F]cyclofoxy in long-term, methadone-treated former heroin addicts. J Pharmacol Exp Ther. 2000;295(3):1070–6.
8. Howlett AC, Breivogel CS, Childers SR, Deadwyler SA, Hampson RE, Porrino LJ. Cannabinoid physiology and pharmacology: 30 years of progress. Neuropharmacology. 2004;47(Suppl 1):345–58.
9. Hasin DS, Fenton MC, Beseler C, Park JY, Wall MM. Analyses related to the development of DSM-5 criteria for substance use related disorders: 2. Proposed DSM-5 criteria for alcohol, cannabis, cocaine and heroin disorders in 663 substance abuse patients. Drug Alcohol Depend. 2012;122(1–2):28–37.
10. Spangler R, Unterwald EM, Kreek MJ. 'Binge' cocaine administration induces a sustained increase of prodynorphin mRNA in rat caudate-putamen. Brain Res Mol Brain Res. 1993;19(4):323–7.
11. Gorelick DA, Kim YK, Bencherif B, Boyd SJ, Nelson R, Copersino ML, et al. Brain mu-opioid receptor binding: relationship to relapse to cocaine use after monitored abstinence. Psychopharmacology. 2008;200(4):475–86.
12. Fagergren P, Smith HR, Daunais JB, Nader MA, Porrino LJ, Hurd YL. Temporal upregulation of prodynorphin mRNA in the primate striatum after cocaine self-administration. Eur J Neurosci. 2003;17(10):2212–8.
13. Smith HR, Beveridge TJ, Nader MA, Porrino LJ. Effects of abstinence from chronic cocaine self-administration on nonhuman primate dorsal and ventral noradrenergic bundle terminal field structures. Brain Struct Funct. 2016;221(5):2703–15.
14. Kwako LE, Bickel WK, Goldman D. Addiction biomarkers: dimensional approaches to understanding addiction. Trends Mol Med. 2018;24:121–8.
15. Butelman ER, Chen CY, Brown KG, Kreek MJ. Escalation of drug use in persons dually diagnosed with opioid and cocaine dependence: gender comparison and dimensional predictors. Drug Alcohol Depend. 2019;205:107657.
16. Kirisci L, Tarter RE, Reynolds M, Vanyukov MM. Item response theory analysis to assess dimensionality of substance use disorder abuse and dependence symptoms. Int J Pers Cent Med. 2016;6(4):260–73.
17. Cuthbert BN. The RDoC framework: facilitating transition from ICD/DSM to dimensional approaches that integrate neuroscience and psychopathology. World Psychiatry. 2014;13(1):28–35.
18. Chen CY, Storr CL, Anthony JC. Early-onset drug use and risk for drug dependence problems. Addict Behav. 2009;34(3):319–22.
19. Morin JG, Afzali MH, Bourque J, Stewart SH, Seguin JR, O'Leary-Barrett M, et al. A population-based analysis of the relationship between substance use and adolescent cognitive development. Am J Psychiatry. 2018. https://doi.org/10.1176/appi.ajp.2018.18020202.
20. Rodriguez-Cintas L, Daigre C, Grau-Lopez L, Barral C, Perez-Pazos J, Voltes N, et al. Impulsivity and addiction severity in cocaine and opioid dependent patients. Addict Behav. 2016;58:104–9.
21. Moses TEH, Woodcock EA, Lister JJ, Lundahl LH, Greenwald MK. Developing a scale of domains of negative consequences of chronic heroin use. Addict Behav. 2018;77:260–6.
22. Compton WM, Jones CM, Baldwin GT. Relationship between nonmedical prescription-opioid use and heroin use. N Engl J Med. 2016;374(2):154–63.

23. Zhang Y, Picetti R, Butelman ER, Schlussman SD, Ho A, Kreek MJ. Behavioral and neurochemical changes induced by oxycodone differ between adolescent and adult mice. Neuropsychopharmacology. 2009;34(4):912–22.
24. Corongiu S, Dessi C, Cadoni C. Adolescence versus adulthood: differences in basal mesolimbic and nigrostriatal dopamine transmission and response to drugs of abuse. Addict Biol. 2020;25(1):e12721.
25. Zhang Y, Windisch K, Altschuler J, Rahm S, Butelman ER, Kreek MJ. Adolescent oxycodone self administration alters subsequent oxycodone-induced conditioned place preference and anti-nociceptive effect in C57BL/6J mice in adulthood. Neuropharmacology. 2016;111:314–22.
26. Sanchez V, Carpenter MD, Yohn NL, Blendy JA. Long-lasting effects of adolescent oxycodone exposure on reward-related behavior and gene expression in mice. Psychopharmacology. 2016;233(23–24):3991–4002.
27. Randesi M, Zhou Y, Mazid S, Odell SC, Gray JD, Correa da Rosa J, et al. Sex differences after chronic stress in the expression of opioid-, stress- and neuroplasticity-related genes in the rat hippocampus. Neurobiol Stress. 2018;8:33–41.
28. Becker JB, Chartoff E. Sex differences in neural mechanisms mediating reward and addiction. Neuropsychopharmacology. 2019;44(1):166–83.
29. Egenrieder L, Mitricheva E, Spanagel R, Noori HR. No basal or drug-induced sex differences in striatal dopaminergic levels: a cluster and meta-analysis of rat microdialysis studies. J Neurochem. 2020;152(4):482–92.
30. Collins D, Reed B, Zhang Y, Kreek MJ. Sex differences in responsiveness to the prescription opioid oxycodone in mice. Pharmacol Biochem Behav. 2016;148:99–105.
31. Hernandez-Avila CA, Rounsaville BJ, Kranzler HR. Opioid-, cannabis- and alcohol-dependent women show more rapid progression to substance abuse treatment. Drug Alcohol Depend. 2004;74(3):265–72.
32. McCance-Katz EF, Carroll KM, Rounsaville BJ. Gender differences in treatment-seeking cocaine abusers--implications for treatment and prognosis. Am J Addict. 1999;8(4):300–11.
33. Wagner FA, Anthony JC. Male-female differences in the risk of progression from first use to dependence upon cannabis, cocaine, and alcohol. Drug Alcohol Depend. 2007;86(2–3):191–8.
34. Hasin DS, Grant BF. The National Epidemiologic Survey on Alcohol and Related Conditions (NESARC) Waves 1 and 2: review and summary of findings. Soc Psychiatry Psychiatr Epidemiol. 2015;50:1609–40.
35. Cheng HG, Anthony JC. Female-male differences in alcohol dependence levels: evidence on newly incident adolescent and young-adult drinkers in the United States, 2002-2014. Int J Methods Psychiatr Res. 2018;27:e1717.
36. Townsend EA, Negus SS, Caine SB, Thomsen M, Banks ML. Sex differences in opioid reinforcement under a fentanyl vs. food choice procedure in rats. Neuropsychopharmacology. 2019;44(12):2022–9.
37. Diester CM, Banks ML, Neigh GN, Negus SS. Experimental design and analysis for consideration of sex as a biological variable. Neuropsychopharmacology. 2019;44(13):2159–62.
38. Ahmed SH, Koob GF. Transition from moderate to excessive drug intake: change in hedonic set point. Science (New York, NY). 1998;282(5387):298–300.
39. Mantsch JR, Yuferov V, Mathieu-Kia AM, Ho A, Kreek MJ. Effects of extended access to high versus low cocaine doses on self-administration, cocaine-induced reinstatement and brain mRNA levels in rats. Psychopharmacology. 2004;175(1):26–36.
40. Epstein D, Preston K, Stewart J, Shaham Y. Toward a model of drug relapse: an assessment of the validity of the reinstatement procedure. Psychopharmacology. 2006;189(1):1–16.
41. Zernig G, Ahmed SH, Cardinal RN, Morgan D, Acquas E, Foltin RW, et al. Explaining the escalation of drug use in substance dependence: models and appropriate animal laboratory tests. Pharmacology. 2007;80(2–3):65–119.
42. Rockman MV, Hahn MW, Soranzo N, Zimprich F, Goldstein DB, Wray GA. Ancient and recent positive selection transformed opioid cis-regulation in humans. PLoS Biol. 2005;3(12):e387.
43. Rouault M, Nielsen DA, Ho A, Kreek MJ, Yuferov V. Cell-specific effects of variants of the 68-base pair tandem repeat on prodynorphin gene promoter activity. Addict Biol. 2011;16(2):334–46.
44. Liu-Chen LY. Agonist-induced regulation and trafficking of kappa opioid receptors. Life Sci. 2004;75(5):511–36.
45. Berger B, Rothmaier AK, Wedekind F, Zentner J, Feuerstein TJ, Jackisch R. Presynaptic opioid receptors on noradrenergic and serotonergic neurons in the human as compared to the rat neocortex. Br J Pharmacol. 2006;148(6):795–806.
46. Waters RP, Moorman DE, Young AB, Feltenstein MW, See RE. Assessment of a proposed "three-criteria" cocaine addiction model for use in reinstatement studies with rats. Psychopharmacology. 2014;231(16):3197–205.
47. Smith MA. Nonhuman animal models of substance use disorders: translational value and utility to basic science. Drug Alcohol Depend. 2019;206:107733.
48. Singer BF, Fadanelli M, Kawa AB, Robinson TE. Are cocaine-seeking "habits" necessary for the development of addiction-like behavior in rats? J Neurosci. 2018;38(1):60–73.
49. Everitt BJ, Giuliano C, Belin D. Addictive behaviour in experimental animals: prospects for translation. Philos Trans R Soc Lond B Biol Sci. 2018;373(1742):20170027.
50. Girardeau P, Navailles S, Durand A, Vouillac-Mendoza C, Guillem K, Ahmed SH. Relapse to cocaine use persists following extinction

of drug-primed craving. Neuropharmacology. 2019;155:185–93.
51. Venniro M, Zhang M, Shaham Y, Caprioli D. Incubation of methamphetamine but not heroin craving after voluntary abstinence in male and female rats. Neuropsychopharmacology. 2017;42(5):1126–35.
52. Zhang Y, Picetti R, Butelman ER, Ho A, Blendy JA, Kreek MJ. Mouse model of the OPRM1 (A118G) polymorphism: differential heroin self-administration behavior compared with wild-type mice. Neuropsychopharmacology. 2015;40(5):1091–100.
53. Mague SD, Isiegas C, Huang P, Liu-Chen LY, Lerman C, Blendy JA. Mouse model of OPRM1 (A118G) polymorphism has sex-specific effects on drug-mediated behavior. Proc Natl Acad Sci U S A. 2009;106(26):10847–52.
54. Elliott Robinson J, Vardy E, DiBerto JF, Chefer VI, White KL, Fish EW, et al. Receptor reserve moderates mesolimbic responses to opioids in a humanized mouse model of the OPRM1 A118G polymorphism. Neuropsychopharmacology. 2015; 40(11):2614–22.
55. Everitt BJ, Robbins TW. Drug addiction: updating actions to habits to compulsions ten years on. Annu Rev Psychol. 2016;67(1):23–50.
56. Volkow ND, Wang GJ, Ma Y, Fowler JS, Wong C, Ding YS, et al. Activation of orbital and medial prefrontal cortex by methylphenidate in cocaine-addicted subjects but not in controls: relevance to addiction. J Neurosci. 2005;25(15):3932–9.
57. Unterwald EM, Rubenfeld JM, Kreek MJ. Repeated cocaine administration upregulates kappa and mu, but not delta, opioid receptors. Neuroreport. 1994;5(13):1613–6.
58. Mantsch JR, Baker DA, Funk D, Le AD, Shaham Y. Stress-induced reinstatement of drug seeking: 20 years of progress. Neuropsychopharmacology. 2016;41:335–56.
59. Li X, Venniro M, Shaham Y. Translational research on incubation of cocaine craving. JAMA Psychiat. 2016;73(11):1115–6.
60. Zubieta J-K, Gorelick DA, Stauffer R, Ravert HT, Dannals RF, Frost JJ. Increased mu opioid receptor binding detected by PET in cocaine-dependent men is associated with cocaine craving. Nat Med. 1996;2(11):1225–9.
61. Parvaz MA, Moeller SJ, Goldstein RZ. Incubation of Cue-induced craving in adults addicted to cocaine measured by electroencephalography. JAMA Psychiat. 2016;73(11):1127–34.
62. Volkow ND, Fowler JS, Wang GJ, Baler R, Telang F. Imaging dopamine's role in drug abuse and addiction. Neuropharmacology. 2009;56(Suppl 1):3–8.
63. Butelman ER, Chen CY, Fry RS, Kimani R, Levran O, Ott J, et al. Re-evaluation of the KMSK scales, rapid dimensional measures of self-exposure to specific drugs: gender-specific features. Drug Alcohol Depend. 2018;190:179–87.
64. Becker JA, Kieffer BL, Le Merrer J. Differential behavioral and molecular alterations upon protracted abstinence from cocaine versus morphine, nicotine, THC and alcohol. Addict Biol. 2017;22:1205–17.
65. Larochelle MR, Bernson D, Land T, Stopka TJ, Wang N, Xuan Z, et al. Medication for opioid use disorder after nonfatal opioid overdose and association with mortality: a cohort study. Ann Intern Med. 2018;169(3):137–45.
66. Bart G, Schluger JH, Borg L, Ho A, Bidlack JM, Kreek MJ. Nalmefene induced elevation in serum prolactin in normal human volunteers: partial kappa opioid agonist activity? Neuropsychopharmacology. 2005;30(12):2254–62.
67. Wentland MP, Lu Q, Lou R, Bu Y, Knapp BI, Bidlack JM. Synthesis and opioid receptor binding properties of a highly potent 4-hydroxy analogue of naltrexone. Bioorg Med Chem Lett. 2005;15(8):2107–10.
68. Lile JA, Johnson AR, Banks ML, Hatton KW, Hays LR, Nicholson KL, et al. Pharmacological validation of a translational model of cocaine use disorder: effects of d-amphetamine maintenance on choice between intravenous cocaine and a nondrug alternative in humans and rhesus monkeys. Exp Clin Psychopharmacol. 2019;28(2):169–80.
69. Levin FR, Mariani JJ, Specker S, Mooney M, Mahony A, Brooks DJ, et al. Extended-release mixed amphetamine salts vs placebo for comorbid adult attention-deficit/hyperactivity disorder and cocaine use disorder: a randomized clinical trial. JAMA Psychiat. 2015;72(6):593–602.
70. Kreek MJ, Nielsen DA, Butelman ER, LaForge KS. Genetic influences on impulsivity, risk taking, stress responsivity and vulnerability to drug abuse and addiction. Nat Neurosci. 2005;8(11):1450–7.
71. Koob GF, Volkow ND. Neurobiology of addiction: a neurocircuitry analysis. Lancet Psychiatry. 2016;3(8):760–73.
72. Koob G, Kreek MJ. Stress, dysregulation of drug reward pathways, and the transition to drug dependence. Am J Psychiatry. 2007;164(8):1149–59.
73. Yu L. The mu opioid receptor: from molecular cloning to functional studies. Addict Biol. 1996;1(1):19–30.
74. Mansour A, Fox CA, Thompson RC, Akil H, Watson SJ. Mu-opioid receptor mRNA expression in the rat CNS: comparison to mu-receptor binding. Brain Res. 1994;643(1–2):245–65.
75. Di Chiara G, Imperato A. Drugs abused by humans preferentially increase synaptic dopamine concentrations in the mesolimbic system of freely moving rats. Proc Natl Acad Sci U S A. 1988;85(14):5274–8.
76. Di Chiara G, Imperato A. Opposite effects of mu and kappa opiate agonists on dopamine release in the nucleus accumbens and in the dorsal caudate of freely moving rats. J Pharmacol Exp Ther. 1988;244:1067–80.
77. Zhang Y, Liang Y, Randesi M, Yuferov V, Zhao C, Kreek MJ. Chronic oxycodone self-administration altered reward-related genes in the ventral and dorsal

striatum of C57BL/6J mice: an RNA-seq analysis. Neuroscience. 2018;393:333–49.
78. Pettit HO, Ettenberg A, Bloom FE, Koob GF. Destruction of dopamine in the nucleus accumbens selectively attenuates cocaine but not heroin self-administration in rats. Psychopharmacology. 1984;84(2):167–73.
79. Koob GF. Neurobiology of opioid addiction: opponent process, hyperkatifeia, and negative reinforcement. Biol Psychiatry. 2020;87(1):44–53.
80. Schluger JH, Borg L, Ho A, Kreek MJ. Altered HPA axis responsivity to metyrapone testing in methadone maintained former heroin addicts with ongoing cocaine addiction. Neuropsychopharmacology. 2001;24(5):568–75.
81. McClung CA, Nestler EJ, Zachariou V. Regulation of gene expression by chronic morphine and morphine withdrawal in the locus ceruleus and ventral tegmental area. J Neurosci. 2005;25(25):6005–15.
82. Negus SS, Banks ML. Modulation of drug choice by extended drug access and withdrawal in rhesus monkeys: implications for negative reinforcement as a driver of addiction and target for medications development. Pharmacol Biochem Behav. 2018;164:32–9.
83. Cooper ZD, Truong YN, Shi YG, Woods JH. Morphine deprivation increases self-administration of the fast- and short-acting mu-opioid receptor agonist remifentanil in the rat. J Pharmacol Exp Ther. 2008;326(3):920–9.
84. Chartoff EH, Carlezon WA Jr. Drug withdrawal conceptualized as a stressor. Behav Pharmacol. 2014;25(5–6):473–92.
85. Torralva PR, Janowsky A. Noradrenergic mechanisms in fentanyl-mediated rapid death explain failure of naloxone in the opioid crisis. J Pharmacol Exp Ther. 2019;371(2):453–75.
86. Varga AG, Reid BT, Kieffer BL, Levitt ES. Differential impact of two critical respiratory centers in opioid-induced respiratory depression in awake mice. J Physiol. 2019;598(1):189–205.
87. Yuferov V, Zhang Y, Liang Y, Zhao C, Randesi M, Kreek MJ. Oxycodone self-administration induces alterations in expression of integrin, semaphorin and ephrin genes in the mouse striatum. Front Psych. 2018;9:257.
88. Zhang Y, Liang Y, Levran O, Randesi M, Yuferov V, Zhao C, et al. Alterations of expression of inflammation/immune-related genes in the dorsal and ventral striatum of adult C57BL/6J mice following chronic oxycodone self-administration: a RNA sequencing study. Psychopharmacology. 2017;234(15):2259–75.
89. Lutz PE, Ayranci G, Chu-Sin-Chung P, Matifas A, Koebel P, Filliol D, et al. Distinct mu, delta, and kappa opioid receptor mechanisms underlie low sociability and depressive-like behaviors during heroin abstinence. Neuropsychopharmacology. 2014;39(11):2694–705.
90. Welsch L, Bailly J, Darcq E, Kieffer BL. The negative affect of protracted opioid abstinence: progress and perspectives from rodent models. Biol Psychiatry. 2020;87(1):54–63.
91. Browne CJ, Godino A, Salery M, Nestler EJ. Epigenetic mechanisms of opioid addiction. Biol Psychiatry. 2020;87(1):22–33.
92. Wang XM, Zhou Y, Spangler R, Ho A, Han JS, Kreek MJ. Acute intermittent morphine increases preprodynorphin and kappa opioid receptor mRNA levels in the rat brain. Brain Res Mol Brain Res. 1999;66(1–2):184–7.
93. Piechota M, Korostynski M, Sikora M, Golda S, Dzbek J, Przewlocki R. Common transcriptional effects in the mouse striatum following chronic treatment with heroin and methamphetamine. Genes Brain Behav. 2012;11(4):404–14.
94. Lalanne L, Ayranci G, Filliol D, Gaveriaux-Ruff C, Befort K, Kieffer BL, et al. Kappa opioid receptor antagonism and chronic antidepressant treatment have beneficial activities on social interactions and grooming deficits during heroin abstinence. Addict Biol. 2016;22:1010–21.
95. Ritz MC, Cone EJ, Kuhar MJ. Cocaine inhibition of ligand binding at dopamine, norepinephrine and serotonin transporters: a structure-activity study. Life Sci. 1990;46(9):635–45.
96. Zhang Y, Butelman ER, Schlussman SD, Ho A, Kreek MJ. Effect of the endogenous kappa opioid agonist dynorphin A(1-17) on cocaine-evoked increases in striatal dopamine levels and cocaine-induced place preference in C57BL/6J mice. Psychopharmacology. 2004;172(4):422–9.
97. Sora I, Hall FS, Andrews AM, Itokawa M, Li XF, Wei HB, et al. Molecular mechanisms of cocaine reward: combined dopamine and serotonin transporter knockouts eliminate cocaine place preference. Proc Natl Acad Sci U S A. 2001;98(9):5300–5.
98. Lazenka MF, Suyama JA, Bauer CT, Banks ML, Negus SS. Sex differences in abuse-related neurochemical and behavioral effects of 3,4-methylened ioxymethamphetamine (MDMA) in rats. Pharmacol Biochem Behav. 2017;152:52–60.
99. Wang GJ, Wiers CE, Shumay E, Tomasi D, Yuan K, Wong CT, et al. Expectation effects on brain dopamine responses to methylphenidate in cocaine use disorder. Transl Psychiatry. 2019;9(1):93.
100. Keiflin R, Janak PH. Dopamine prediction errors in reward learning and addiction: from theory to neural circuitry. Neuron. 2015;88(2):247–63.
101. Lecca D, Cacciapaglia F, Valentini V, Acquas E, Di Chiara G. Differential neurochemical and behavioral adaptation to cocaine after response contingent and noncontingent exposure in the rat. Psychopharmacology. 2006;191(3):653–67: online publication.
102. Zhang Y, Schlussman SD, Rabkin J, Butelman ER, Ho A, Kreek MJ. Chronic escalating cocaine exposure, abstinence/withdrawal, and chronic re-exposure: effects on striatal dopamine and opioid systems in C57BL/6J mice. Neuropharmacology. 2012;67:259–66.

103. Schmitt KC, Reith ME. Regulation of the dopamine transporter: aspects relevant to psychostimulant drugs of abuse. Ann N Y Acad Sci. 2010;1187:316–40.
104. Daunais JB, Roberts DC, McGinty JF. Cocaine self-administration increases preprodynorphin, but not c-fos, mRNA in rat striatum. Neuroreport. 1993;4(5):543–6.
105. Hurd YL, Brown EE, Finlay JM, Fibiger HC, Gerfen CR. Cocaine self-administration differentially alters mRNA expression of striatal peptides. Brain Res Mol Brain Res. 1992;13(1–2):165–70.
106. Wang JQ, McGinty JF. Dose-dependent alteration in zif/268 and preprodynorphin mRNA expression induced by amphetamine or methamphetamine in rat forebrain. J Pharmacol Exp Ther. 1995;273(2):909–17.
107. Spencer S, Scofield M, Kalivas PW. The good and bad news about glutamate in drug addiction. J Psychopharmacol. 2016;30(11):1095–8.
108. Valenza M, Butelman ER, Kreek MJ. Effects of the novel relatively short-acting kappa opioid receptor antagonist LY2444296 in behaviors observed after chronic extended-access cocaine self-administration in rats. Psychopharmacology. 2017;234:2219–31.
109. Chartoff E, Sawyer A, Rachlin A, Potter D, Pliakas A, Carlezon WA. Blockade of kappa opioid receptors attenuates the development of depressive-like behaviors induced by cocaine withdrawal in rats. Neuropharmacology. 2012;62:167–76.
110. Valenza M, Windisch K, Butelman ER, Reed B, Kreek MJ. Effects of Kappa opioid receptor blockade by LY2444296 HCl, a selective short-acting antagonist, during chronic extended-access cocaine self-administration and re-exposure in rat. Psychopharmacology. 2020;237(4):1147–60.
111. Beardsley PM, Howard JL, Shelton KL, Carroll FI. Differential effects of the novel kappa opioid receptor antagonist, JDTic, on reinstatement of cocaine-seeking induced by footshock stressors vs cocaine primes and its antidepressant-like effects in rats. Psychopharmacology. 2005;183(1):118–26.
112. Weiss F, Lorang MT, Bloom FE, Koob GF. Oral alcohol self-administration stimulates dopamine release in the rat nucleus accumbens: genetic and motivational determinants. J Pharmacol Exp Ther. 1993;267(1):250–8.
113. Urban NB, Kegeles LS, Slifstein M, Xu X, Martinez D, Sakr E, et al. Sex differences in striatal dopamine release in young adults after oral alcohol challenge: a positron emission tomography imaging study with [^{11}C]raclopride. Biol Psychiatry. 2010;68(8):689–96.
114. Aalto S, Ingman K, Alakurtti K, Kaasinen V, Virkkala J, Någren K, et al. Intravenous ethanol increases dopamine release in the ventral striatum in humans: PET study using bolus-plus-infusion administration of [(11)C]raclopride. J Cereb Blood Flow Metab. 2015;35(3):424–31.
115. Hall FS, Sora I, Uhl GR. Ethanol consumption and reward are decreased in mu-opiate receptor knockout mice. Psychopharmacology. 2001;154(1):43–9.
116. Bencherif B, Wand GS, McCaul ME, Kim YK, Ilgin N, Dannals RF, et al. Mu-opioid receptor binding measured by [11C]carfentanil positron emission tomography is related to craving and mood in alcohol dependence. Biol Psychiatry. 2004;55(3):255–62.
117. Hermann D, Hirth N, Reimold M, Batra A, Smolka MN, Hoffmann S, et al. Low mu-opioid receptor status in alcohol dependence identified by combined positron emission tomography and post-mortem brain analysis. Neuropsychopharmacology. 2017;42(3):606–14.
118. Colombo G, Serra S, Brunetti G, Atzori G, Pani M, Vacca G, et al. The GABA(B) receptor agonists baclofen and CGP 44532 prevent acquisition of alcohol drinking behaviour in alcohol-preferring rats. Alcohol Alcohol. 2002;37(5):499–503.
119. Walker BM, Koob GF. The gamma-aminobutyric acid-B receptor agonist baclofen attenuates responding for ethanol in ethanol-dependent rats. Alcohol Clin Exp Res. 2007;31(1):11–8.
120. Lingford-Hughes A, Reid AG, Myers J, Feeney A, Hammers A, Taylor LG, et al. A [11C]Ro15 4513 PET study suggests that alcohol dependence in man is associated with reduced α5 benzodiazepine receptors in limbic regions. J Psychopharmacol. 2012;26(2):273–81.
121. Hwa L, Besheer J, Kash T. Glutamate plasticity woven through the progression to alcohol use disorder: a multi-circuit perspective. F1000Research. 2017;6:298.
122. Chen G, Cuzon Carlson VC, Wang J, Beck A, Heinz A, Ron D, et al. Striatal involvement in human alcoholism and alcohol consumption, and withdrawal in animal models. Alcohol Clin Exp Res. 2011;35(10):1739–48.
123. Windisch KA, Czachowski CL. Effects of group II metabotropic glutamate receptor modulation on ethanol- and sucrose-seeking and consumption in the rat. Alcohol (Fayetteville, NY). 2018;66:77–85.
124. Cannady R, Fisher KR, Graham C, Crayle J, Besheer J, Hodge CW. Potentiation of amygdala AMPA receptor activity selectively promotes escalated alcohol self-administration in a CaMKII-dependent manner. Addict Biol. 2017;22(3):652–64.
125. Cannady R, Fisher KR, Durant B, Besheer J, Hodge CW. Enhanced AMPA receptor activity increases operant alcohol self-administration and cue-induced reinstatement. Addict Biol. 2013;18(1):54–65.
126. Yin HH, Park BS, Adermark L, Lovinger DM. Ethanol reverses the direction of long-term synaptic plasticity in the dorsomedial striatum. Eur J Neurosci. 2007;25(11):3226–32.
127. Blitzer RD, Gil O, Landau EM. Long-term potentiation in rat hippocampus is inhibited by low concentrations of ethanol. Brain Res. 1990;537(1–2):203–8.
128. Edwards S, Guerrero M, Ghoneim OM, Roberts E, Koob GF. Evidence that vasopressin V1b receptors mediate the transition to excessive drinking in ethanol-dependent rats. Addict Biol. 2012;17(1):76–85.

129. Lindholm S, Rosin A, Dahlin I, Georgieva J, Franck J. Ethanol alters the effect of kappa receptor ligands on dopamine release in the nucleus accumbens. Physiol Behav. 2007;92(1–2):167–71.
130. Zhou Y, Franck J, Spangler R, Maggos CE, Ho A, Kreek MJ. Reduced hypothalamic POMC and anterior pituitary CRF1 receptor mRNA levels after acute, but not chronic, daily "binge" intragastric alcohol administration. Alcohol Clin Exp Res. 2000;24(10):1575–82.
131. Zhou Y, Colombo G, Carai MA, Ho A, Gessa GL, Kreek MJ. Involvement of arginine vasopressin and V1b receptor in alcohol drinking in Sardinian alcohol-preferring rats. Alcohol Clin Exp Res. 2011;35(10):1876–83.
132. Benowitz NL. Pharmacology of nicotine: addiction, smoking-induced disease, and therapeutics. Annu Rev Pharmacol Toxicol. 2009;49:57–71.
133. Picciotto MR, Zoli M, Rimondini R, Léna C, Marubio LM, Pich EM, et al. Acetylcholine receptors containing the beta2 subunit are involved in the reinforcing properties of nicotine. Nature. 1998;391(6663):173–7.
134. Tapper AR, McKinney SL, Nashmi R, Schwarz J, Deshpande P, Labarca C, et al. Nicotine activation of alpha4* receptors: sufficient for reward, tolerance, and sensitization. Science (New York, NY). 2004;306(5698):1029–32.
135. Grieder TE, Besson M, Maal-Bared G, Pons S, Maskos U, van der Kooy D. β2* nAChRs on VTA dopamine and GABA neurons separately mediate nicotine aversion and reward. Proc Natl Acad Sci U S A. 2019;116(51):25968–73.
136. Husson M, Harrington L, Tochon L, Cho Y, Ibañez-Tallon I, Maskos U, et al. β4-nicotinic receptors are critically involved in reward-related behaviors and self-regulation of nicotine reinforcement. J Neurosci. 2020;40(17):3465–77.
137. Wonnacott S. Presynaptic nicotinic ACh receptors. Trends Neurosci. 1997;20(2):92–8.
138. Quarta D, Ciruela F, Patkar K, Borycz J, Solinas M, Lluis C, et al. Heteromeric nicotinic acetylcholine-dopamine autoreceptor complexes modulate striatal dopamine release. Neuropsychopharmacology. 2007;32(1):35–42.
139. Marchi M, Risso F, Viola C, Cavazzani P, Raiteri M. Direct evidence that release-stimulating alpha7* nicotinic cholinergic receptors are localized on human and rat brain glutamatergic axon terminals. J Neurochem. 2002;80(6):1071–8.
140. Jackson KJ, Carroll FI, Negus SS, Damaj MI. Effect of the selective kappa-opioid receptor antagonist JDTic on nicotine antinociception, reward, and withdrawal in the mouse. Psychopharmacology. 2010;210(2):285–94.
141. Jackson KJ, Muldoon PP, De Biasi M, Damaj MI. New mechanisms and perspectives in nicotine withdrawal. Neuropharmacology. 2015;96(Pt B):223–34.
142. Grieder TE, Herman MA, Contet C, Tan LA, Vargas-Perez H, Cohen A, et al. VTA CRF neurons mediate the aversive effects of nicotine withdrawal and promote intake escalation. Nat Neurosci. 2014;17(12):1751–8.
143. Fride E, Barg J, Levy R, Saya D, Heldman E, Mechoulam R, et al. Low doses of anandamides inhibit pharmacological effects of delta 9-tetrahydrocannabinol. J Pharmacol Exp Ther. 1995;272(2):699–707.
144. Yamaguchi F, Tokuda M, Hatase O, Brenner S. Molecular cloning of the novel human G protein-coupled receptor (GPCR) gene mapped on chromosome 9. Biochem Biophys Res Commun. 1996;227(2):608–14.
145. Picone RP, Fournier DJ, Makriyannis A. Ligand based structural studies of the CB1 cannabinoid receptor. J Pept Res. 2002;60(6):348–56.
146. Tanda G, Pontieri FE, Di Chiara G. Cannabinoid and heroin activation of mesolimbic dopamine transmission by a common mu1 opioid receptor mechanism. Science (New York, NY). 1997;276(5321):2048–50.
147. Justinova Z, Tanda G, Redhi GH, Goldberg SR. Self-administration of delta9-tetrahydrocannabinol (THC) by drug naive squirrel monkeys. Psychopharmacology. 2003;169(2):135–40.
148. Wakeford AGP, Wetzell BB, Pomfrey RL, Clasen MM, Taylor WW, Hempel BJ, et al. The effects of cannabidiol (CBD) on Delta(9)-tetrahydrocannabinol (THC) self-administration in male and female Long-Evans rats. Exp Clin Psychopharmacol. 2017;25(4):242–8.
149. Ghozland S, Matthes HW, Simonin F, Filliol D, Kieffer BL, Maldonado R. Motivational effects of cannabinoids are mediated by mu-opioid and kappa-opioid receptors. J Neurosci. 2002;22(3):1146–54.
150. Zimmer A, Valjent E, Konig M, Zimmer AM, Robledo P, Hahn H, et al. Absence of delta-9-tetrahydrocannabinol dysphoric effects in dynorphin-deficient mice. J Neurosci. 2001;21(23):9499–505.
151. Mensen VT, Vreeker A, Nordgren J, Atkinson A, de la Torre R, Farré M, et al. Psychopathological symptoms associated with synthetic cannabinoid use: a comparison with natural cannabis. Psychopharmacology. 2019;236(9):2677–85.
152. Mechoulam R, Shvo Y, Hashish I. The structure of cannabidiol. Tetrahedron. 1963;19(12):2073–8.
153. Elsaid S, Kloiber S, Le Foll B. Effects of cannabidiol (CBD) in neuropsychiatric disorders: a review of pre-clinical and clinical findings. Prog Mol Biol Transl Sci. 2019;167:25–75.
154. Freeman AM, Petrilli K, Lees R, Hindocha C, Mokrysz C, Curran HV, et al. How does cannabidiol (CBD) influence the acute effects of delta-9-tetrahydrocannabinol (THC) in humans? A systematic review. Neurosci Biobehav Rev. 2019;107:696–712.
155. Parrott AC, Hayley AC, Downey LA. Recreational stimulants, herbal, and spice cannabis: the core psy-

chobiological processes that underlie their damaging effects. Hum Psychopharmacol. 2017 32(3).
156. Bart G, Kreek MJ, Ott J, LaForge KS, Proudnikov D, Pollak L, et al. Increased attributable risk related to a functional mu-opioid receptor gene polymorphism in association with alcohol dependence in Central Sweden. Neuropsychopharmacology. 2005;30(2):417–22.
157. Edenberg HJ, Foroud T. Genetics of alcoholism. Handb Clin Neurol. 2014;125:561–71.
158. Yuferov V, Ji F, Nielsen DA, Levran O, Ho A, Morgello S, et al. A functional haplotype implicated in vulnerability to develop cocaine dependence is associated with reduced PDYN expression in human brain. Neuropsychopharmacology. 2009;34(5):1185–97.
159. Agrawal A, Verweij KJ, Gillespie NA, Heath AC, Lessov-Schlaggar CN, Martin NG, et al. The genetics of addiction-a translational perspective. Transl Psychiatry. 2012;2:e140.
160. Zhang H, Largent-Milnes TM, Vanderah TW. Glial neuroimmune signaling in opioid reward. Brain Res Bull. 2020;155:102–11.
161. Massart R, Barnea R, Dikshtein Y, Suderman M, Meir O, Hallett M, et al. Role of DNA methylation in the nucleus accumbens in incubation of cocaine craving. J Neurosci. 2015;35(21):8042–58.
162. Unterwald EM, Kreek MJ, Cuntapay M. The frequency of cocaine administration impacts cocaine-induced receptor alterations. Brain Res. 2001;900(1):103–9.
163. Sloan ME, Gowin JL, Yan J, Schwandt ML, Spagnolo PA, Sun H, et al. Severity of alcohol dependence is associated with the fatty acid amide hydrolase Pro129Thr missense variant. Addict Biol. 2018;23(1):474–84.
164. Agrawal A, Lynskey MT, Bucholz KK, Kapoor M, Almasy L, Dick DM, et al. DSM-5 cannabis use disorder: a phenotypic and genomic perspective. Drug Alcohol Depend. 2014;134:362–9.

3 Psychological Antecedents and Correlates of Substance Use and Addiction

Ralph E. Tarter and Maureen D. Reynolds

Introduction

Diminished capacity to deter onset or discontinue a behavior is a ubiquitous feature of addiction. The etymology, *addictus*, refers to a once-free person reduced to slave which, in the vernacular, reflects loss or sharply limited "free-will." Within a neuropsychological framework, addictive behavior indicates deficient functioning of the executive control system evinced as poor modulation of behavior and emotions during goal-directed motivation and social interactions [1]. Low psychological self-regulation is not only a cardinal feature of addiction but also, as will be discussed in this chapter, the main characteristic heightening risk for this outcome.

Addictive behaviors, appetitive (sex, food) and non-appetitive (gambling, video gaming, etc.), are genetically correlated and have the same neurobiological underpinnings [2–7]. Addiction consequent to consumption of addictive chemicals (ACs) is unique, however, in two key respects. First, regular consumption of most ACs leads to neuroadaptation. Hence, an increasingly larger amount or a more potent product needs to be consumed over time to experience the desired subjective effect. As dependence is established, consumption motivation shifts toward averting punishment, namely, withdrawal syndrome. Accordingly, mental effort commonly rising in severity to ruminative preoccupation is devoted to ensuring a reliable AC supply. AC consumption at this juncture is, therefore, obsessive-compulsive behavior. Second, ACs and their metabolites are toxins. Consequently, habitual AC use disrupts neurological functioning as well as injures vital organs that are essential for servicing the brain's metabolic requirements. For example, lung disease in smokers and liver disease in alcohol consumers may cause, respectively, hypoxia and portal systemic encephalopathy manifesting as impaired cognitive capacity along with behavior and emotion disturbances. These psychological sequelae of AC toxicity increase the likelihood of interpersonal problems and social maladjustment which, without intervention, may accelerate progression to addiction. In sum, the prodrome stage associated with consumption of ACs is distinctly different from other addictions notwithstanding substantially genetic and phenotypic commonality prior to onset of the particular addictive behavior.

The label *mania* currently denotes a state of heightened behavior activity concomitant with

R. E. Tarter (✉)
Department of Pharmaceutical Sciences, School of Pharmacy, University of Pittsburgh, Pittsburgh, PA, USA
e-mail: tarter@pitt.edu

M. D. Reynolds
Pharmaceutical Sciences, University of Pittsburgh School of Pharmacy, Pittsburgh, PA, USA
e-mail: maureen@pitt.edu

M. M. Vanyukov (ed.), *Genetics of Substance Use*, https://doi.org/10.1007/978-3-030-95350-8_3

intense excitement. Historically, mania has been affixed to behaviors to designate *excess* such as *erotomania* (sexual desire), *mythomania* (lying), dipsomania (alcohol consumption), narcomania (drug use), and heliomania (sunbathing). Consumption of ACs indicating excess is commonly evinced as a violation of sociocultural mores and secular laws (e.g., underage alcohol use, cocaine use, prescription drug use without physician oversight) presaged by poor self-control. Hence, to understand the etiology of addiction, it is essential to conjointly take into account the psychological disposition in the social environment leading to AC use onset, escalation to a pattern of regular consumption, and addiction.

Psychological Characteristics Predisposing to AC Use and Addiction

Many psychological characteristics heighten the probability of AC use and addiction. The large majority aggregate within the rubric of self-regulation, defined as the cognitive control of behavior and emotions during goal-directed motivation and social interactions. Notably, scores on cognitive, emotion, and behavior indicators of psychological self-regulation constitute a continuous trait, and the score on this trait in children and adolescents forecasts addiction [8]. Relatedly, shared genetic and phenotypic factors are involved in all categories of substance use disorder [9].

Ontogenetic Addiction Suboptimal *acquisition* of psychological self-regulation biases childhood and adolescent development toward deviant socialization marked by indifference to or rejection of sociocultural mores and secular laws. One expression of deviancy is underage consumption of ACs that are legal for adults or consumption of illegal ACs. Contingent on the pattern of interactions with the social environment, AC use may consolidate into a regular habit that segues to addictive (compulsive) behavior during adolescence and adulthood.

Addiction Reaction Stressors diminish psychological self-regulation, that is, the capacity to cognitively modulate emotions and behavior. Whether stimulants or depressants, ACs induce physiological stability and, therefore, enhance well-being. Improved subjective well-being is experienced as euphoria (positive reinforcement) or alleviation of an aversive state (negative reinforcement). Thus, AC use is an expeditious tactic, at least in the short term, to ameliorate stress concomitant with negative emotions (anxiety, panic, depression, etc.) and/or aversive physical condition (pain, insomnia, fatigue, etc.). AC use leading to this variant of addiction is thus motivated by a desire to improve subjective state by consuming a recreational substance or FDA-approved medicament.

In summary, suboptimal psychological self-regulation is the core characteristic associated with elevated risk for respectively ontogenetic addiction and addiction reaction. Prior to AC use onset, these two addiction variants are differentiated according to the origins of low psychological self-regulation, quality of socialization, and role of stressors prompting AC consumption.

Sociocultural Milieu

Numerous public and private behaviors (e.g., diet, dress, manners) along with beliefs and values are deeply ingrained in cultural mores (rules, virtues) and folkways (social conventions). Cultures differ widely with respect to their stridency of negatively sanctioning AC use due in part to the meaning attached to consumption. However, the same core psychological characteristics are exhibited by consumers of proscribed ACs across different cultures. For example, the psychological characteristics of consumers of snake venom in India include behavior undercontrol, sensation seeking, and behavioral overactivity [10]. Furthermore, venom consumers congregate in neglected neighborhoods where socially non-normative behavior is more likely to be tolerated [11]. In western societies, consumers of plant-based ACs exhibit similar characteristics. Regardless of the particular substance, the psychological characteristics of offenders of norms are, therefore, similar across cultures.

Although most cultures negatively sanction recreational AC use, they are accepted, however, as medicine to treat physical and psychological discomfort. Aversive states are stressful, requiring action to obtain relief. Notably, risk for AC use leading to addiction is higher among individuals who have greater susceptibility to stressors [12]. It is also noteworthy that ACs have been used prophylactically in diet, as, for example, drinking wine instead of unsanitary water. Thus, the curative and preventive properties promote the adaptational success of a culture and, accordingly, are endorsed.

In summary, AC use reflecting proneness to violating sociocultural norms emanates from suboptimal acquisition of psychological self-regulation, whereas AC use as a medicament is motivated by the need to alleviate an aversive subjective state associated with reduction of psychological self-regulation. Sociocultural norms and secular laws provide the meaning, purpose, and context associated with AC use consequent to low psychological self-regulation.

Outcome of AC Use

Although AC use does not lead inevitably to problems, a portion of the population develops one or more medical diseases, psychological disturbance, and social adjustment difficulties. Currently, there is a lack of consensus regarding (1) the label designating the problem outcome; (2) the features of the problem; and (3) a schema to quantify severity of the problem, including the threshold that objectively and meaningfully distinguishes the affected and non-affected segments of the AC-consuming population. Three overlapping frameworks specify the problem outcome of AC use: (1) *dependence syndrome* emphasizing the neurobiological consequences of AC use; (2) substance use disorder reflecting a mixture of adverse biological, behavioral, and social sequelae; and (3) addiction denoting obsessive-compulsive AC use behavior. Before examining etiology, it is important to first consider these outcomes of AC use.

Dependence Syndrome

The *dependence* syndrome, first detailed by Edwards and Gross [13], is marked by (1) acquired tolerance, (2) preoccupation with AC consumption, (3) irresistible urge to consume the AC, (4) rumination about ensuring access to the AC, (5) withdrawal symptoms triggered upon cessation of AC consumption, (6) sustaining AC consumption to avoid onset of withdrawal, and (7) reinstatement of these latter six characteristics upon resuming AC consumption after a period of abstinence. These symptoms are inferred to reflect AC-induced alteration of brain functioning.

Substance Use Disorder (SUD)

The dependence syndrome constitutes a subset of the criteria adopted by the American Psychiatric Association to specify the outcome, namely, substance use disorder (SUD). The current fifth edition of the *Diagnostic and Statistical Manual of Mental Disorders* (DSM-5) additionally includes psychological, medical, and social criteria to characterize the outcome of AC use as a polythetic syndrome, that is, a disorder without the presence of an essential required symptom. The affected segment of the AC-using population is, therefore, very heterogenous, especially considering that only 2 of 11 criteria need to be present to qualify for SUD diagnosis. Indeed, the affected population consists of individuals who do not have any symptoms in common, thereby challenging research aimed at delineating an etiological psychological trait.

The SUD categories constitute two genetically correlated classes distinguished according to whether the AC is legal or illegal [9]. In effect, the type of AC that was used resulting in SUD reflects, at least in part, a proclivity to engage in illegal behavior. Relatedly, the SUD categories can be scaled as a continuous variable denoting severity of social sanction of the AC. Legal substances (for adults) such as alcohol are located at the low end of the scale, whereas "hard" drugs such as cocaine are located at the high end of the scale [14]. Significantly, low and high externalizing severity, respectively, portends using legal and illegal ACs that culminated in their corresponding SUD. In a complementary line of research, the transmissible liability index (TLI) measuring the component of SUD risk that has intergenerational continuity consists almost entirely of items that depict disruptive and socially deviant behavior [15]. The TLI score also predicts membership in all SUD categories [16]. Overall, these studies indicate that (1) the SUD categories are scalable as a continuous trait varying in severity according to social acceptability and legal status of the AC; (2) the characteristics presaging all SUDs consist in varying severity of undercontrolled behavior and proneness to social deviancy; and (3) all SUDs have shared genetic predisposition.

Violating the law, at least with respect to using ACs, has high prevalence. Notably, 58.5% and 22.3% of high school seniors in the USA have used alcohol and tobacco at least one time [17]. Whereas alcohol and tobacco use are status offenses, marijuana use is currently a Federal offense, and a first offense is punishable by incarceration of up to 1 year. Nevertheless, lifetime prevalence of marijuana use among high school seniors exceeds 40%. Indeed, lifetime use of any illicit drug exceeds 45%. This propensity for rule-breaking, either persisting since childhood or emerging during adolescence [18], is a major factor causing youths to transition into the criminal justice system. Drug use disorder in the incarcerated population has high prevalence, estimated in one study to constitute 30% of men and 51% of women [19].

Antisocial personality disorder prominently featured by behavior undercontrol and more prevalent in men [20] and borderline personality disorder prominently featured by intense negative emotion reactivity and more prevalent in women [21] have shared genetic risk with and frequently co-occur with addiction [22, 23]. Moreover, these three disorders are featured by a mixture of internalizing (e.g., anxiety, mood) and externalizing (e.g., impulsivity, hyperactivity) characteristics [15, 24, 25] along with suboptimum executive capacity [26] integral to planning, implementing, and persisting in goal-directed activities and self-monitoring behavior and emotions during social interactions [1]. It is also noteworthy that variation in the amplitude of the P300 component of the event-related potential, a neurophysiological correlate of attention capacity, is strongly influenced by genetics and is attenuated in youths at heightened risk for addiction based on family history of addiction, childhood conduct disorder, or antisocial personality disorder [27–30]. A key component of the executive control system is, therefore, impaired in disorders that share genetic risk with addiction.

Other factors besides suboptimal psychological self-regulation also, however, promote the onset of AC use. Considering that adolescence is the phase of development linking childhood and adulthood, AC use may reflect a mimicking of normative adult behavior. AC consumption may also constitute one feature of adolescent-limited antisociality [18]. In this circumstance, normatively socialized childhood development is succeeded in adolescence by rule-breaking behavior that ceases in adulthood. Furthermore, culturally inculcated beliefs about the benefits of ACs may catalyze onset of AC use. While AC use can be triggered by numerous factors, segueing to SUD is potentiated in individuals who obtain persisting benefits so as to establish a pattern of regular consumption. As will be discussed later, AC use embedded in social deviancy or intended to ameliorate stress with concomitant negative emotions elevates the likelihood of establishing a pattern of habitual consumption leading to SUD.

Addiction

As defined by the American Society for Addiction Medicine [31], "Addiction is a treatable, chronic medical disease involving complex interactions among brain circuits, genetics, the environment, and an individual's life experiences. People with addiction use substances or engage in behaviors that become compulsive and often continue despite harmful consequences." The hallmark features of addictive behavior are the irresistible urge to initiate AC use and the diminished capacity to cease consumption. Addiction, therefore, is a behavioral phenomenon. The compulsive quality of AC seeking is often, but not necessarily, potentiated by the need to avert onset of withdrawal symptoms. Hence, sustained mental effort is required to ensure an uninterrupted AC supply. Accordingly, addictive behavior (or addiction) can be specified on a dimension quantifying obsessive-compulsive motivation. The overarching task in etiology research involves delineating the pathway from low psychological self-regulation (vulnerability phenotype) to obsessive-compulsive (addictive) AC use. Accordingly, this chapter utilizes the terms *addictive behavior and addiction*. One advantage of this framework is that it aligns etiology and outcome on the same empirical plane, namely, psychological processes.

Sociocultural Contexts of AC Use Leading to Ontogenetic Addiction and Addiction Reaction

Many animal species consume plants, fungi, and soil products to prevent and treat diseases [32]. Most medicaments are contained in the stems, leaves, flowers, seeds, and fruit of angiosperms which represent over 90% of terrestrial plants species. Their evolutionary success is largely due to a capacity to manufacture chemicals that attract animals to promote pollination, assist seed dispersal, and thwart predation. Consumption of many of these chemicals by humans produces a subjective experience of augmented well-being. So much so, the plant may be seen as a resource for rapture. The etymology (Sumerian) of opium, for example, is *plant of joy*. Many plants, or their products, having psychoactive properties are exalted. For instance, distilled wine (i.e., brandy) is often still referred to as *aqua vitae* (water of life). Not surprisingly, many plants or their products that produce pleasure are valued as medicines (e.g., lavender, peppermint, rosemary, basil) even though disease-modifying properties are limited or absent. This subset of plants, due to possessing strong reinforcement properties – and accordingly the potential to lead to addictive behavior – are most prized. Prior to the modern era, addictive and non-addictive plant products were agglomerated into the single category of medicament. To this day, the armamentarium of empirical, traditional, and alternative medicines contains many of these latter botanical products.

Medicines advance the adaptation of a culture. Caregiving with medicines also promotes interdependence, cooperation, and social cohesiveness [33]. Thus, a perception that a plant has curative properties is rapidly inculcated into a culture-wide belief [34] and readily incorporated into its medical and cultural practices. Not coincidentally, ACs (alcohol, cocaine, morphine, etc.) were the principal ingredients in nostrums peddled to a uninformed and unprotected population during the patent medicine era in the USA (circa 1850–1920). In the modern era, many over-the-counter (OTC) medicines contain psychoactive chemicals, indicating that their valued benefits, at least in part, are owed to enhancing subjective experience. Alcohol concentrations (%) in *Benadryl Liquid Elixir* (14%), *Contac Severe Cold* (25%), and *Anbesol Liquid* (70%) are higher than many alcoholic beverages. Other popular OTC medicines that contain chemicals with psychoactive properties include *Robitussin* (dextromethorphan) to treat cough, *Imodium* (loperamide) to treat diarrhea, and *Dramamine* (dimenhydrinate) to treat dizziness and motion sickness. Indeed, an AC, regardless of its actual disease-modifying benefits, may acquire panacea status. For example, cannabis is currently widely claimed without strong supporting empirical evidence to have therapeutic benefit for dozens of medical conditions. Cultures with few exceptions (e.g., Christian Scientists) sanction the consumption of medicines, including remedies that are exclusively ACs or contain AC ingredients. However, consumption of ACs other than for utilitarian benefit, such as food or medicine, often remains proscribed.

In his seminal treatise, *The Protestant Ethic*, Max Weber described the attributes of a virtuous person, namely, ascetic lifestyle, disposition marked by deliberative restraint, and life-fulfilling calling or commitment to a vocation (i.e., *berufsmensch*) [35]. These qualities are required for afterlife in paradise. Hence, engaging in activities that are pleasurable but without utilitarian benefit (e.g., eating, sex, drinking alcohol) violates a core cultural ethos. Offenders are immoral sybarites.

The Reformation in the sixteenth and seventeenth centuries had a transformative impact on uplifting the wealth of the population. The reasons for this outcome are numerous; however, one driving factor was that Protestants were prepared to participate in and prosper in the industrial revolution by possessing cognitive skills, especially literacy. Although literacy, specifically reading the Bible, was mandated as the path to salvation, this skill competitively advantaged Protestants in the new era favoring innovation and entrepreneurial activity [36]. Mandatory publicly funded education, widespread growth in printing and publishing, and new mercantile activities such as founding the first stock market in 1613 in Amsterdam further fostered economic success in Protestant countries. Increased wealth provided leisure time and resources to lapse into immorality, including indulging in the capital vices (or seven deadly sins) such as lust and gluttony. Prior to the Reformation, massive poverty restrained opportunities for indulgent pleasure.

This ethos of joining restraint from pleasure with morality arrived in the American colonies with the Pilgrims in 1620 and subsequently the Puritans a decade later. During the next two centuries, their descendants, buttressed by immigrants from largely Protestant regions in Western and Northern Europe who shared this ethos, exercised unchallenged political control. However, the ethos that pleasure without utilitarian value is sin was not subscribed to by subsequent immigrants representing multiple religions and cultures (e.g., Orthodox Christian, Roman Catholic, and non-Christian European and Chinese).

One of the first perceived threats to the Protestant ethos and hegemony mirrored the prior two centuries of brutal religious conflict in Europe. Irish immigration beginning in the 1820s and accelerating during The Famine (1845–1849) reactivated hostility to Catholics that exploded into violence in the Philadelphia Nativist Riot (1844). At around this time, decades before the Civil War and continuing afterward, home-grown Protestant denominations emerged such as the Southern Baptist Convention founded in 1845, Seventh-day Adventist Church founded in 1863, and Jehovah's Witnesses founded in the 1870s, which additionally diluted demographic representation and power of the founding culture from Western/Northern Europe. These new denominations nevertheless largely conformed with the ethos of proscribing self-indulgent pleasure.

Liberation of millions of slaves, continuing conflict with indigenous tribes (concomitant with westward expansion), and anxiety about foreigners, especially Chinese and European immigrants, had an unsettling effect on American society after the Civil War. Traditional cultural norms, values, and authority were perceived to be threatened. Toward the end of short-lived Reconstruction (1865–1877), the grassroots evangelical Women's Christian Temperance Union (WCTU) was founded (1873) having the mission of restoring national piety and moral purity that adherents believed had been degraded by alien cultures favoring, or at least tolerating, alcohol use. Notably, alcohol use was deemed a morality problem. Campaigning against alcohol use, therefore, primed perception of the threat to fulfillment of America's God-given special status (i.e., manifest destiny) posed by foreigners and wayward Americans. Weaponizing ACs thus aroused religious, nativist, and xenophobic sentiments; this tactic was to be repeated several times in the ensuing two centuries. The first federal legislation focused on protecting America from opium was the Chinese Exclusion Act (1882), which mandated termination of immigration, disallowing citizenship among current residents, and prohibiting ownership of real estate or a business.

Prohibition of pleasure was not confined to consuming ACs. The Comstock Law (1873), for example, banned the distribution and use of contraceptives and sex paraphernalia as well as private communications deemed obscene by the post office. Five years of hard labor faced offenders of this law. To this day, paying as well as receiving payment for sexual pleasure is punishable with fines or incarceration and, in some jurisdictions, with added public humiliation. The Blue Laws banned recreation, entertainment, and shopping on Sunday even though, for many, it was the only non-workday. The Food and Drug Administration (FDA) delayed approval of *Enovid*, the first oral contraceptive, even though it had already been available for several years to treat menstrual disorders. Once approval was granted in 1960, "*the Pill*" was authorized for only 2 years use to ostensibly protect safety. The point made is that there is a long history in the USA in which political power effected in laws and regulations ensured conformance with the Protestant ethos prohibiting pleasure. Denying access to pleasure, in some cases, appears to be a higher priority than protecting public safety. For example, an 18-year-old cannot drink a glass of wine at home in the USA but can own and carry a semi-automatic rifle in public. And despite ineffectiveness, sex education, a persisting contentious issue in the USA, is largely anchored to themes exhorting abstinence; thus, the USA continues to have the highest teen pregnancy rate of all developed nations.

The Progressive Era (1890–1929) was marked by intensifying xenophobia. Fears about national security were aroused by the Spanish-American War (1898), Pancho Villa's incursion into the USA (1916), and World War I (1917–1918). The first Red Scare (1917) was followed by the Palmer Raids (1919–1920) in which putative leftists, anarchists, and communists (most of whom were Italians and Jews) were rounded up for deportation. Subsequently, the Johnson-Reed Act (1924) denied immigration to all Asians and limited entry of immigrants from southern and Eastern Europe to 2% of the size of their respective ethnic populations that was admitted in 1890. In keeping with wide acceptance at that time of eugenics, these actions were partly guided by the belief that "inferior races" threatened the strength, character, and vitality of America. Immigration policy once again was aimed at protecting against perceived societal degradation.

Societal unrest was further amplified by relocation of a large portion of the population from farms to cities concurrent with rapid industrialization. Reforms were enacted to protect public welfare such as the Meat Inspection Act (1906), the Pure Food Act (1906), the Keating-Owen Act prohibiting child labor (1916), and the Sheppard-Towner Maternity and Infancy Protection Act (1921). Grassroots organizations were founded to redress social inequality, such as the National Association for the Advancement of Colored People (1909), the Urban League (1910), Women's Suffrage Association (1890), and the Socialist Party of America (1901).

Undesirable segments of the population domiciling either outside or inside the USA were, as in the past, portrayed as leaders in the manufacture and distribution of ACs: beer (Germans), wine (Italians), spirits (Jews), marijuana (Mexicans), and opium (Chinese). The Harrison Act in (1914) banned opioids and cocaine. The 18th Amendment of the US Constitution ratified in 1919 and enforced by the Volstead Act prohibited the manufacture, transportation, and consumption of alcohol beverages. Consumption of wine confined to religious rituals was, however, protected. Also, some alcohol products remained commercially available for use as medicaments. Alcohol, for example, was a commonly used treatment for influenza (1918–1919). Although not having any impact on pathology, the reinforcement properties nevertheless provided temporary subjective enhancement of well-being. But consuming alcohol with the intention of experiencing pleasure was now prohibited by federal law, thereby effectively transitioning millions of law-abiding citizens to criminals. The Volstead Act reinterpreted AC use from immorality to criminality.

The onset of the prohibition era coincided with a broad sociocultural transformation of American society. Behaviors that violated mores and folkways were rapidly gaining acceptance as normative in a large portion of the population.

One factor catalyzing relaxation of adherence to long-standing norms was the experience of military veterans who had been exposed in Europe to behaviors that were disapproved and, in some cases, severely negatively sanctioned in America such as sexual relationships before marriage and socializing across racial and gender boundaries. Newly acquired independence of women was another factor propelling the change in norms. After obtaining suffrage, partly as a reward for contributing to the war effort, many women continued to remain in the labor force and independently participate in social activities such as frequenting the speakeasy where they could drink alcohol and smoke cigarettes in a tolerant environment. With fiscal resources and social independence, the behavior repertoire expanded into other areas as well such as choosing to dress in rakish attire, joining social clubs, and interacting with men without a chaperone. Nevertheless, progress in the 1920s toward an egalitarian society was slow, beset with racial violence and discrimination against women. Marijuana use was legal and becoming a drug of choice among the avant-garde.

The Great Depression, beginning in August 1929 following a decade of prosperity, ripped the American Dream from much of the population. Economic collapse and media reports of rampant violent crime ramped up societal stress. Both left- and right-wing nationalism further amplified anxiety. In 1930 the Federal Bureau of Narcotics (FBN) was established with J. Harry Anslinger installed as its first Commissioner. Marijuana was a high priority, hyped as more dangerous than the evidence indicated. Also, this drug was asserted to be the steppingstone to using "hard" drugs. Not coincidentally, the Marijuana Tax Act (1937) essentially terminated previously legal consumption corresponding with growing visibility and acceptance of marginalized segments of the population into mainstream society. Marijuana use was associated with African Americans and the growing popularity of jazz. The pleasures of marijuana use have been long extolled in such jazz hits as *Reefer Man* (1932) by Cab Calloway, *Viper's Drag (1930)* by Fats Waller, and *When I Get Low I Get High* (1937) by Ella Fitzgerald and Chick Webb. Criminalizing marijuana use was thus directed at protecting traditional culture from degradation, including the influence of non-conformists (hipsters, libertines, etc.) [37] by legislation that connected this drug with social undesirables.

The zeitgeist of American society after World War II was captured in W.H. Auden's Pulitzer prize-winning poem, *The Age of Anxiety* (1947). The setting is a New York City bar where four strangers, three men and a woman, meet, talk, and drink. They then go to the woman's apartment, and after a brief interlude, two of the men leave, while the one remaining is intoxicated and unconscious. This outcome is disappointing for the woman who had an expectation of intimacy. Themes such as anxiety, social isolation, and purposelessness are examined and concluded to reflect weakened commitment to traditional religion. The message is that anxiety and alienation are costs for disengagement from traditional culture.

Anxiety and apprehension were exacerbated by events occurring during the first decade after the War, particularly the second Red Scare (1947–1957), establishment of the People's Republic of China (1949), Korean Conflict (1950–1953), and early Soviet dominance in space exploration. The Cold War adversaries stumbling into nuclear war was an ever-present threat. Preparation for this war included expanding the military infrastructure (e.g., installation of the North American Aerospace Defense Command) and participation of the general population in civil defense (e.g., building a bomb shelter in the home, practicing crouching under the desk at school). The aftermath of nuclear war was portrayed in popular films such as *The Day After (1983)*, *Dr. Strangelove (1964)*, and *On the Beach (1959)*. The impending end of civilization remained a cause of persisting angst.

Using an animal model, the first empirical study showing that alcohol alleviated stress was published in 1951 [38]. The first anxiolytic medicine meprobamate (Milltown) marketed as a "minor tranquilizer" started a transformation of psychiatry in 1955. Negative emotions (phobia, anxiety, depression, panic, anger, etc.) previously considered to be manifestations of psychic conflicts were now interpreted to be mental illness caused by a biochemical disorder or "imbalance." In effect, meprobamate began the transition of psychiatry from treatment of inner conflicts to basic disorder. The position that a putative biochemical disturbance was responsible for causing negative emotions brought the key stakeholders into alignment: the pharmaceutical industry having the mission of synthesizing and selling drugs, the American Psychiatric Association having the mission of treating mental illness, and consumers eager to alleviate stress with concomitant negative emotions without stigma of character weakness, immorality, or social deviancy. Consuming medicaments that may have addictive properties under Aesculapian authority of a physician to alleviate negative emotions is, therefore, embraced. Also, consumption of "recreational" ACs (e.g., alcohol, nicotine) as self-medication is legally tolerated within specified constraints such as the person's age, type of drug, and vendor. The point made is that while ACs have been long consumed to alleviate stress, the associated negative emotions were reinterpreted to indicate mental illness having biological determinants. Whether physician-directed or self-directed, ACs are, therefore, medications to ameliorate an aversive subjective state.

The number and variety of stress-related disorders have been expanded through successive editions of the *Diagnostic and Statistical Manual of Mental Disorders*. Excluding eating and somatic disorders, anxiety disorders alone comprise over 20 diagnostic categories in the DSM-5. Designating stress-related negative emotions as mental illnesses has, however, been met in some quarters with sardonic skepticism. Referring to meprobamate (the little yellow pill), the song *Mother's Little Helper* (1966 by the Rolling Stones) mocks the claim that stress is illness.

> And though she's not really ill,
> there's a little yellow pill.
> She goes running for the shelter
> of a mother's little helper.

Meprobamate did not establish the precedent of using chemicals having psychoactive properties to alleviate stress and concomitant negative emotions. Other chemicals (e.g., barbiturates, antihistamines) as well as "recreational" ACs have a long history of use to ameliorate stress. Rather, it was the reinterpretation of negative emotions as mental illness that was novel. This conceptual shift away from psychodynamic psychiatry beginning in the1950s continues to drive the practice of administering medication as the first line of treatment. Emotions are, however, psychological phenomena quantifiable as continuous traits. Magnitude of deviation from a neutral point on a trait denotes intensity of positive (e.g., happy) or negative (e.g., sad) emotion. The threshold in the DSM at which point emotion is mental illness is arbitrary, and it is important to note that ACs attenuate negative emotions across the full spectrum of severity. In contemporary sociocultural context, the "happy hour" is a folkway providing a sanctioned opportunity to alleviate stress with concomitant negative emotions among the largely non-affected portion of the population. Drinking alcohol is similarly common among individuals who have an anxiety disorder.

Chlordiazepoxide (Librium), the first blockbuster anxiolytic drug, was introduced in 1960 coinciding roughly with renewed fears of war after the downing of a U.S. spy airplane in Russia. Numerous events and factors contributed to sustaining societal stress throughout the 1960s. The Cuban missile crisis (1962) brought civilization perilously close to extinction. Vigorous social activism by segments of society outside the cultural mainstream threatened adherents of traditional norms and the established social order. The National Organization for Women, African-American movements (Black Panthers, Nation of Islam, etc.), and political activism on college campuses energized by the Vietnam War rattled mainstream society amplified by assassinations of political and religious leaders, arson directed at African-American churches, murder of civil rights advocates, and violence in response to court-mandated racial desegregation. In 1964

Bob Dylan exhorted rebellion in the song *The Times They Are A-Changin'*:

> *Come mothers and fathers throughout the land and don't criticize what you can't understand.*
> *Your sons and your daughters are beyond your command.*
> *Your old road is rapidly agin'.*
> *Please get out of the new one if you can't lend your hand.*
> *For the times they are a-changin.*

In 1966, to escape unrelenting stress, Timothy Leary exhorted 30,000 hippies at Golden State Park in San Francisco: to "turn on, tune in, drop out."

Thus, by the mid-1960s, AC use had elements of striving for cultural independence and stress relief. Consumption was linked to rebellious nonconformists challenging traditional norms. Richard Nixon mobilized the so-called silent majority as a bulwark against this threat to traditional norms and hegemony to win the presidential election. While putatively protecting America from drugs, he declared on June 18, 1971, a *War on Drugs* and subsequently had legislation enacted to expand the number of federal drug crimes, increase the budget for intelligence operations, boost interdiction activities, and ramp up criminal prosecution. Rather than addressing AC use as a public health or social problem, the War on Drugs was an expedient political strategy to marginalize the "other" under the umbrella of federal law. Notwithstanding the absence of independent veracity of the following quote by John Ehrlichman, senior advisor to President Nixon, the views expressed are consistent with recorded positions:

> "You want to know what this was really all about?" he asked with the bluntness of a man who, after public disgrace and a stretch in federal prison, had little left to protect. "The Nixon campaign in 1968, and the Nixon White House after that, had two enemies: the antiwar left and black people. You understand what I am saying? We knew we couldn't make it illegal to be either against the war or blacks, but by getting the public to associate the hippies with marijuana and blacks with heroin, and then criminalizing both heavily, we could disrupt those communities. We could arrest their leaders, and their homes, break up their meetings, and vilify them night after night on the evening news. Did we know we were lying about the drugs? Of course we did". (en.m.wikipedia.org)

Consumption of ACs for pleasure had gained wide acceptance among the baby boomer generation before the War on Drugs was launched. For example, the Woodstock Festival attended by 300,000 youths and young adults provided the opportunity to peacefully enjoy "three days of music, companionship, and in many cases, drugs" (N.Y. Times, August 19th, 1968). A year before the "war" declaration, four Vietnam War protesters were killed and nine others wounded by the Ohio National Guard on the campus of Kent State University. As in the WCTU's drive for alcohol prohibition, ACs were polarizing, weaponizing, and linked to segments by society that were putatively different from and outside the cultural mainstream. Jerry Garcia, leader of the *Grateful Dead* band, states: "And as far as I am concerned, it's like I say, drugs are not the problem. Other stuff is the problem" (inspiringquotes.us).

Although the sociocultural milieu has substantially changed since 1970, the two main reasons remain the same for using ACs that have the highest likelihood of transitioning to addictive behavior, whether medicine or recreational substances. First, as discussed below, deviant socialization predisposed by suboptimal acquisition of psychological self-regulation prompts AC use onset as one facet of non-adherence with sociocultural mores and secular laws. The outcome, ontogenetic addiction, thus reflects rejection of or indifference to societal rules. Second, AC use can be triggered by psychological or physical discomfort caused by stressors. The outcome, addiction reaction, reflects an attempt (i.e., coping tactic) to alleviate an aversive state by using a medication under physician supervision or as self-medication.

Psychological Self-Regulation Trait and Risk for Addiction

Findings obtained in a groundbreaking genetic epidemiology study revealed that alcoholism manifests before completing neuromaturation (that is, prior to approximately 25 years of age) [39, 40], it is transmissible, it is associated with an elevated rate of antisociality in parents [41] and with a history of rule-breaking behavior since childhood [42]. Many studies corroborate the finding that early age onset alcoholism (and other addictive behaviors) is preceded by disruptive, socially non-conforming and rule-breaking behavior that commonly co-occurs with negative affect, deficient social competence, and deviant socialization [43–48].

Antisocial behavior genetically overlaps with and commonly antedates as well as co-occurs with AC use and addictive behavior [41, 42]. Moreover, conduct disorder during childhood frequently precedes and shares genetic risk with addiction during adolescence and adulthood [49–53]. Disinhibitory behaviors presaging and concurrent with antisociality, particularly impulsivity and sensation (or thrill) seeking, elevate risk for developing addiction [54–56]. Complementing these findings, intense negative emotion reactivity and behavior overactivity biases development toward both antisociality and addiction [57, 58]. These latter psychological propensities have a strong genetic influence and constitute the key features of *difficult temperament* [59] during infancy which frequently segues to disruptive behavior disorder, deviant socialization, and substance use [60–63]. Significantly, suboptimal executive cognitive functioning also portends antisociality and addictive behavior [64–66]. Overall, these findings indicate that genetic factors predispose to disruptive and rule-breaking social behavior which portends early age onset AC use and addiction.

Low socioeconomic status (SES) of the family is associated with elevated risk for antisociality in the child [67]. Education and income constituting the SES index in parents are usually associated with quality of neighborhood in which the family domiciles. Thus, low SES is related to domiciling in an economically depressed neighborhood. Disadvantaged neighborhoods are marked by a paucity of social capital, easy access to illegal ACs from street peddlers, omnipresent stressors (e.g., violence), and weak compliance with the law. These adversities in social environment singly and in combination potentiate the likelihood of underage use of ACs that are legal for adults as well as consuming illegal ACs. Notably, low SES, a proxy indicator of heightened stress concomitant with domicile, is associated with suboptimal neurodevelopment [67] which, as reviewed later, manifests as suboptimal executive control of emotions and behavior. Another common stressor, maltreatment (abuse and neglect), also impedes neurodevelopment [68, 69]. In sum, genetic factors and stressors hamper development of cognitive capacities integral to modulating behavior and emotions reflected overall as quality of psychological self-regulation [70].

Scores on tests of executive cognitive capacity, emotion stability, and behavior control are constituents of a unidimensional trait [8], termed herein *psychological self-regulation*. The American Psychological Association definition of self-regulation is:

> the control of one's own behavior through self-monitoring of the conditions that evoke desired and undesired behaviors, structuring the personal environment to facilitate desired behavior and circumvent situations that tend to elicit undesired behavior, self-evaluation, and self-administration of punishments and rewards, or some combination of these [71].

The executive cognitive processes subserved by neural circuits distributed along the prefrontal cortex-limbic-midbrain axis oversee and modulate emotions and behavior during goal-directed motivation and social interactions [1, 72–75]. Accordingly, the psychological self-regulation trait is heuristic for elucidating addiction etiology within a neuropsychological framework. Notably, executive functioning in 3- and 4-year-old children mediates the association between temperament indicators of emotion and subsequent emergence of attention deficit hyperactivity disorder (ADHD) [76] which, as discussed later, shares genetic risk with and frequently segues to addiction. Moreover, the psychological self-regulation trait parsimoniously quantifies addiction vulnerability. In this regard, it is noteworthy that the score on this trait in children and adolescents forecasts addiction up to 10 years later [77].

In the next section, the empirical literature is reviewed showing that suboptimal *acquisition* of psychological self-regulation portends norm-violating behavior leading to ontogenetic addiction, whereas stressor-induced *reduction* of psychological self-regulation leads to addiction reaction.

Psychological Etiology of Addiction

Ontogenetic Addiction

Suboptimal psychological self-regulation during early and middle childhood potentiates conflictual interpersonal interactions with parents, teachers, and peers and consequently augurs social maladjustment and marginalization. Friendships are established, therefore, with similar youths, thereby providing an environmental context for catalyzing non-normative behavior. Underage use of an AC that is legal for adults or consumption of illicit ACs is embedded, therefore, in developmental patterning marked by deviant socialization. In effect, suboptimal acquisition of psychological self-regulation interacting with social contextual (e.g., deviant friends, poor relationship with and inadequate supervision from parents) biases progression from AC use onset to escalation into regular habit resulting in neuroadaptation that in turn amplifies consumption consequent to addictive (i.e., compulsive) motivation. Termed ontogenetic addiction, the etiology has its origins during gestation.

Fetus Maternal stress during pregnancy exerts a deleterious effect on neurodevelopment [78] that is postnatally evinced as elevated risk of internalizing (e.g., anxiety, depression) and externalizing (oppositional and disruptive behavior) psychopathology [79, 80], including "unsociable" behavior [81]. Moreover, stress increases sensitivity to the acute effects of ACs during adolescence [81]. One mechanism underlying these psychological propensities for addiction may involve epigenetic modulation of serotoninergic transmission [82–84] displayed phenotypically as negative emotions and behavior undercontrol [84, 85] and syndromally as attention deficit hyperactivity disorder (ADHD) [86]. Also, nutrition deprivation inferred from small body size at birth presages poor regulation of mood and behavior up to 6 years later [87]. It has been shown that severe nutrition deficiency in survivors of the Dutch Hunger Winter in 1944 has elevated risk (OR = 2.5) for antisociality [88] that usually co-occurs with regular AC use during late adolescence and adulthood. Significantly, ACs and their metabolites impede maturation of dopamine-rich circuitry that functionally connects prefrontal cortex and striatum [89] integral to executive modulation of emotions and behavior along with reward processing.

Besides multiple adverse effects on the fetus, stressors (violence, housing insecurity, etc.) disrupt the capacity of the prospective mother to cognitively regulate emotions and behavior. One consequence is reduced motivation for self-care that in turn hinders fetal development. Stress and negative emotions associated with pregnancy that is unplanned or awaiting an unwanted baby weaken maternal concern for welfare of the fetus that mitigates bonding [90]. Even relatively benign factors have an outsized deleterious impact on the fetus that continues after birth. For example, insufficient sleep continuing after birthing causes daytime fatigue resulting in reduced caregiving effectiveness [91]. Emotional development in the infant is accordingly jeopardized, especially establishing a stable circadian routine and emotional attachment with the caregiver [92–94]. In sum, acquiring optimal psychological self-regulation begins during fetal development.

Infancy Physiological reactivity during the neonatal period influences the potential to acquire psychological self-regulation. Intense crying, fussiness, stiff limbs, clenched hands, and tense abdomen are indicators of severe distress, usually referred to as colic. Attempts to comfort the baby do not readily alleviate the distress, thereby frustrating caregivers, especially considering that a colic episode often occurs in the evening and frequently after parents retired for the night. The baby is effectively a stressor. Depending on caregiver characteristics (e.g., psychiatric or medical illness) and circumstances (e.g., available social support), the baby will either receive the extra parenting needed to be soothed or otherwise experience sustained stress. In severe circumstances, caregiver behavior may rise to maltreatment, namely, avoidance (neglect) or harshness (abuse). Thus, the infant learns whether caregivers are a reliable resource to ease distress. In circumstances where caregivers inadequately respond to the baby's needs, accomplishing the main developmental task of infancy – establishing secure attachment to the primary caregiver – is jeopardized.

Thus, characteristics of both the caregiver and the infant determine the prospect and quality of attachment. An "easy" temperament in each member of the infant-caregiver dyad facilitates developing a harmonious relationship resulting in secure emotional attachment [95]. A mismatch or where both members of the dyad have a difficult temperament leads to a stressful relationship between caregiver and baby. Hence, extra parenting effort and skill are required to promote the child's healthy psychological development. Weak, disorganized, and insecure attachment has long-term negative consequences, including stress hypersensitivity [96] and an admixture of internalizing and externalizing psychological disturbances in later childhood and thereafter [97–101]. These outcomes of suboptimal attachment increase the probability of AC use onset at a young age.

Low parental engagement, besides impeding attachment, shapes the infant's early psychological development. One manifestation is sleep problems [102] which is often embedded in difficult temperament that amplifies risk for internalizing and externalizing psychopathology during later childhood [103, 104]. Low parental involvement may also contribute to suboptimal cognitive development. Without caregivers to reliably dampen stress, persistent crying during infancy impedes cognitive development [100, 105]. As noted earlier, cognitive processes modulate emotions and behavior during goal-directed motivation and social interactions; hence, parenting quality is critical to acquisition of psychological self-regulation and, accordingly, biasing the developmental trajectory toward or away from AC use.

Early Childhood Transitioning from externally supported (i.e., caregiver) to self-regulated stress management begins during toddlerhood. Genetic factors largely account for variation in the quality of psychological self-regulation measured as temperament [106–108]. Notably, difficult temperament (slow adaptability, intense emotion reaction, irregular sleep and eating rhythmicity, negative mood, high behavioral activity) in preschool children mediates the association between parental addiction and the transmissible liability index (TLI) score at 10–12 years of age. This latter measure consists almost entirely of items documenting behavior undercontrol and social deviancy proneness [60]. In effect, temperament during early childhood indicating low self-regulation presages disruptive behavior concomitant with deviant socialization in late childhood. Significantly, 75–85% of variance in TLI scores is accounted for by genetics [109, 110]. Although research has yet to be conducted to determine whether the genetic variance predisposing to difficult temperament maps to the transmissible liability index, it is noteworthy that both traits quantify self-regulation using age-appropriate psychological indicators. Thus, it can be tentatively concluded that the same genetic factors largely underlie the temperament phenotype [106–108] during early childhood and subsequently the TLI [109, 110], predisposing to addiction. Notably, the genetic component of TLI variance in late childhood accounts for most of genetic variance in the risk for addiction in adulthood [110].

A difficult temperament disposition challenges parenting motivation and competence and therefore is a stressor to caregivers. Consequently, they may react negatively to their children [111, 112], especially if compromised by elevated stress associated with medical illness, psychiatric disturbance, or domiciling in an unsafe or adverse environment. It is thus noteworthy that difficult temperament is prominent among infants and young children of addicted parents [113] and most severe where parents have co-occurring antisociality [61]. In this circumstance, intergenerational transmission of difficult temperament compounded by reduced parenting motivation and competence concomitant with addiction [114] potentiates a disruptive and conflictual caregiver-child relationship which subsequently facilitates the child's disengagement from the family.

Difficult temperament in preschool children foreshadows addiction two decades later [60] as well as its intermediate outcomes such as internalizing and externalizing psychopathology [115–117]. Suboptimal emotion and behavior self-regulation may manifest in part from deficient internal language [73] (thinking in words) as the mechanism to *access* the executive control system. This capacity begins to consolidate at approximately 14 months of age when communications with the caregiver transitions from gestures to vocalized speech [118]. Ongoing interactions with caregivers inculcate the mores, values, and beliefs of the culture [119]. When not engaged with the caregiver or others, self-regulation is managed by private speech that is *audible to others but not intended to communicate* with them. By approximately 7 years of age, internal language replaces private speech as the mechanism to access the executive control system [120]. At this juncture, as pointed out by Tomasello [121], "the child executively monitoring her communication with others is a form of social self-regulation" (p. 132–133).

Variation in executive cognitive capacity in the population is largely accounted for by genetic factors [73, 74]. Research has not been conducted on young children to learn whether acquisition of language competence, the mechanism to access the executive control system, is directly related to risk for and speed of development of ontogenetic addiction. However, several lines of evidence indirectly indicate that this may be the case. Environmental factors such as poverty and maltreatment heighten risk for addiction and disrupt the neurological substrate underpinning maturation of language [122, 123]. Suboptimal language competence has also been shown to be associated with impulsive aggression and antisociality which portend underage AC use [124–126]. Furthermore, adolescents with a speech and language disorder are more likely than their peers to qualify for diagnosis of substance use disorder [127]. Considering that internal language intermediates stimulus reception and response selection, suboptimal capacity to think in words hinders contemplating "if-then" contingencies required to appraise risk [128]. Based on these findings, it is plausible to conclude that both suboptimal language and executive capacities lead to low emotion and behavior self-regulation during goal-directed activity and social interactions.

Observation of parental behavior instills in children as young as 2 years of age beliefs about the effects of alcohol [129–131]. This age corresponds with emergent language processes for accessing the executive control system and accordingly regulating interpersonal interactions. Although not yet submitted to empirical investigation, it is reasonable to conjecture that acquiring false beliefs about the effects of ACs may emanate from and correlate with suboptimal executive functioning.

Low harm avoidance and high sensation seeking increase the probability of using ACs [132]. These disinhibitory behaviors in severe circumstances are ubiquitous features of externalizing psychiatric disorders such as ADHD and conduct disorder during childhood and antisocial and borderline personality disorders during adolescence and thereafter. These later disorders share genetic risk with addiction, commonly presage and co-occur with addiction, and are marked by suboptimal executive cognitive functioning and an admixture of externalizing and internalizing symptoms, displayed overall as low psychological self-regulation [76, 133–139].

Middle and Late Childhood Impulsivity, low threshold for emotion reaction, aggressivity, and low goal persistence comprise several of the core features of low psychological self-regulation which fosters stressful and conflictual interactions with parents, teachers, and peers. Disruptive interpersonal interactions and social adjustment difficulties are especially prominent in offspring of addicted parents [140] who, as noted above, exhibit low psychological self-regulation disposition. Addiction in parents at this stage of the child's development has especially deleterious effects inasmuch as insufficient oversight and inadequate communication [141, 142] increase the child's opportunities for risky behavior that lower the threshold for onset of AC use [143]. Hence, the consequences of mutual dissatisfaction leading to the child's disengagement from the family are more egregious when one or more parents have addiction [144].

Aggression in response to mild provocation is more likely in youths with suboptimal executive cognitive capacity [145–148] and potentiates disruptive and conflictual interpersonal interactions. Friendships are formed with peers who have similar characteristics, namely, suboptimal psychological self-regulation, aggressivity, and indifference to mores and laws. Thus, at the cusp of adolescence, coinciding with entering high school where ACs are more readily available, psychological disposition and social environment conjointly catalyze underage use of an AC that is legal for adults or consumption of an illegal AC.

Adolescence The main sphere of influence shifts from parents to peers during adolescence. Without effective parental oversight, low psychological self-regulation facilitated by socially non-normative peers increases the probability of AC consumption. The results of one study show that quality of parent-child relationship and characteristics of peers account for 77% of variance on a measure of substance use severity in 14-year-old youths [149].

Adolescence, a critical developmental period that shapes the life course of social adjustment and health, is marked by onset of "adult" behaviors, including AC use. A habit of regular AC use that segues to addictive (compulsive consumption) behavior often occurs during this period of transitioning from childhood to adulthood. As discussed earlier, non-normative socialization is the proximal trigger for AC use onset in ontogenetic addiction. One prospective study using machine learning methods found that the strongest predictor of AC use and addiction from over two thousand variables is a propensity for obscene language or swearing [150]. This finding is intriguing since it reflects both deviancy-proneness and crude language to access the executive control system integral to modulating emotions and behavior during social interactions.

Adolescence is marked by ongoing neuromaturation that continues up to almost 30 years of age along with completion of sexual maturation and physical growth. These maturational processes are associated with increased susceptibility to stress concomitant with emotion and behavior disturbances that heightens risk for AC use [12, 14, 18, 27, 151]. These risk-enhancing factors for addiction are not effectively buffered by the law in a large portion of the population. National survey data results indicate that 17.4% of high school seniors have used an illegal drug [17].

The most reliable and strongest physiological harbinger of antisociality is hypoarousal in the sympathetic component of the autonomic nervous system [152–154]. Hypoarousal has also been documented with respect to addiction risk evinced as attenuated cardiovascular response to a stressor [155] and lower salivary cortisol level [156]. Indeed, low cortisol level portends early age onset AC (alcohol) use [157]. It is also noteworthy that low attention control (e.g., P300 amplitude of the event-related potential antisaccade) and arousal (heart rate, skin conductance) are associated with elevated risk for addiction [158–161]. Although these findings should be viewed as tentative, they indicate that biochemical and physiological processes reflecting activation essential to sustained attention and arousal are dampened in antisociality and ontogenetic addiction.

Adolescents are primed to engage in behaviors that produce intense hedonic experience.

Motivation is potentiated by the especially strong social facilitating effects of ACs during adolescence [162–164]. Moreover, compared to adults, adolescents are reportedly able to consume a larger amount of alcohol without impairment caused by intoxication [164]. It has also been shown that magnitude of stress covaries negatively with interval to addiction [165]. Inasmuch as adolescents are exposed to manifold stressors, high susceptibility to stress additionally primes motivation for AC use leading to addiction [12]. In summary, adolescence is a critical developmental stage in the etiology of addiction owing to the interplay of maturational processes, easy availability of numerous inexpensive ACs, quality of psychological self-regulation, manifold stressors, social (friendships, parents) relationships, and pharmacological effects of ACs, notably, dependence. Addiction manifest during adolescence occurs on average less than 3 years after AC use onset [163].

Four main tasks need to be accomplished during adolescence for long-term adjustment in adulthood [166]. These tasks are (1) acquire secure sexual identity, (2) learn to protect personal safety, (3) learn to navigate social hierarchies, and (4) learn skills necessary for independence. Suboptimal psychological self-regulation hinders accomplishing these tasks which amplifies the propensity for AC use and risk for addiction.

1. *Acquire Secure Sexual Identity.* Prevalence of smoking cigarettes, drinking alcohol, using illicit drugs, and substance use disorder is higher among sexual minorities [165]. Early pubertal sexual maturation places both males and females at risk for AC use [167–171].
2. *Learn to Protect Personal Safety.* Quality of the parent-child relationship, particularly parental monitoring or oversight of their children, strongly influences the likelihood of AC use [172]. Androgens modulate dopaminergic signaling in mesocorticolimbic circuitry [173] underpinning motivation, emotion regulation, and reward processing [174]. Sex steroids in the brain also impact language competence [175] which, as discussed earlier, is the mechanism to access the executive control system integral to regulating emotions and behavior. Diminished capacity to cognitively regulate emotions and behavior during social interactions exacerbates conflicts with parents, thereby diminishing opportunity to acquire knowledge pertaining to protecting personal safety.

   A strong positive relationship with parents is especially important when puberty begins at a young age and sexual maturation progresses rapidly. Precocious display of secondary sex characteristics conveys a false signal of more advanced age which in the absence of caregiver oversight and control augments the likelihood of affiliating with older peers. Consequently, the likelihood of initiating "adult" behaviors is increased, including AC use. This risk is especially high among youths with low psychological self-regulation inasmuch as executive cognitive capacities are not deployed to appraise risk and restrain behavior. The probability of AC use onset at a young age is further augmented in youths having a developmental history of non-normative socialization. Furthermore, a strong desire for acceptance diminishes the prospect of averting AC use and other risky behaviors.

   Maltreatment (neglect and abuse) during childhood accelerates puberty onset as well as hampers neurodevelopment [176, 177] manifest as poor cognitive control of behavior and emotions [178]. Hence, failure to protect personal safety, evinced as risky sexual behavior, may have its origins during a stressful childhood. Notably, stressors such as maltreatment in early childhood potentiate risk of developing ADHD in childhood which shares genetic risk with addiction and increases the probability of early age onset AC use and risk for addiction [179, 180]. Notably, a history of maltreatment is associated with reduced performance on tests measuring executive cognitive capacities in children [170] and adolescents [168]. In effect, the capacity to acquire an executive control system to modulate behavior and emotions during social interactions is compromised. These findings demonstrate that childhood stressors potentiate emergence of intermediate outcomes that hamper acquisition of capacities required for protection of personal safety. One manifestation is early age onset AC use and accompanying elevated risk for addiction [181–183].

3. *Learn to Navigate Social Hierarchies.* Adolescents are acutely aware of their social status and are preoccupied with approval from their peers [184]. Social standing, displayed as popularity, encompasses a constellation of desired attributes encompassing physical appearance (fashionable clothes, attractiveness, etc.) and competencies (social, academic, athletic, etc.) along with possessions (car, PlayStation, etc.).

   Youths having high or low social status are more likely to use ACs [185]. Also, a change in social status, elevation or decline, increases the probability of consuming ACs [186]. Owing to a paucity of research on this topic, it is not possible to confidently explain these findings; however, it is plausible to conjecture that the common feature is elevated stress. High and low social rank for different reasons is stressful. Constant vigilance of the social environment and energy are required to protect high status and elevate low status. Adolescents are not only faced with manifold social stressors; they have heightened sensitivity to glucocorticoids [81]. Consequently, the adverse effects of stressors are potentiated by susceptibility to stress navigating the social environment. It is noteworthy in this regard that compared to adults AC use during adolescence has a stronger social facilitating benefit [164]; hence, a socially deviant friendship cluster catalyzes consumption in an environment that amplifies the likelihood inculcating a habit of frequent consumption leading to neuroadaptation and addictive (compulsive) behavior.

   Low social rank influences motivation for AC use beyond the peer environment. Demise of the industrial sector of the US economy has led to reduction (or cessation) of air, rail, and bus services resulting in status decline, marginalization, and isolation of once prosperous communities. According to Case and Deaton [186], residents are susceptible to "diseases of despair," including hazardous AC use, drug overdose, and addiction.

   Poverty is associated with suboptimal neurodevelopment [187], most likely the consequence of chronic stress. Volume of the cingulum and caudate nucleus correlates negatively with social stressors [188]. It is also noteworthy that the same frontal-subcortical structures are activated by social rejection and physical pain [189]. Social exclusion disrupts ventrolateral prefrontal cortex (Brodmann's areas 44, 45, 47) subserving emotion, which is adjacent to and communicates with dorsolateral prefrontal cortex underpinning the executive cognitive functions [188].

   Endocrinological mechanisms in context of social disadvantage also impact addiction risk via development of intermediate phenotypes. Elevated testosterone level in boys (age 12–14) living in disadvantaged neighborhoods portends in mid-adolescence (age 16) dominance striving, norm-violating behavior, and AC use which forecast addiction in young adulthood [171]. Although elevated testosterone level is widely thought to potentiate aggressive behavior, it appears that this steroid hormone is more closely related to motivation for ascendance in the social hierarchy [190, 191]. Thus, in disadvantaged or resource-poor environments, high testosterone level biases adolescents toward AC use via social dominance striving in concert with norm-violating behavior.

4. *Learn Skills Necessary for Independence.* Caregivers provide protection, mentoring, and resources for two decades or longer to prepare their children for assuming multiple roles and responsibilities in adulthood. Disengagement from parents too early, resulting in inadequate competence required for independent living, may therefore lead to lasting social maladjustment.

   Preparing for independent socially adjusted adulthood requires the capacity for telescopic thinking to enable goal setting and formulation of an action plan. Hence, efficient access to the executive via internal language is critical to successful transition into adulthood. One study reports that language deficiency increases in severity throughout adolescence in youths who are at elevated risk for addiction [192]. Moreover, adolescent offenders of the law, typically also AC users, exhibit suboptimal oral language competence [193, 194]. These findings suggest that suboptimal language, by mitigating efficient access to the executive control system, augments addiction risk. Relatedly, it has been reported that scores on a learning disability test and severity of behavior problems in 12-year-old children forecast substance use disorder at 19 years of age [195]. The rate of substance use disorder in this sample of youths is three times higher than youths without learning and behavior problems. Furthermore, it was found in this latter study that language deficiency at 5 years of age predicts learning disability severity at 12 years of age, prompting the authors to theorize that learning impairment mediates the relationship between suboptimal language capacity and risk for substance use disorder. The dearth of research on this topic notwithstanding, the available findings suggest that language competence, the mechanism for accessing the executive control system, is deficient in youths at elevated risk for ontogenetic addiction. Suboptimal language development, therefore, mitigates acquiring skills required for independent adulthood.

This impairment during adolescence has its most damaging influence in the academic setting. Impaired capacity to satisfy grade-appropriate education standards fosters disinterest in academic achievement and lowers motivation for school attendance. Hence, problems in school lead to marginalization or rejection by achievement-oriented peers and catalyze affiliation with similar maladjusted peers. The constellation of underachievement, truancy, and friendships with problem behavior youths promote delinquency which strongly increases risk of AC use [195]. In effect, education achievement essential for successful independent adulthood may be compromised by the same neurocognitive processes that are associated with risk for addiction.

Summary Suboptimal psychological self-regulation (1) impedes goal-directed motivation; (2) predisposes to disruptive interactions with parents, peers, and teachers; and (3) lowers the threshold for engaging in behaviors that violate sociocultural mores and folkways and secular laws. The developmental outcome, deviant socialization, manifests as underage use of ACs that are legal for adults or consumption of illicit ACs as one facet of non-adherence with rules. Low psychological self-regulation and deviant socialization biases the developmental trajectory toward disengagement from parents and affiliations with similarly poorly regulated socially non-normative youths. During late childhood or early adolescence, AC use is initiated which escalates to a habit of regular consumption potentiated by a motivational bias toward intense hedonic experience and robust pharmacological and social facilitating effects of ACs. Neuroadaptation (chronic tolerance) thus develops rapidly which consequent to large quantity consumption segues to addictive (i.e., obsessive compulsive) AC use. This developmental outcome is termed herein ontogenetic addiction.

Addiction Reaction

An 18-year-old in the USA can vote but not legally drink a glass of wine until 21 years of age. In 1960, these age thresholds were reversed. Raising the age of alcohol (and tobacco) consumption extended the duration of legally defined immaturity even though at 18 years of age other dangerous behaviors such as carrying a weapon or piloting an airplane are legal. The consequence of raising the legal age of AC use is an increase in the size of the population qualifying as offenders of the law even though most individuals are normatively socialized. A key question, therefore, pertains to understanding the predisposing factors and pathway to addiction in this normatively socialized segment of the population compared to individuals who develop ontogenetic addiction ensuing from deviant socialization.

Adolescents are inclined for many reasons to begin consumption of an AC. A portion of normatively socialized youths shifts to "adolescent-limited" antisociality that resolves in adulthood [18]. AC use onset during adolescence may, therefore, constitute a facet of a transitory inclination for norm-violating behavior. Relatedly, AC use may be an expression of rebellion against traditional cultural norms, especially mores proscribing pleasures. This propensity is not restricted to AC use. For example, consensual sex is legal at 16 years of age; nevertheless, approximately 20% of 13–14-year-olds [196] and 30% of 15–16-year-olds [197] report having had intercourse. In addition, AC use onset during adolescence may mimic normative adult behavior. As noted above, a main developmental task during adolescence is to inculcate competencies required to assume adult roles and responsibilities. Inasmuch as AC use is woven tightly into many types of social interactions (business, recreation, gifting, etc.), consumption during adolescence may thus reflect precocious behavior.

Motivation for consumption is strongest, however, among individuals who benefit from the negative reinforcement properties of ACs; that is, obtain relief from psychological (negative emotions) and/or physical (pain, insomnia, etc.) discomfort. AC use in this segment of the population is, therefore, a coping tactic which has high probability of developing into a regular habit. During peak production 70 million Valium tablets were manufactured every 15 h [198]. One long-term effect of repetitive reinforcement is a reduction of intensity of subjective experience [199] which, with respect to AC use, is exacerbated by chronic tolerance. Consequently, a progressively larger dose of the particular AC, or shifting to a more potent AC, is required to sustain the reward experience. Furthermore, memories of positive experiences during the earlier period drive motivation to re-experiencing previous reward intensity [200]. Under these circumstances, motivation may transition from voluntary AC use to addictive (compulsive) behavior. Risk for addiction reaction remains throughout life inasmuch as stressors may emerge any time before or after AC use onset.

Summary AC use may be uneventful throughout life. A subset of consumers, however, segue to addictive behavior. These individuals most likely constitute the portion of the population that has a strong motivation to use ACs for improving subjective well-being. Accordingly, the probability of transitioning from AC use to addictive behavior is highest among individuals experiencing stressor-induced *reduction* in self-regulation manifesting primarily as negative emotions (anxiety, panic, sadness, etc.) and/or their physiological precursors and correlates (pain, insomnia, fatigue, etc.). In severe circumstances, defined in the DSM as impaired adaptation, negative emotions are deemed mental illnesses. ACs are, however, effective at reducing emotional and/or physical discomfort across the entire range of severity, that is, below and above diagnostic threshold. AC use is, therefore, in the short term a coping tactic whether physician-prescribed or alternatively self-directed and whether the product is an FDA-approved medicament or a recreational substance. Once a pattern of AC use is established, neuroadaptation may develop which subsequently leads to addictive (obsessive compulsive) consumption behavior.

Etiology of Addiction: Neuropsychological Perspective

Performance on tests such as attention control, goal planning, goal persistence, problem-solving, and abstract thinking measuring executive functioning is poorer among youths with a family history of addiction [18, 26, 145] or a personal history of psychiatric disorder such as ADHD, disruptive behavior disorder, and antisocial personality disorder that shares genetic risk with as well as frequently precedes or co-occurs with addiction [15, 29, 66, 145, 154, 201–206].

Variation in executive cognitive capacity in the population is largely accounted for by genetics [207, 208], and as discussed throughout this chapter, suboptimal functioning manifests as suboptimal modulation of emotions and behavior during goal-directed motivation and social interactions. Notably, the cognitive, emotion, and behavior processes constitute a continuous unidimensional trait.

The executive control system, subserved largely in dorsolateral prefrontal cortex, is one component of complex neural circuitry distributed along the frontal cortex-midbrain axis. Other components of the circuitry involved in addiction vulnerability include the septum (social cooperation and emotional attachment) [209, 210], nucleus accumbens (reward processing and effortful motivation) [211, 212], amygdala (emotion and fear processing) [213], hippocampus (approach/avoidance conflict resolution) [214], and brainstem nuclei (cortical and autonomic activation) [215]. In that as yet unknown, but most likely individually variable fashion, these components synergistically interact with the components mediating psychological self-regulation so as to bias motivation toward onset of AC use and development of a consumption habit leading to addictive (compulsive) behavior.

Conclusions

This chapter describes two variants of addiction. One variant, ontogenetic addiction, is the developmental outcome of deficient *acquisition* of psychological self-regulation during child and adolescent development. The other variant, addiction reaction, ensues from stressor-induced *diminution* of psychological self-regulation. Low psychological self-regulation although having different etiologies predisposes to both addiction variants. The two variants do not, however, constitute mutually exclusive types of addiction since low psychological self-regulation is the result in varying degree of both developmental patterning and current stressors. However, a differentiation of addiction into two variants is justified because AC use has different meanings in each variant. Consumption leading to ontogenetic addiction is a feature of an identity marked by non-adherence with sociocultural mores and secular laws. In addiction reaction, ACs are a coping tactic to ameliorate stress. Once repetitive consumption is established, whether embedded in deviancy proneness or a coping tactic, neuroadaptation develops, thereby shifting AC use from voluntary to compulsive (addiction) behavior.

Specifying etiological variants of addiction within a lifespan framework provides the rubric for designing and deploying targeted preventions. Toward this goal, it is essential to document intermediate age-specific outcomes that bias the trajectory to addictive behavior. Examples of intermediate outcomes discussed in this chapter include attachment with caregiver during infancy, attention deficit hyperactivity disorder during middle childhood, and social rank during adolescence. Averting or lowering severity of these outcomes reduces, therefore, the likelihood of advancing to AC use onset and addiction.

Vanyukov and colleagues proposed a theoretical framework [216] and corresponding measurement scheme [217] in which risk-promoting and risk-attenuating factors are specified as vectors that in aggregate constitute an overall or resultant vector that biases the individual toward or away from the subsequent intermediate outcomes increasing or decreasing risk for AC use and addiction. A strength of this model is that it is amenable to explicating addiction etiology within a lifespan developmental framework. In preschool children low executive capacity portends externalizing behaviors [218] which commonly segues to early age onset AC use and addiction. It is also noteworthy that low capacity to sustain attention can be measured within a few weeks after birth. This cardinal feature of ADHD shares genetic risk with and often segues to addiction. Hence, age-appropriate assessment tools can quantify and monitor addiction risk. Risk assessment is especially important in young children so that intermediate adverse outcomes can be averted while there is neurobehavioral plasticity. Thus, it is noteworthy that promising neuropsychological interventions for young children have recently been developed which may improve executive functioning [219–221].

Potentiating development of executive capacities in early childhood may, therefore, instill cognitive resources for modulating behavior and emotions during goal-directed motivation and social interactions. Accordingly, interpersonal interactions are optimized so that development proceeds toward normative socialization, thereby lowering the probability of early age onset AC use and ontogenetic addiction. Optimal executive cognitive resources also enhance the capacity to anticipate and manage stressors so that the likelihood of leading to addiction reaction is also reduced.

References

1. Luria A. Higher cortical functions in man. New York: Basic Books; 1966.
2. Albayrak O, Wölfle SM, Hebebrand J. Does food addiction exist? A phenomenological discussion based on the psychiatric classification of substance-related disorders and addiction. Obes Facts. 2012;5(2):165–79.
3. Grall-Bronnec M, et al. Attention deficit hyperactivity disorder among pathological and at-risk gamblers seeking treatment: a hidden disorder. Eur Addict Res. 2011;17(5):231–40.
4. Grant JE, Brewer JA, Potenza MN. The neurobiology of substance and behavioral addictions. CNS Spectr. 2006;11(12):924–30.
5. Han DH, et al. Dopamine genes and reward dependence in adolescents with excessive internet video game play. J Addict Med. 2007;1(3):133–8.
6. Lobo DS, Kennedy JL. The genetics of gambling and behavioral addictions. CNS Spectr. 2006;11(12):931–9.
7. Zhang Y, et al. Similarities and differences in genetics. In: Zhang X, Shi J, Tao R, editors. Substance and non-substance addiction. Singapore: Springer; 2017. p. 59–71.
8. Tarter RE, et al. Neurobehavior disinhibition in childhood predisposes boys to substance use disorder by young adulthood: direct and mediated etiologic pathways. Drug Alcohol Depend. 2004;73(2):121–32.
9. Kendler KS, et al. Specificity of genetic and environmental risk factors for use and abuse/dependence of cannabis, cocaine, hallucinogens, sedatives, stimulants, and opiates in male twins. Am J Psychiatry. 2003;160(4):687–95.
10. Katshu MZ, et al. Snake bite as a novel form of substance abuse: personality profiles and cultural perspectives. Subst Abus. 2011;32(1):43–6.
11. Wilcox C. Venomous: how earth's deadliest creatures mastered biochemistry. 1st ed. New York: Scientific American/Farrar, Straus and Giroux; 2016.
12. Milivojevic V, Sinha R. Central and peripheral biomarkers of stress response for addiction risk and relapse vulnerability. Trends Mol Med. 2018;24(2):173–86.
13. Edwards G, Gross MM. Alcohol dependence: provisional description of a clinical syndrome. Br Med J. 1976;1(6017):1058–61.
14. Krueger RF, et al. Etiologic connections among substance dependence, antisocial behavior, and personality: modeling the externalizing spectrum. J Abnorm Psychol. 2002;111(3):411–24.
15. Vanyukov MM, et al. Measurement of the risk for substance use disorders: phenotypic and genetic analysis of an index of common liability. Behav Genet. 2009;39(3):233–44.
16. Ridenour TA, et al. Could a continuous measure of individual transmissible risk be useful in clinical assessment of substance use disorder? Findings from the National Epidemiological Survey on Alcohol and Related Conditions. Drug Alcohol Depend. 2011;119(1–2):10–7.
17. Miech RA, et al. Monitoring the future national survey results on drug use, 1975–2019; volume I, secondary school students. Ann Arbor: Institute for Social Research, University of Michigan; 2020.
18. Moffitt TE. Adolescence-limited and life-course-persistent antisocial behavior: a developmental taxonomy. Psychol Rev. 1993;100(4):674–701.
19. SAMHSA. Behavioral health barometer: United States. Rockville: Substance Abuse and Mental Health Services Administration; 2015.
20. DeBrita S, Hodgins S. Antisocial personality disorder. In: McMurran M, Howard R, editors. Personality, personality disorders and violence: an evidence-based approach. Hoboken: Wiley; 2009.
21. Grant BF, et al. Prevalence, correlates, disability, and comorbidity of DSM-IV borderline personality disorder: results from the Wave 2 National Epidemiologic Survey on Alcohol and Related Conditions. J Clin Psychiatry. 2008;69(4):533–45.
22. Becker DF, et al. Comorbidity of borderline personality disorder with other personality disorders in hospitalized adolescents and adults. Am J Psychiatry. 2000;157(12):2011–6.
23. Fu Q, et al. Shared genetic risk of major depression, alcohol dependence, and marijuana dependence: contribution of antisocial personality disorder in men. Arch Gen Psychiatry. 2002;59(12):1125–32.
24. Fazel S, Yoon IA, Hayes AJ. Substance use disorders in prisoners: an updated systematic review and meta-regression analysis in recently incarcerated men and women. Addiction. 2017;112(10):1725–39.

25. Eaton NR, et al. Borderline personality disorder co-morbidity: relationship to the internalizing-externalizing structure of common mental disorders. Psychol Med. 2011;41(5):1041–50.
26. Chang S, et al. Shared polygenic risk for ADHD, executive dysfunction and other psychiatric disorders. Transl Psychiatry. 2020;10(1):182.
27. Bauer LO, Hesselbrock VM. P300 decrements in teenagers with conduct problems: implications for substance abuse risk and brain development. Biol Psychiatry. 1999;46(2):263–72.
28. Carlson SR, Iacono WG, McGue M. P300 amplitude in nonalcoholic adolescent twin pairs who become discordant for alcoholism as adults. Psychophysiology. 2004;41(6):841–4.
29. Costa L, et al. Frontal P300 decrements, alcohol dependence, and antisocial personality disorder. Biol Psychiatry. 2000;47(12):1064–71.
30. Iacono WG, Malone SM. Developmental endophenotypes: indexing genetic risk for substance abuse with the P300 brain event-related potential. Child Dev Perspect. 2011;5(4):239–47.
31. ASAM. Definition of addiction. Rockville: American Society of Addiction Medicine; 2019.
32. Raman R, Kandula S. Zoopharmacognosy. Resonance. 2008;13(3):245.
33. Laland KN. Darwin's unfinished symphony. How culture made the human mind. Princeton: Princeton University Press; 2018. p. 464.
34. Dawkins R. The selfish gene. New ed. Oxford: Oxford University Press; 1989.
35. Weber M. The Protestant ethic and the spirit of capitalism. New York: Penguin Classics; 2002. p. 464.
36. Henrich JP. The WEIRDest people in the world: how the west became psychologically peculiar and particularly prosperous. 1st ed. New York: Farrar, Straus and Giroux; 2020.
37. Booth M. Cannabis: a history. 1st ed. New York: Thomas Dunne Books/St. Martin's Press; 2004.
38. Conger JJ. The effects of alcohol on conflict behavior in the albino rat. Q J Stud Alcohol. 1951;12(1):1–29.
39. Giedd JN, et al. Brain development during childhood and adolescence: a longitudinal MRI study. Nat Neurosci. 1999;2(10):861–3.
40. Huttenlocher PR. Morphometric study of human cerebral cortex development. Neuropsychologia. 1990;28(6):517–27.
41. Cloninger CR, Sigvardsson S, Bohman M. Childhood personality predicts alcohol abuse in young adults. Alcohol Clin Exp Res. 1988;12(4):494–505.
42. Shoal GD, et al. Delinquency as a mediator of the relation between negative affectivity and adolescent alcohol use disorder. Addict Behav. 2007;32(12):2747–65.
43. Hussong AM, et al. Social competence in children of alcoholic parents over time. Dev Psychol. 2005;41(5):747–59.
44. Jackson C, et al. The early use of alcohol and tobacco: its relation to children's competence and parents' behavior. Am J Public Health. 1997;87(3):359–64.
45. Kirisci L, et al. Individual differences in childhood neurobehavior disinhibition predict decision to desist substance use during adolescence and substance use disorder in young adulthood: a prospective study. Addict Behav. 2006;31(4):686–96.
46. Masten AS, Burt KB, Coatsworth JD. Competence and psychopathology in development. In: Cicchetti D, Cohen DJ, editors. Developmental psychopathology. Hoboken: Wiley; 2006.
47. Poudel A, Gautam S. Age of onset of substance use and psychosocial problems among individuals with substance use disorders. BMC Psychiatry. 2017;17(1):10.
48. von Knorring L, et al. Personality traits in subtypes of alcoholics. J Stud Alcohol. 1987;48(6):523–7.
49. Goldman D, Oroszi G, Ducci F. The genetics of addictions: uncovering the genes. Nat Rev Genet. 2005;6(7):521–32.
50. Grove WM, et al. Heritability of substance abuse and antisocial behavior: a study of monozygotic twins reared apart. Biol Psychiatry. 1990;27(12):1293–304.
51. Slutske WS, et al. Common genetic risk factors for conduct disorder and alcohol dependence. J Abnorm Psychol. 1998;107(3):363–74.
52. Werner KB, Few LR, Bucholz KK. Epidemiology, comorbidity, and behavioral genetics of antisocial personality disorder and psychopathy. Psychiatr Ann. 2015;45(4):195–9.
53. Young SE, et al. Genetic and environmental influences on behavioral disinhibition. Am J Med Genet. 2000;96(5):684–95.
54. Fillmore MT, Weafer J. Impaired inhibitory control as a mechanism of drug abuse. In: Bardo MT, Fishbein DH, Milich R, editors. Inhibitory control and drug abuse prevention: from research to translation. New York: Springer; 2011. p. 85–100.
55. Portnoy J, et al. Heart rate and antisocial behavior: the mediating role of impulsive sensation seeking. Criminology. 2014;52(2):292–311.
56. Zuckerman M. Sensation seeking and risky behavior. Washington, DC: American Psychological Association; 2007.
57. Caspi A, et al. Behavioral observations at age 3 years predict adult psychiatric disorders. Longitudinal evidence from a birth cohort. Arch Gen Psychiatry. 1996;53(11):1033–9.
58. DeLisi M, Vaughn MG. Foundation for a temperament-based theory of antisocial behavior and criminal justice system involvement. J Crim Just. 2014;42(1):10–25.
59. Thomas A, Chess S. Temperament and development. New York: Brunner/Mazel; 1977.
60. Horner MS, et al. Temperament disturbances measured in infancy progress to substance use disorder 20 years later. Pers Individ Dif. 2015;82:96–101.
61. Jansen RE, et al. Pathways into risk: temperament and behavior problems in three- to five-year-old sons of alcoholics. Alcohol Clin Exp Res. 1995;19(2):501–9.

62. Martel MM, et al. Temperament pathways to childhood disruptive behavior and adolescent substance abuse: testing a cascade model. J Abnorm Child Psychol. 2009;37(3):363–73.
63. Micalizzi L, Wang M, Saudino KJ. Difficult temperament and negative parenting in early childhood: a genetically informed cross-lagged analysis. Dev Sci. 2017;20(2):e12355.
64. Raine A. Annotation: the role of prefrontal deficits, low autonomic arousal, and early health factors in the development of antisocial and aggressive behavior in children. J Child Psychol Psychiatry. 2002;43(4):417–34.
65. Moffitt TE, et al. A gradient of childhood self-control predicts health, wealth, and public safety. Proc Natl Acad Sci U S A. 2011;108(7):2693–8.
66. Morgan AB, Lilienfeld SO. A meta-analytic review of the relation between antisocial behavior and neuropsychological measures of executive function. Clin Psychol Rev. 2000;20(1):113–36.
67. Hackman DA, Farah MJ. Socioeconomic status and the developing brain. Trends Cogn Sci. 2009;13(2):65–73.
68. Glaser D. Child abuse and neglect and the brain--a review. J Child Psychol Psychiatry. 2000;41(1):97–116.
69. Long M, et al. A functional neuro-anatomical model of human attachment (NAMA): insights from first- and second-person social neuroscience. Cortex. 2020;126:281–321.
70. Baumeister RF, Vohs KD, Tice DM. The strength model of self-control. Curr Dir Psychol Sci. 2007;16(6):351–5.
71. VandenBos GR. APA dictionary of psychology. 1st ed. Washington, DC: American Psychological Association; 2007.
72. Collette F, et al. Exploration of the neural substrates of executive functioning by functional neuroimaging. Neuroscience. 2006;139(1):209–21.
73. Lezak MD. The problem of assessing executive functions. Int J Psychol. 1982;17(1–4):281–97.
74. McKenna R, Rushe T, Woodcock KA. Informing the structure of executive function in children: a meta-analysis of functional neuroimaging data. Front Hum Neurosci. 2017;11:154.
75. Otero TM, Barker LA. The frontal lobes and executive functioning. In: Goldstein S, Naglieri JA, editors. Handbook of executive functioning. New York: Springer; 2014. p. 29–44.
76. Rabinovitz BB, et al. Temperament, executive control, and attention-deficit/hyperactivity disorder across early development. J Abnorm Psychol. 2016;125(2):196–206.
77. Tarter RE, et al. Neurobehavioral disinhibition in childhood predicts early age at onset of substance use disorder. Am J Psychiatry. 2003;160(6):1078–85.
78. Stott DH. Follow-up study from birth of the effects of prenatal stresses. Dev Med Child Neurol. 1973;15(6):770–87.
79. Glover V. Prenatal stress and its effects on the fetus and the child: possible underlying biological mechanisms. Adv Neurobiol. 2015;10:269–83.
80. MacKinnon N, et al. The association between prenatal stress and externalizing symptoms in childhood: evidence from the avon longitudinal study of parents and children. Biol Psychiatry. 2018;83(2):100–8.
81. Lupien SJ, et al. Effects of stress throughout the lifespan on the brain, behaviour and cognition. Nat Rev Neurosci. 2009;10(6):434–45.
82. Seckl JR, Meaney MJ. Glucocorticoid programming. Ann N Y Acad Sci. 2004;1032:63–84.
83. Archer T, et al. Epigenetic modulation of mood disorders. J Genet Syndr Gene Ther. 2013;4(120):1000120.
84. Nestler EJ, et al. Neurobiology of depression. Neuron. 2002;34(1):13–25.
85. Mueller BR, Bale TL. Sex-specific programming of offspring emotionality after stress early in pregnancy. J Neurosci. 2008;28(36):9055–65.
86. Archer T, Oscar-Berman M, Blum K. Epigenetics in developmental disorder: ADHD and endophenotypes. J Genet Syndr Gene Ther. 2011;2(104):1000104.
87. Pesonen AK, et al. Fetal programming of temperamental negative affectivity among children born healthy at term. Dev Psychobiol. 2006;48(8):633–43.
88. Neugebauer R, Hoek HW, Susser E. Prenatal exposure to wartime famine and development of antisocial personality disorder in early adulthood. JAMA. 1999;282(5):455–62.
89. Derauf C, et al. Neuroimaging of children following prenatal drug exposure. Semin Cell Dev Biol. 2009;20(4):441–54.
90. Mikulincer M, Florian V. Maternal-fetal bonding, coping strategies, and mental health during pregnancy : the contribution of attachment style. J Soc Clin Psychol. 1999;18(3):255–76.
91. White CP, White MB, Fox MA. Maternal fatigue and its relationship to the caregiving environment. Fam Syst Health. 2009;27(4):325–45.
92. Dennis CL, Ross L. Relationships among infant sleep patterns, maternal fatigue, and development of depressive symptomatology. Birth. 2005;32(3):187–93.
93. Cannella BL. Maternal-fetal attachment: an integrative review. J Adv Nurs. 2005;50(1):60–8.
94. Siddiqui A, Hägglöf B. Does maternal prenatal attachment predict postnatal mother-infant interaction? Early Hum Dev. 2000;59(1):13–25.
95. Vaughn BE, Bost KK, van IJzendoorn MH. Attachment and temperament: additive and interactive influences on behavior, affect, and cognition during infancy and childhood. In: Cassidy J, Shaver PR, editors. Handbook of attachment : theory, research, and clinical applications. New York: Guilford Press; 2008. p. 192–216.

96. Pietromonaco PR, Powers SI. Attachment and health-related physiological stress processes. Curr Opin Psychol. 2015;1:34–9.
97. DeKlyen M, Greenberg MT. Attachment and psychopathology in childhood. In: Cassidy J, Shaver PR, editors. Handbook of attachment : theory, research, and clinical applications. New York: Guilford Press; 2008. p. 637–65.
98. Green JG, et al. Childhood adversities and adult psychiatric disorders in the national comorbidity survey replication I: associations with first onset of DSM-IV disorders. Arch Gen Psychiatry. 2010;67(2):113–23.
99. McLaughlin KA, Sheridan MA, Lambert HK. Childhood adversity and neural development: deprivation and threat as distinct dimensions of early experience. Neurosci Biobehav Rev. 2014;47:578–91.
100. Rao MR, et al. Long term cognitive development in children with prolonged crying. Arch Dis Child. 2004;89(11):989–92.
101. Schmid G, et al. Predictors of crying, feeding and sleeping problems: a prospective study. Child Care Health Dev. 2011;37(4):493–502.
102. Morrell J, Steele H. The role of attachment security, temperament, maternal perception, and care-giving behavior in persistent infant sleeping problems. Infant Ment Health J. 2003;24(5):447–68.
103. Green J, Goldwyn R. Annotation: attachment disorganisation and psychopathology: new findings in attachment research and their potential implications for developmental psychopathology in childhood. J Child Psychol Psychiatry. 2002;43(7):835–46.
104. Guttmann-Steinmetz S, Crowell JA. Attachment and externalizing disorders: a developmental psychopathology perspective. J Am Acad Child Adolesc Psychiatry. 2006;45(4):440–51.
105. Out D, et al. Intended sensitive and harsh caregiving responses to infant crying: the role of cry pitch and perceived urgency in an adult twin sample. Child Abuse Negl. 2010;34(11):863–73.
106. Planalp EM, Goldsmith HH. Observed profiles of infant temperament: stability, heritability, and associations with parenting. Child Dev. 2020;91(3):e563–80.
107. Saudino KJ. Behavioral genetics and child temperament. J Dev Behav Pediatr. 2005;26(3):214–23.
108. Silberg JL, Bulik CM. The developmental association between eating disorders symptoms and symptoms of depression and anxiety in juvenile twin girls. J Child Psychol Psychiatry. 2005;46(12):1317–26.
109. Hicks BM, Iacono WG, McGue M. Index of the transmissible common liability to addiction: heritability and prospective associations with substance abuse and related outcomes. Drug Alcohol Depend. 2012;123(Suppl 1):S18–23.
110. Vanyukov M, et al. Genetic relationship between the addiction diagnosis in adults and their childhood measure of addiction liability. Behav Genet. 2015;45(1):1–11.
111. Ganiban JM, et al. Understanding child-based effects on parenting: temperament as a moderator of genetic and environmental contributions to parenting. Dev Psychol. 2011;47(3):676–92.
112. Liu C, et al. Child effects on parental negativity: the role of heritable and prenatal factors. Child Dev. 2020;91(5):e1064–81.
113. Edwards EP, Leonard KE, Eiden RD. Temperament and behavioral problems among infants in alcoholic families. Infant Ment Health J. 2001;22(3):374–92.
114. Munn-Chernoff MA, et al. Shared genetic risk between eating disorder- and substance-use-related phenotypes: evidence from genome-wide association studies. Addict Biol. 2021;26(1):e12880.
115. Fitzgerald HE, et al. Predictors of behavior problems in three-year-old sons of alcoholics: early evidence for the onset of risk. Child Dev. 1993;64(1): 110–23.
116. Mesman J, et al. Predicting growth curves of early childhood externalizing problems: differential susceptibility of children with difficult temperament. J Abnorm Child Psychol. 2009;37(5):625–36.
117. Nigg JT. Temperament and developmental psychopathology. J Child Psychol Psychiatry. 2006;47(3–4):395–422.
118. Carpenter M, Nagell K, Tomasello M. Social cognition, joint attention, and communicative competence from 9 to 15 months of age. Monogr Soc Res Child Dev. 1998;63(4):i–vi, 1–143.
119. Newman F, Holzman L. Lev Vygotsky : revolutionary scientist. In: Critical psychology. London: Routledge; 1993.
120. Fernyhough C, Fradley E. Private speech on an executive task: relations with task difficulty and task performance. Cogn Dev. 2005;20(1):103–20.
121. Tomasello M. Becoming human : a theory of ontogeny. Cambridge, MA: Harvard University Press; 2019.
122. Farah MJ, et al. Childhood poverty: specific associations with neurocognitive development. Brain Res. 2006;1110(1):166–74.
123. Raizada RD, Kishiyama MM. Effects of socioeconomic status on brain development, and how cognitive neuroscience may contribute to levelling the playing field. Front Hum Neurosci. 2010;4:3.
124. Winstanley M, Webb RT, Conti-Ramsden G. More or less likely to offend? Young adults with a history of identified developmental language disorders. Int J Lang Commun Disord. 2018;53(2):256–70.
125. Bryan K, Freer J, Furlong C. Language and communication difficulties in juvenile offenders. Int J Lang Commun Disord. 2007;42(5):505–20.
126. Snow PC, Powell MB. Oral language competence in incarcerated young offenders: links with offending severity. Int J Speech Lang Pathol. 2011;13(6):480–9.
127. Beitchman JH, et al. Adolescent substance use disorders: findings from a 14-year follow-up of speech/language-impaired and control children. J Clin Child Psychol. 1999;28(3):312–21.

128. Baird AA, Fugelsang JA. The emergence of consequential thought: evidence from neuroscience. Philos Trans R Soc Lond Ser B Biol Sci. 2004;359(1451):1797–804.
129. Kuntsche E, Kuntsche S. Even in early childhood offspring alcohol expectancies correspond to parental drinking. Drug Alcohol Depend. 2018;183: 51–4.
130. Smit K, et al. Exposure to drinking mediates the association between parental alcohol use and preteen alcohol use. Addict Behav. 2018;87:244–50.
131. Voogt C, et al. Alcohol-related cognitions in children (aged 2-10) and how they are shaped by parental alcohol use: a systematic review. Drug Alcohol Depend. 2017;177:277–90.
132. Màsse LC, Tremblay RE. Behavior of boys in kindergarten and the onset of substance use during adolescence. Arch Gen Psychiatry. 1997;54(1):62–8.
133. Arcos-Burgos M, et al. A common genetic network underlies substance use disorders and disruptive or externalizing disorders. Hum Genet. 2012;131(6):917–29.
134. Guerin DW, Gottfried AW, Thomas CW. Difficult temperament and behaviour problems: a longitudinal study from 1.5 to 12 years. Int J Behav Dev. 1997;21(1):71–90.
135. Maziade M, et al. Value of difficult temperament among 7-year-olds in the general population for predicting psychiatric diagnosis at age 12. Am J Psychiatry. 1985;142(8):943–6.
136. Maziade M, et al. Psychiatric status of adolescents who had extreme temperaments at age 7. Am J Psychiatry. 1990;147(11):1531–6.
137. Nigg JT, Goldsmith HH, Sachek J. Temperament and attention deficit hyperactivity disorder: the development of a multiple pathway model. J Clin Child Adolesc Psychol. 2004;33(1):42–53.
138. Walcott CM, Landau S. The relation between disinhibition and emotion regulation in boys with attention deficit hyperactivity disorder. J Clin Child Adolesc Psychol. 2004;33(4):772–82.
139. Wichstrøm L, et al. Explaining the relationship between temperament and symptoms of psychiatric disorders from preschool to middle childhood: hybrid fixed and random effects models of Norwegian and Spanish children. J Child Psychol Psychiatry. 2018;59(3):285–95.
140. Tarter RE, et al. Mutual dissatisfaction between mother and son in substance-abusing and normal families. Am J Addict. 1993;2(2):116–25.
141. Blackson TC, Tarter RE. Individual, family, and peer affiliation factors predisposing to early-age onset of alcohol and drug use. Alcohol Clin Exp Res. 1994;18(4):813–21.
142. Blackson TC, Tarter RE, Mezzich AC. Interaction between childhood temperament and parental discipline practices on behavioral adjustment in preadolescent sons of substance abuse and normal fathers. Am J Drug Alcohol Abuse. 1996;22(3):335–48.
143. Blackson TC, et al. Individual traits and family contexts predict sons' externalizing behavior and preliminary relative risk ratios for conduct disorder and substance use disorder outcomes. Drug Alcohol Depend. 1999;56(2):115–31.
144. Zhai ZW, et al. Psychological dysregulation during adolescence mediates the association of parent-child attachment in childhood and substance use disorder in adulthood. Am J Drug Alcohol Abuse. 2014;40(1):67–74.
145. Giancola PR, et al. Executive cognitive functioning predicts reactive aggression in boys at high risk for substance abuse: a prospective study. Alcohol Clin Exp Res. 1996;20(4):740–4.
146. Giancola PR, et al. Cognitive distortions, aggressive behavior, and drug use in adolescent boys with and without a family history of a substance use disorder. Psychol Addict Behav. 1999;13(1):22–32.
147. Waschbusch DA, et al. Reactive aggression in boys with disruptive behavior disorders: behavior, physiology, and affect. J Abnorm Child Psychol. 2002;30(6):641–56.
148. Kirisci L, et al. Relation between cognitive distortions and neurobehavior disinhibition on the development of substance use during adolescence and substance use disorder by young adulthood: a prospective study. Drug Alcohol Depend. 2004;76(2):125–33.
149. Walden B, et al. Identifying shared environmental contributions to early substance use: the respective roles of peers and parents. J Abnorm Psychol. 2004;113(3):440–50.
150. Jing Y, et al. Analysis of substance use and its outcomes by machine learning I. Childhood evaluation of liability to substance use disorder. Drug Alcohol Depend. 2020;206:107605.
151. Spear LP. The adolescent brain and age-related behavioral manifestations. Neurosci Biobehav Rev. 2000;24(4):417–63.
152. Baker LA, et al. Resting heart rate and the development of antisocial behavior from age 9 to 14: genetic and environmental influences. Dev Psychopathol. 2009;21(3):939–60.
153. Ortiz J, Raine A. Heart rate level and antisocial behavior in children and adolescents: a meta-analysis. J Am Acad Child Adolesc Psychiatry. 2004;43(2):154–62.
154. Raine A, et al. Low heart rate as a risk factor for child and adolescent proactive aggressive and impulsive psychopathic behavior. Aggress Behav. 2014;40(4):290–9.
155. Evans BE, et al. Blunted heart rate response as a potential endophenotype of substance use disorders: evidence from high-risk youth. Front Pediatr. 2015;3:66.
156. Taylor J, et al. Individual differences in electrodermal responsivity to predictable aversive stimuli and substance dependence. Psychophysiology. 1999;36(2):193–8.

157. Iacono WG, et al. P3 event-related potential amplitude and the risk for disinhibitory disorders in adolescent boys. Arch Gen Psychiatry. 2002;59(8):750–7.
158. Iacono WG. Identifying psychophysiological risk for psychopathology: examples from substance abuse and schizophrenia research. Psychophysiology. 1998;35(6):621–37.
159. Iacono WG, Carlson SR, Malone SM. Identifying a multivariate endophenotype for substance use disorders using psychophysiological measures. Int J Psychophysiol. 2000;38(1):81–96.
160. Zapolski TC, Cyders MA, Smith GT. Positive urgency predicts illegal drug use and risky sexual behavior. Psychol Addict Behav. 2009;23(2):348–54.
161. Spear LP. The behavioral neuroscience of adolescence. 1st ed. New York: W. W. Norton; 2010.
162. Spear LP, Varlinskaya EI. Adolescence. In: Galanter M, et al., editors. Recent developments in alcoholism: alcohol problems in adolescents and young adults. Boston: Springer; 2005. p. 143–59.
163. Clark DB, Kirisci L, Tarter RE. Adolescent versus adult onset and the development of substance use disorders in males. Drug Alcohol Depend. 1998;49(2):115–21.
164. Del Valle Tena O, et al. Chronic childhood adversity and speed of transition through stages of alcohol involvement. Drug Alcohol Depend. 2019;205:107669.
165. Medley G, et al. Sexual orientation and estimates of adult substance use and mental health: Results from the 2015 National Survey on Drug Use and Health. Rockville: Substance Abuse and Mental Health Services Administration; 2016. p. 54.
166. Natterson-Horowitz B, Bowers K. Wildhood: the epic journey from adolescence to adulthood in humans and other animals. New York: Scribner; 2019. p. 3681501164694.
167. Costello EJ, et al. Pubertal maturation and the development of alcohol use and abuse. Drug Alcohol Depend. 2007;88(Suppl 1):S50–9.
168. Horner MS, et al. Modeling the association between sexual maturation, transmissible risk, and peer relationships during childhood and adolescence on development of substance use disorder in young adulthood. Am J Addict. 2013;22(5):474–80.
169. Kirillova G, et al. Familiality of addiction and its developmental mechanisms in girls. Drug Alcohol Depend. 2014;143:213–8.
170. Marceau K, Kirisci L, Tarter RE. Correspondence of pubertal neuroendocrine and Tanner stage changes in boys and associations with substance use. Child Dev. 2019;90(6):e763–82.
171. Reynolds MD, et al. Testosterone levels and sexual maturation predict substance use disorders in adolescent boys: a prospective study. Biol Psychiatry. 2007;61(11):1223–7.
172. Marceau K, et al. Lability in parent- and child-based sources of parental monitoring is differentially associated with adolescent substance use. Prev Sci. 2020;21(4):568–79.
173. Tobiansky DJ, Fuxjager MJ. Sex steroids as regulators of gestural communication. Endocrinology. 2020;161(7):bqaa064.
174. Mendle J, et al. Associations between early life stress, child maltreatment, and pubertal development among girls in foster care. J Res Adolesc. 2011;21(4):871–80.
175. Negriff S, Blankson AN, Trickett PK. Pubertal timing and tempo: associations with childhood maltreatment. J Res Adolesc. 2015;25(2):201–13.
176. Kavanaugh BC, et al. Neurocognitive deficits in children and adolescents following maltreatment: neurodevelopmental consequences and neuropsychological implications of traumatic stress. Appl Neuropsychol Child. 2017;6(1):64–78.
177. Dinkler L, et al. Maltreatment-associated neurodevelopmental disorders: a co-twin control analysis. J Child Psychol Psychiatry. 2017;58(6):691–701.
178. Norman RE, et al. The long-term health consequences of child physical abuse, emotional abuse, and neglect: a systematic review and meta-analysis. PLoS Med. 2012;9(11):e1001349.
179. Nikulina V, Widom CS. Child maltreatment and executive functioning in middle adulthood: a prospective examination. Neuropsychology. 2013;27(4):417–27.
180. Mothes L, et al. Childhood maltreatment and executive functions in adolescents. Child Adolesc Ment Health. 2015;20(1):56–62.
181. Mendle J. Why puberty matters for psychopathology. Child Dev Perspect. 2014;8(4):218–22.
182. Somerville LH. Special issue on the teenage brain: sensitivity to social evaluation. Curr Dir Psychol Sci. 2013;22(2):121–7.
183. Ennett ST, et al. The peer context of adolescent substance use: findings from social network analysis. J Res Adolesc. 2006;16(2):159–86.
184. Moody J, et al. Popularity trajectories and substance use in early adolescence. Soc Networks. 2011;33(2):101–12.
185. Evans GW, English K. The environment of poverty: multiple stressor exposure, psychophysiological stress, and socioemotional adjustment. Child Dev. 2002;73(4):1238–48.
186. Case A, Deaton A. Deaths of despair and the future of capitalism. Princeton: Princeton University Press; 2021. p. 336.
187. Cohen RA, et al. Early life stress and morphometry of the adult anterior cingulate cortex and caudate nuclei. Biol Psychiatry. 2006;59(10):975–82.
188. Masten CL, et al. Neural correlates of social exclusion during adolescence: understanding the distress of peer rejection. Soc Cogn Affect Neurosci. 2009;4(2):143–57.
189. Eisenberger NI, Lieberman MD, Williams KD. Does rejection hurt? An FMRI study of social exclusion. Science. 2003;302(5643):290–2.

190. Mazur A, Booth A. Testosterone and dominance in men. Behav Brain Sci. 1998;21(3):353–63; discussion 363–97.
191. Tremblay RE, et al. Male physical aggression, social dominance and testosterone levels at puberty. In: Raine A, et al., editors. Biosocial bases of violence. New York: Plenum Press; 1997. p. 359.
192. Najam N, Tarter RE. Language deficits in children at high risk for drug abuse. J Child Adolesc Subst Abuse. 1997;6(2):69.
193. Snow PC, Powell MB. Oral language competence, social skills and high-risk boys: what are juvenile offenders trying to tell us? Child Soc. 2008;22(1):16–28.
194. Beitchman JH, et al. Substance use disorders in young adults with and without LD: predictive and concurrent relationships. J Learn Disabil. 2001;34(4):317–32.
195. Brunelle N, Cousineau MM, Brochu S. Juvenile drug use and delinquency: youths' accounts of their trajectories. Subst Use Misuse. 2005;40(5):721–34.
196. Boyer J. New name, same harm: rebranding of federal abstinence-only programs. In: Reproductive health in crisis: a special series. Guttmacher Institute Inc, Washington, DC; 2018.
197. Finer LB, Philbin JM. Sexual initiation, contraceptive use, and pregnancy among young adolescents. Pediatrics. 2013;131(5):886–91.
198. Posner GL. Pharma: greed, lies, and the poisoning of America, First avid reader press hardcover edition. ed. ed. New York: Avid Reader Press, an imprint of Simon & Schuster, Inc; 2020.
199. Alba JW, Williams EF. Pleasure principles: a review of research on hedonic consumption. J Consum Psychol. 2013;23(1):2–18.
200. Kahneman D. Thinking, fast and slow. 1st ed. New York: Farrar, Straus and Giroux; 2011.
201. Martel M, Nikolas M, Nigg JT. Executive function in adolescents with ADHD. J Am Acad Child Adolesc Psychiatry. 2007;46(11):1437–44.
202. Hummer TA, et al. Executive functioning characteristics associated with ADHD comorbidity in adolescents with disruptive behavior disorders. J Abnorm Child Psychol. 2011;39(1):11–9.
203. Dolan M, Park I. The neuropsychology of antisocial personality disorder. Psychol Med. 2002;32(3):417–27.
204. Haaland V, Esperaas L, Landrø NI. Selective deficit in executive functioning among patients with borderline personality disorder. Psychol Med. 2009;39(10):1733–43.
205. Chen Y, et al. Accessing the development and heritability of the capacity of cognitive control. Neuropsychologia. 2020;139:107361.
206. Baliousis M, et al. Executive function, attention, and memory deficits in antisocial personality disorder and psychopathy. Psychiatry Res. 2019;278:151–61.
207. Friedman NP, et al. Individual differences in executive functions are almost entirely genetic in origin. J Exp Psychol Gen. 2008;137(2):201–25.
208. Polderman TJ, et al. Genetic analyses of the stability of executive functioning during childhood. Biol Psychol. 2007;76(1–2):11–20.
209. Moll J, et al. Impairment of prosocial sentiments is associated with frontopolar and septal damage in frontotemporal dementia. NeuroImage. 2011;54(2):1735–42.
210. Moll J, et al. Opinion: the neural basis of human moral cognition. Nat Rev Neurosci. 2005;6(10):799–809.
211. Salamone JD, et al. Effort-related functions of nucleus accumbens dopamine and associated forebrain circuits. Psychopharmacology. 2007;191(3):461–82.
212. Floresco SB. The nucleus accumbens: an interface between cognition, emotion, and action. Annu Rev Psychol. 2015;66:25–52.
213. Sergerie K, Chochol C, Armony JL. The role of the amygdala in emotional processing: a quantitative meta-analysis of functional neuroimaging studies. Neurosci Biobehav Rev. 2008;32(4):811–30.
214. Bach DR, et al. Human hippocampus arbitrates approach-avoidance conflict. Curr Biol. 2014;24(5):541–7.
215. Fuller PM, et al. Reassessment of the structural basis of the ascending arousal system. J Comp Neurol. 2011;519(5):933–56.
216. Vanyukov MM, et al. Liability to substance use disorders: 1. Common mechanisms and manifestations. Neurosci Biobehav Rev. 2003;27(6):507–15.
217. Vanyukov MM, et al. Liability to substance use disorders: 2. A measurement approach. Neurosci Biobehav Rev. 2003;27(6):517–26.
218. Schoemaker K, et al. Executive functions in preschool children with externalizing behavior problems: a meta-analysis. J Abnorm Child Psychol. 2013;41(3):457–71.
219. Fishbein DH, et al. Short-term intervention effects of the PATHS curriculum in young low-income children: capitalizing on plasticity. J Prim Prev. 2016;37(6):493–511.
220. Flook L, et al. Promoting prosocial behavior and self-regulatory skills in preschool children through a mindfulness-based kindness curriculum. Dev Psychol. 2015;51(1):44–51.
221. Tamm L, et al. Generating attention, inhibition, and memory: a pilot randomized trial for preschoolers with executive functioning deficits. J Clin Child Adolesc Psychol. 2019;48(sup1):S131–s145.

Part II

Biometric Genetic Studies in Substance Use

Twin Studies of Substance Use

4

Michael C. Neale, Daniel Bustamante, Yi Zhou Daniel, and Nathan A. Gillespie

Background

For centuries, twins have been thought to be useful in inferring the origins of individual differences. Perhaps the earliest recorded reference to twins in this context was the remarks made by St. Augustine (Book 5, City of God) in the fourth century of the current era. He noted that a person's destiny could not be entirely due to the alignment of the planets and stars, per astrological beliefs popular at the time, because twins were born at the same time and yet had different destinies. The astrological zeitgeist that it challenged was much older, perhaps 2300 years BCE or earlier, as lunar almanacs existed some 25,000 years ago.

Formalization of the idea to use twins to quantify the relative effects of biology and environmental conditions on health and other outcomes did not emerge for almost another 1500 years. In part, the delay was due to the need to develop probability theory, which came surprisingly late in the history of mathematics, with major contributions in the seventeenth and eighteenth centuries. Even then, it was not until the 1860s that the potential utility of twins to discern genetic from environmental etiologies was described by Sir Francis Galton, a half cousin of Charles Darwin. These ideas and the statistical theory described by Sir Ronald Fisher in 1918 have been the basis of heritability estimation, which inspired the direct biological measurement of polymorphisms in the genome. Perhaps the most important aspect of heritability is that it isn't a constant associated with a trait, but it varies with the characteristics of the population being assayed. One of the clearest examples of this concerns the heritability of nicotine use across the lifespan. As one might expect, individual differences in use at ages 9–13 years are largely associated with shared environmental factors (such as access to tobacco in the home or neighborhood, parental guidance). In adulthood, when personal choice has a greater influence on

M. C. Neale (✉)
Department of Psychiatry, Virginia Institute for Psychiatric and Behaviour Genetics, Virginia Commonwealth University, Richmond, VA, USA
e-mail: michael.neale@vcuhealth.org

D. Bustamante
Integrative Life Sciences – Virginia Institute for Psychiatric and Behavioral Genetics, Richmond, VA, USA
e-mail: bustamanted@vcu.edu

Y. Zhou Daniel
Virginia Institute for Psychiatric and Behavioral Genetics, Virginia Commonwealth University, Richmond, VA, USA
e-mail: zhouy33@vcu.edu

N. A. Gillespie
Department of Psychiatry, Virginia Institute for Psychiatric and Behaviour Genetics, Virginia Commonwealth University, Richmond, VA, USA

QIMR Berghofer Medical Research Institute, Brisbane, QLD, Australia
e-mail: nathan.gillespie@vcuhealth.org

M. M. Vanyukov (ed.), *Genetics of Substance Use*, https://doi.org/10.1007/978-3-030-95350-8_4

behavior, additive genetic factors emerge as a substantial component of variation, and the effects of the rearing environment diminish [1].

Galton was a proponent of positive eugenics, in which those with positive traits should self-select to reproduce more than those with less positive traits. Darwin saw the use of eugenics as having significant practical difficulties – especially negative eugenics, in which those perceived as having less desirable traits were discouraged or prevented from reproduction. The Nazis used eugenics as a rationale for the attempted genocide of the Jews in World War II, where the atrocities and human rights violations associated with eugenics became rightly vilified throughout much of the world.

Twin studies, therefore, come with undesirable historical associations with individuals and political movements that are now considered to be inhumane and immoral. However, to abandon scientific methods because of their associations with individuals who held heinous socio-political beliefs would be foolish. Twin studies are simply a tool with which some insight into nature-nurture debates and causation can be obtained. Like any tool, statistical methods and twin studies may be used for beneficent purposes as well as for destructive ones. Over the past 50 years, twin studies have delivered a huge array of research findings (e.g., for variance component estimates of over 17,000 traits, see [2]). Many of these research studies were medically motivated, to understand the causes of human afflictions to reduce human suffering. Studies of the genetics of substance use are a part of this effort to create positive change with science.

Methods

General Principles

The classical twin design (CTD) involves measuring pairs of identical (monozygotic, MZ) and fraternal (dizygotic, DZ) twins on traits of interest. Our interest stems from the desire to understand the origins of individual differences. For example, we wish to improve our understanding of why some are susceptible to a disorder when others appear immune. To do so, measurements are taken independently from both members of many twin pairs. Summary statistics, consisting of the means and variances of each twin and the covariance between the twins, can provide a useful impression of the genetic architecture of a trait in a particular population at a particular time. Usually, this impression is summarized as the relative proportions of additive genetic (A), common environment shared by twins reared together in the same home (C), or unique environment (E) not shared by twins. A graphical view of this variance decomposition is shown in Fig. 4.1, where twin phenotypic correlations, calculated as cov(twins)/sqrt(var(Twin1)*var(Twin2), are plotted against their genetic correlation.

The x-axis shows the degree of additive genetic correlation (rG), which on average is 0.5 for DZ pairs and almost exactly 1.0 for MZ pairs. Somatic mutations make the genomes of MZ twins differ at a median number of 5.4 nucleotides[2], with some pairs differing at hundreds of loci, but these within-pair differences are only a

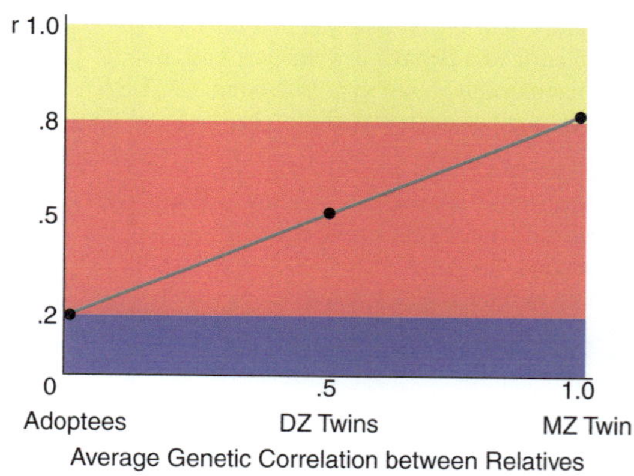

Fig. 4.1 Graphical representation of variance component estimation with MZ and DZ twin pair correlations. Unrelated adoptees are shown as predicted correlation based on the linear genetic model of additive genetic (A), common environment (C), and individual environment (E) variance components. Colored blocks represent proportions of variance: A, red; C, blue; and E, yellow

drop in the bucket of 3.1 billion base pairs along the genome, so rG = 1 for MZ twins is a very good approximation. Also illustrated, for reference, is the intercept with the y-axis, which is the expected resemblance for unrelated persons reared together in the same family. In the example shown, MZ and DZ pairs correlate 0.8 and 0.5, respectively. The intercept on the y-axis (where genetic relatedness is zero) is 0.2, which is the *predicted* covariance of unrelated persons reared together. This quantity is also the proportion of variation associated with the shared environment, shown as the blue-shaded area. Twice the difference between the MZ and DZ correlations yields 0.6, shown as the red area, and is an estimate of the variance associated with additive genetic effects. Lastly, 1-rMZ, the yellow area at the top of the figure, estimates the variance associated with environmental factors that are not shared by MZ twins (E), which includes phenotypic variation resulting from measurement error. Note that all three components of variance may be estimated from data exclusively on MZ and DZ twin pairs. The resemblance between unrelated persons reared together is a prediction that can be made from this study. Subsequent observation of pairs of adoptees (ideally of the same age and reared in the same family since birth, to match the conditions of the twins) can provide a test of the model, particularly its assumptions concerning additivity. Although this test with adoptees seems simple, it has several practical difficulties: (i) adoptees are rarely the same age (though some are close in age to a biological child within the adopting family); (ii) neither parents who adopt children nor those who give theirs up for adoption are representative of the population of parents as a whole; and (iii) maintaining the confidentiality of the identities of an adoptee's biological parents can be a practical ethical challenge.

Perhaps unsurprisingly, modern statistical treatments of data collected from twins or other relatives do not use a simple method such as 2(rMZ – rDZ) to estimate variance components from a twin study. The rationale for this divergence was described by Neale [3] in an encyclopedia article, which listed eight primary reasons. These are as follows: (1) it is possible to obtain nonsensical estimates of the heritability, both greater than 1.0 and less than zero; (2) it takes no account of the relative precision of the MZ and DZ means, variances, and covariances, which may be unequal if the sample sizes differ or if the magnitude of the correlation is different, or (as is usually the case) both; (3) there is no assessment of whether the correlations are consistent with the additive genetic model; (4) it does not easily generalize to the multivariate case to permit the examination of why variables correlate with each other; (5) there is no easy way to correct estimates for the effects of covariates such as age, race, or sex; (6) it does not generalize to extended twin studies that involve other relatives; (7) it is inefficient when there are missing data; and (8) it is not suitable for selected samples of twins. As a result, improved statistical estimation via maximum likelihood has become a popular approach. First, there are useful generic properties common to all maximum likelihood estimates (MLEs): they are asymptotically unbiased (i.e., with a large enough sample, there is no bias) and of all estimators with this property, MLEs have the smallest variance (so on average they are expected to be most accurate). For situations such as twin studies, where there is more than one dependent variable (both twins have a dependent variable, their phenotype), or latent variables are desired (the A, C, and E variance components are latent variables because they are not directly observed), structural equation models (SEMs) provide a useful statistical framework. Better still, Full Information Maximum Likelihood (FIML) has become available in many SEM packages since it was first implemented in Mx in 1990. FIML does not use summary statistics such as means and covariances to fit models, but directly calculates the likelihood of each row of data, based on the model's parameter estimates, which in turn generate predictions about means, variances, and covariances. A primary advantage of FIML is that it makes less restrictive assumptions (compared to fitting models to pre-calculated variance-covariance matrices) about why some of the data are missing. As long as data are missing completely at random, or as a function of variables that have been measured, FIML will recover asymptotically unbiased estimates. For example, if the second twin is more likely to be missing when their co-twin has a low score (or due to other factors unrelated to their own score), FIML can still yield unbiased estimates as long as pairs in which only one twin has provided data are included in the analysis [4]. The method is especially useful in longitudinal and multivariate analyses, where missing data are common.

Structural Equation Models for Univariate Twin Data

Structural equation modeling is very widely used for the analysis of data collected from twins and other relatives. One source of its popularity is that a SEM can be represented as a path diagram, which can be a mathematically complete description of the model (sufficient for model fitting), as long as it is drawn correctly. Sadly, many path diagrams fail in this regard, with a resulting ambiguity as to how they should be implemented, which in turn can contribute to the so-called reproducibility crisis [5]. We hope that, over time, most diagrams will be drawn in an unambiguous way that minimizes guesswork in their implementation. Here we describe the elegant and minimal method due to McArdle and McDonald [6] and illustrate it with path diagrams for the ACE model for twin data. The increasingly popular Onyx software [7] is consistent with this approach.

Three types of nodes are commonly used in path diagrams: squares, representing observed variables; circles, representing latent variables; and triangles, which are used to specify models for the means. The information needed to estimate A, C, and E variance components comes from the variances and covariances, so the model for the means is not strictly required, but in FIML estimation and for fitting, e.g., growth curve models (which make predictions about mean changes over time), they are necessary.

Two types of relationships between variables are usually specified in SEMs. First are single-headed arrows that denote a relationship where one variable (at the tail of a single-headed arrow) causes another variable (at the pointed end of the arrow). It is important to note that these paths are used to estimate partial regression coefficients; in a twin study, we aim to estimate the partial regressions of phenotype on each of the A, C, and E latent variables, as shown in Fig. 4.2a. However, simply drawing a causal arrow from, e.g., X to Y, does not unequivocally state that X is a cause of Y – just as in simple linear regression one can regress Y on X or X on Y, but in both cases, a perfect fit to the data may be found. It is the research design that determines the degree of confidence with which causal inferences can be drawn. As always, many different models may be consistent with a particular set of data. In some cases, reversing a causal path in a structural equation model may yield the same fit to the data, whereas in others it may not. As we describe below, data from relatives can often help to differentiate between models that fit equally well when applied to data from unrelated individuals.

There are many ways in which the information in a mathematically complete path diagram may be used to derive the model's predicted variances and covariances. There exist tracing rules to derive the expected covariance between two variables in a diagram. These rules are useful for simple models and can generate equations sufficient for model-fitting purposes. However, in the authors' experience, adding the possibility for human error to enter between the model and its implementation in software is generally not recommended. Better, it seems, is to use the McDonald-McArdle RAM notation [6], for which a little matrix algebra is required. The idea is to gather all the one-headed Asymmetric arrows in one matrix named **A** and all the two-headed Symmetric arrows in a second matrix named **S**. Only one matrix algebra formula is

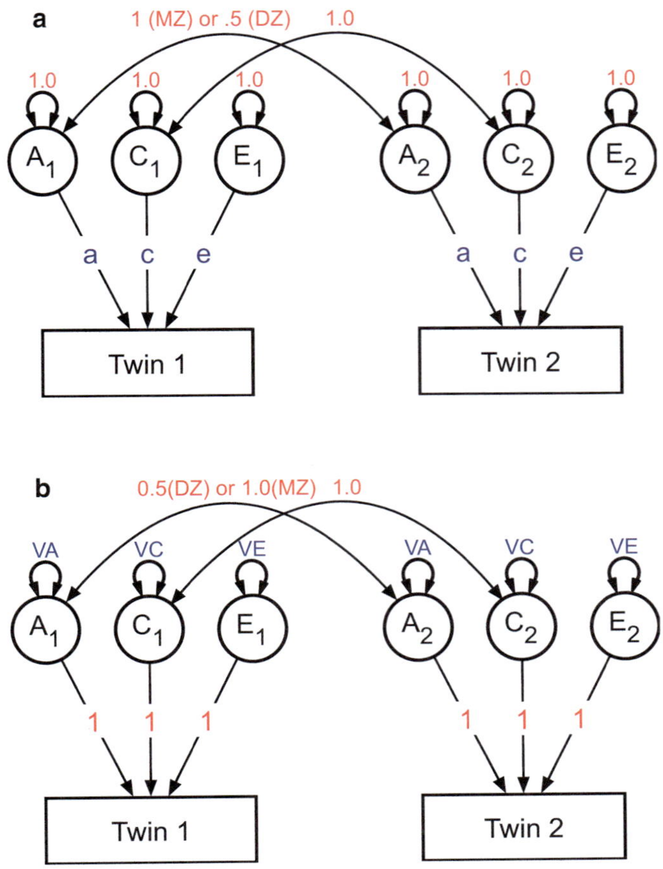

Fig. 4.2 Path diagrams for the ACE model of twin resemblance. Free parameters are shown in blue, and fixed quantities are shown in red. (**a**) Path coefficients model for the resemblance between twins. (**b**) Variance components model

needed to generate the expected variances and covariances between all the latent and observed variables ($\boldsymbol{\Sigma}_{LO}$) in the model. This formula is:

$$\sum_{LO} = (I - A)^{-1} S (I - A)^{-1'}.$$

For model fitting, only the expected variances and covariances of the observed variables are required, which can be extracted by pre-multiplying and post-multiplying this expression by a filter matrix named **F**:

$$\sum_{O} = F(I - A)^{-1} S (I - A)^{-1'} F'.$$

To put this in concrete terms, the three matrices (zero entries left blank) for the model in Fig. 4.2a are:

A matrix

	A_1	C_1	E_1	A_2	C_2	E_2	P_1	P_2
A_1								
C_1								
E_1								
A_2								
C_2								
E_2								
P_1	a	c	e					
P_2				a	c	e		

S matrix

	A_1	C_1	E_1	A_2	C_2	E_2	P_1	P_2
A_1	1			1 or 0.5				
C_1		1			1			
E_1			1					
A_2	1 or 0.5			1				
C_2		1			1			
E_2						1		
P_1								
P_2								

F matrix

	A_1	C_1	E_1	A_2	C_2	E_2	P_1	P_2
P_1							1	
P_2								1

Figure 4.2b shows a reparameterization of the model in Fig. 4.2a. Those unfamiliar with path analysis may wish to update the matrices **A**, **S**, and **F** for this version of the model. Here, rather than estimating the path coefficients *a, c*, and *e*, they are fixed at the value 1.0, while the variances of the latent factors are estimated instead. Quite often, but not always, these two models will give an identical fit to the data. The rationale for presenting this alternative model is statistical rather than conceptual. The expected variance of an individual is $a^2 + c^2 + e^2$ in the path coefficient model, but VA + VC + VE in the variance components model. Similarly, the MZ and DZ covariances are $a^2 + c^2$ and $0.5a^2 + c^2$ in the path model, but VA + VC and 0.5VA + VC in the variance components specification. These seem identical, with VA = a^2, VC = c^2, and VE = e^2, but they differ in one important respect. As long as *a*, *c*, and *e* are the parameters being estimated (as real numbers), none of their squares, i.e., the variance component estimates, can be negative. However, by estimating VA, VC, and VE directly, their estimates can be negative. This approach has several advantages [8], particularly that it avoids the accumulation of upward bias of estimates of *a* and *c* due to their having a lower bound of zero. In the multivariate case especially, likelihood ratio tests for whether a particular component is zero are biased in the direction of too frequently accepting the null hypotheses of no VC and no VA components. In practice, there is often more evidence for VA than for VC. Consequently, analyses where all VC parameters have been set to zero because doing so affects the fit less than removing all VA should be interpreted with caution. This issue becomes increasingly problematic with the number of variables in a multivariate analysis.

Assumptions of the Classical Twin Design

Many of the assumptions of the classical twin design can be seen in the path diagrams used to illustrate the model. The lack of a double-headed arrow between A_1 and C_1, for example, represents the assumption that genotypes and the family environment are not correlated. Similarly, their absences between A_1 and E_1 and between C_1 and E_1 embody assumptions that there is no gene-environment covariance and no covariance between the common and random environments, respectively. The model is also additive: both $A \times E$ interaction and $A \times A$ additive-by-additive genetic interaction (epistasis) are assumed to be absent. Perhaps the most commonly questioned assumption of twin studies is that the extent to which environments are shared by twins is the same, regardless of whether they are MZ or DZ twins. The equal environments assumption (EEA) is simply expressed by setting the value of 1.0 between C_1 and C_2, regardless of zygosity. Studies of environmental exposures such as stressful life events typically show greater similarity for MZ than for DZ twins (e.g. [9]), and the same is true of exposure to substances of abuse [10]. Although these findings suggest that the equal environments assumption is violated, it is still necessary to consider the origin of the violations. To the extent that MZ twin pairs seek out more similar environments than do DZ twin pairs, on account of their greater genetic similarity, the issue becomes one of proximal vs. distal causes. Proximally, the more similar environments of MZs than DZs may result in their phenotypes being more similar on average. Distally, however, the effects of the twins' genotypes may have created this assumption failure by eliciting particular environments. For practical purposes such as intervention, understanding the pathways from genetic factors to phenotypic outcomes is important. High estimates of heritability may partly result from outside-the-body effects of an individual's genotype on their phenotypic outcome. An example of this is the CHRNA5-CHRNA3-CHRNB4 gene cluster, which associates strongly with cigarettes per day [11]. The very same locus is also associated with lung cancer and chronic obstructive pulmonary disorder. Its effects on the latter are very likely mediated by the inhalation of cigarette smoke, which originates outside the body. Further details on these associations may be found in Kendler et al. [12]. An important aspect of heritable variation in human behavior is therefore that it is not immutable, since the pathways from genes to behavior may be open to environmental intervention. For substances of abuse, this is very clear, since availability and access to drugs can in part be controlled. Unfortunately, attempts to control harmful drugs by, e.g., making them illegal have only been partially successful.

Another key assumption of the models in Fig. 4.2 is that the mode of gene action is additive. The effects of genetic dominance or epistasis on the resemblance of MZ pairs are the same as for the additive model because they share essentially all their genetic variants – and this is true no matter how many loci are involved in such interactions. However, DZ pairs' expected correlations for genetic dominance or additive-by-additive epistatic interactions are 0.25 instead of 0.5 and rapidly drop below 0.25 for epistatic interactions involving more than two loci. Substantial non-additive genetic effects of this sort will, in the absence of common environment effects, tend to result in a DZ pair correlation that is less than half that of MZ pairs. In the path coefficient approach, the common environmental variance would be estimated at zero, but the variance component method would yield a negative estimate of V_C. It seems best to acknowledge this confounding of non-additive genetic and common environmental variance by noting that negative estimates of V_C may be due to non-additivity. Arbitrarily switching to an ADE model if V_C is estimated at zero has the statistical disadvantage that it capitalizes on chance so that, on average, the reported fit of ACE/ADE models would be too good.

Structural Equation Models for Multivariate Twin Data

Multivariate twin modeling permits the distinction between genetic and environmental factors that contribute to the covariance of two or more traits. Similar to the univariate case, the additive genetic and shared- and unique-environmental factors associated with covariation between the traits can be estimated. Figure 4.3a shows a path diagram for twin data on two traits. The parameters rA, rC, and rE estimate the covariance between Traits 1 and 2 that is associated with additive genetic, common, and unique environmental sources. Thus the multivariate twin study can address questions such as: Do the same genetic factors influence these two traits? If so, in what direction? Do these factors seem to influence both traits positively or negatively? In twin studies with more than two traits, genetic and environmental covariance matrices can be estimated and further modeled as one or more latent factors that influence traits or a subset of them.

A further valuable aspect of modeling data collected from twins is that certain causal hypotheses can be tested [13, 14]. Figure 4.3b also shows five potential sources of covariation between two traits. The first three (rA, rC, and rE) are the bivariate analogs of the variance components themselves, representing covariation due to these common causes. When the paths b_{12} and b_{21} are fixed to zero, the model is identified and is a direct analog of the A, C, and E variance decomposition but applied to the covariance between traits. The parameters b_{12} and b_{21} are different; they represent direct causal paths between the two phenotypes. Unlike the situation with regression analyses of unrelated persons, a model with path b_{12} as a free parameter and b_{21}, rA, rC, and rE all fixed to zero does not fit the same as a model with b_{21} free and b_{12}, rA, rC, and rE fixed to zero. Consequently, it is possible to draw some inferences about the likely direction of causation between two traits. It is also possible to partly combine the approaches, such that the model is identified with *any three* of the five paths $b_{12,}$ b_{21}, rA, rC, and rE.

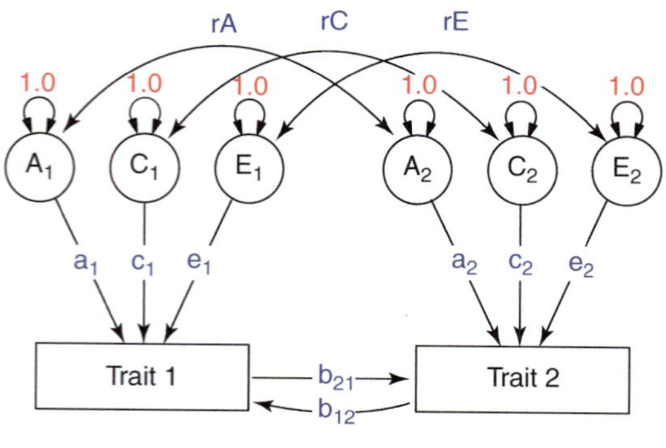

Fig. 4.3 Bivariate path diagram for two traits in one individual, showing additive genetic, common, and unique environmental sources of variance. Model is identified with data from MZ and DZ twin pairs as long as any two of the path coefficient model parameters rA, rC, rE, b21, and b12 are fixed. The model does not test cause in the sense of a randomized experiment, but it can detect whether data are consistent with causal hypotheses. It is useful because randomized experiments and randomized controlled trials are quite often impractical or unethical, especially in substance use

The CCC Model

When testing hypotheses regarding the covariance between SU and SUD, e.g., whether or not the genetic and environmental risks in a particular class of SU are related to the genetic and environmental risks in the SUD, applying the appropriate model is critical. Figure 4.4 shows a

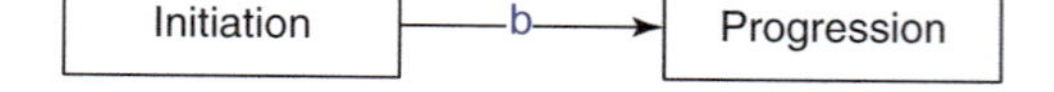

Fig. 4.4 CCC model path diagram. The binary trait Initiation is associated with the ordinal or continuous variable Progression (abuse, dependence, or quantity of use) via the path coefficient b. Since Progression is observed only when Initiation has occurred, no direct estimate of within-person Initiation-Progression is available. This loss of data results in being able to identify only two of the five possible sources of covariance (rA, rC, rE, b21, and b12) shown in Fig. 4.3

path diagram for one member of a twin pair for two stages of substance use, "Initiation" and "Progression" where progression is typically measured by SUD outcomes. This model became known as the CCC model, short for the "Contingent Causal Common" pathway model [15, 16]. It might have been better named as the CCCP model – apart from potentially confusing Russian readers. The diagram is identical to that of Fig. 4.3, except that the paths rA, rC, rE, and b21 have been eliminated (fixed to zero and therefore not shown according to path diagram convention).

The reason that this model is reduced to having one source of covariance is that there is an observed statistic, which is missing when initiation is a yes/no binary variable. Only those who have initiated can progress to regular use or misuse, but the progression status of non-initiators is unknown and coded as missing data. This situation leaves no variation in the initiation variable among those for whom information on progression is available, so the within-person covariance between initiation and progression is unknown. However, the relatives of those who have not initiated may themselves have initiated, and so their progression status would typically be known if they have.

Conceptually, a comparison of rates of progression among relative pairs who are concordant versus discordant for initiation provides information about the within-person initiation-progression covariance. If there is no initiation-progression covariance within-person, we would expect the same rates of progression regardless of whether the pairs are concordant or discordant. Higher rates of progression would be expected for concordant pairs when initiation and progression covary positively. Lower rates of progression would be observed for concordant pairs in the (seemingly unlikely) event that initiation and progression covary negatively. Judging and comparing these rates (by, e.g., odds ratios) would be unsatisfactory because different drugs of abuse have different base rates for both initiation and progression. The great advantage of the SEM model-fitting approach is that the initiation-progression relationship can be quantified as a standardized regression coefficient, which is a consistent index of covariance or association because it is not affected by base rates.

As discussed below in the empirical findings section, most applications to date have found support for positive covariance between initiation and progression, regardless of the drug being studied. Although the CCC model is typically applied with only the causal path b (effectively the same as simply regressing progression on initiation), there is sufficient information to identify the model when one and only one additional source of covariance, due to A, C, or E covariance.

Statistical Considerations

In most modern studies of twins or other close relatives, model parameters are estimated by Maximum Likelihood (ML). Initial starting values for parameter estimates are used to calculate the log-likelihood of each row of data. Data rows are usually organized so that independent observations are on separate rows, with the columns containing different observed measures. The model's parameter estimates are then varied with an algorithm, and the fit values are recalculated until the model parameters that produce the smallest fit function value (usually the minimum of −2 times the log-likelihood) are found. This technique is known as numerical optimization, and there exist many methods for finding the solution, several of which are available in the OpenMx R package [17, 18]. Most algorithms for optimization are based on calculus, in which the first and second derivatives of the fit function are calculated and used to find those parameter values that minimize the fit function.

Once the ideal parameter estimates have been found, several measures of model fit can be obtained that indicate how well the hypothesized model represents the observed data (i.e., how well the model-implied covariances and variances reproduce the empirical/observed covariances and variances). There are many (probably too many) indices of model fit, but they can be grouped into several categories (http://davidakenny.net/cm/fit.htm) including:

- Absolute fit indices (e.g., Chi-square, RMSEA, SRMR)
- Relative fit indices (e.g., NFI, TLI, CFI)
- Parsimony-based fit indices (PBFIs) (e.g., AIC, BIC, SABIC)

Absolute fit indices are derived from the fit function and assess how well the model represents the observed data. These fit indices assume that the best fitting model has a fit of 0 (meaning the model perfectly reproduces the observed variances and covariances) so that the actual fit indices determine how far away the model is from a perfectly fitting one. The fit index is considered a measure of model "badness" so larger values indicate worse fit. One global measure of fit is minus twice the log-likelihood difference in fit (Δ-2lnL) between the hypothesized model and a saturated model, which has a free parameter for every observed variance, covariance, and (where used) mean. Under certain regularity conditions [19], the Δ-2lnL is asymptotically distributed as chi-squared with degrees of freedom equal to the difference in the numbers of free parameters in the two models. In large sample sizes, relatively minor departures from assumptions (such as the data being multivariate normal) can lead to an apparent poor fit of the model. Another commonly used absolute fit index is the Root Mean Square Error Approximation (RMSEA) which was designed to avoid bias due to large sample sizes. Values of RMSEA less than 0.08 are considered a good model fit. However, RMSEA is positively biased, especially with low sample sizes. That is, in models with small sample sizes, the RMSEA fit index tends to be inflated.

Relative fit indices compare the model being tested with a "null" or "independence" model where all the measured variables are uncorrelated. The null model specifies that the measures vary but do not covary with each other at all and thus should fit poorly. Relative fit indices are analogous to R^2 values in that they take on values between 0 and 1, with 0 indicating poor model fit and 1 indicating the best model fit. Typically, values greater than 0.95 are accepted as good fitting models. Commonly used relative fit indices include the Tucker Lewis Index (TLI) and Comparative Fit Index (CFI), both of which penalize models with increased complexity. That is, the more parameters that are specified in the model, the worse the fit will tend to be.

Finally, parsimony-based fit indices (PBFIs) are typically used when two or more different models are being compared. Widely used PBFIs include the Akaike Information Criterion (AIC) and the Bayesian Information Criterion (BIC). For AIC, two formulas are in common use. One, twice the degrees of freedom may be subtracted from the -2lnL, or two, twice the number of free parameters may be added to the -2lnL. These two versions only differ by a constant, but for meta-analyses, it is important to know which has been used. When comparing models, those with lower (or largest negative) comparative fit indices are considered better models. PBFIs are useful because they can be computed for models that are *just identified* or *saturated* (i.e., when their degrees of freedom equal 0). All other fit indices cannot be computed for just-identified/saturated models.

Generally speaking, it is recommended to report several different types of fit measures (e.g., one absolute and one relative measure of fit) as part of the results of model fitting. This is because each category of fit indices can be biased in some way. For example, the chi-squared fit index (an absolute fit index) is known to become very sensitive as sample sizes become large, almost always indicating poor model fit with large sample sizes. Thus, including other measures of fit that are less likely to be biased in this way becomes important to help evaluate model fit.

It is important to note that researchers should decide a priori what fit criteria they will use, to prevent the selection of, or "cherry-picking," indices that make the results look better than they actually are.

While model fit indices give you an idea of how well the model fits the data, one further and very useful step that can be taken is to create different or nested models specifying alternative relationships between the variables in a model. A submodel is called nested when (i) one or more of its parameters is fixed to a particular value, (ii) two or more parameters have been set equal to each other, or (iii) both of these modifications. As noted above, given certain regularity conditions, twice the difference in log-likelihood between a model and a submodel is asymptotically distributed as chi-squared with degrees of freedom equal to the difference in the number of free parameters. This test can be used to evaluate the statistical evidence for specific hypotheses, e.g., whether estimates of variance components differ between males and females.

Empirical Results

Univariate Analyses: Modelling the Sources of Genetic and Environmental Risks Within Each SU and SUD Phenotype

The heritability estimates for substance use disorders are mostly equal to or greater than those for common biomedical diseases [12]. However, the relative contribution of familial environment versus genetic risks changes over time, depending on the stage of use. For example, shared environmental risks account for 40–70% of the risks in nicotine initiation [20, 21], 25–39% in cannabis initiation and use [22], and large portions of variance in alcohol initiation and regular use [23]. As individuals progress to regular substance use and substance use disorders, the role of shared environmental risks declines while heritability increases to 40–79% across all commonly used psychoactive substances including prescription opioids and stimulants [12, 24–27].

Multivariate Analyses: Modelling the Sources of Genetic and Environmental Risks Between Multiple SU and SUD Phenotypes

Use of and dependence on multiple substances occurs frequently. Twin studies provide a way to test alternative hypotheses about the nature of comorbid use. Despite some sex differences in the heritability estimates, multivariate twin studies have shown that comorbidity for substance use is largely explained by shared genetics [12, 21, 22, 28–32]. Two large twin studies examining illicit substances, including illicit opioid dependence, have revealed that most of the observed genetic risks are common across substances [33, 34]. Another twin study [29] found that although the genetic liabilities to licit and illicit SUDs are separable in terms of distinguishable licit and illicit factors, they are nonetheless highly correlated ($r = 0.82$). So, although the degrees of intoxication, tolerance, withdrawal, and physiological effects can differ substantially across substances, twin studies suggest that there is no clear division between licit and illicit SU or SUDs. A model of common genetic risks is consistent with the comorbidity data from relatives. It has been suggested that the common heritability underlying multiple substances is attributable to genes involved in cell adhesion processes required for establishing and maintaining neuronal connections related to the memory-like characteristics of SUDs [35]. Commensurate with these twin studies is the recent evidence from SU and SUD GWAS studies, which also indicate significant pleiotropy [36–38].

We note that while heritability estimates for SUDs are typically higher than those for SU, the importance of environmental risks should not be discounted, especially for initiation. Twin studies have shown that many home and social environments are themselves partly heritable [39–50]; these "environments" can mediate the risk of SU initiation. For example, genetic risks in cannabis dependence are partly mediated by the propensity to affiliate with deviant peers [49]. This propensity is consistent with the theory of non-random selection into risky and protective environments [51] and highlights the impact of genes on home and social environments that are known to confer risk of SU. Such environmental niche selection may also be observed with a longitudinal twin study; see Dolan et al. [52] for a model that could be usefully applied to data on substance use.

CCC Multivariate Analyses: Modelling the Sources of Genetic and Environmental Risks from Initiation to Progression

The initiation of a substance is necessary for developing a substance use disorder. As discussed above, genetic and environmental associations between SU and progression to SUDs should be appropriately modeled as a multistage process using causal-common-contingent (CCC) pathway analyses [16, 53]. By appropriately modeling SUD conditional on SU, the CCC model overcomes the lack of directly measured within-person covariance between initiation and progression. Under the model where initiation causes progression, genetic and environmental factors for progression can be divided into those that are shared with initiation and those that are unique to progression. Twin reports that have applied the CCC have consistently revealed that there is evidence of genetic risks unique to the various classes of SUDs, but that there is also typically a large overlap between risk factors for SU and SUD within substance [29, 34, 54–60]. The same CCC approach has also been applied to model the impact of upstream risk factors such as drug availability on SU and SUD [10]. Here, Gillespie et al. [10] found that the causal impact of the genetic and environmental risks underpinning drug availability on cannabis misuse was entirely mediated by the liability to cannabis initiation. Another multivariate extension of the CCC model [16] permits examination of the relationships between two or more substances of abuse. For example, one could compare a model in which nicotine initiation is associated with progression to marijuana dependence, or vice versa. This is but one example where the multivariate perspectives afforded by structural equation modeling surpass the focus on a single outcome inherent to linear regression.

Multivariate Analyses: Modelling the Sources of Genetic and Environmental Risks Between Multiple SU and SUDs and Other Complex Traits

Twin designs can be used to estimate the covariance and correlation of two or more traits (see sections "Structural Equation Models for Multivariate Twin Data" and "The CCC Model"). In addition to polygenic factors potentially shared by two or more quantitative traits, pleiotropy can also underlie the etiological relation of trait covariance and correlation. Pleiotropy occurs when a single mutation can influence the variation in two or more phenotypes. Biometrical multivariate twin methods can be used to estimate the proportion of shared additive genetic factors influencing two or more phenotypes in addition to shared- and unique-environmental sources of phenotypic variance. The sign of the genetic correlation between the phenotypes gives insights into the direction of their polygenic and/or pleiotropic relationship. Their shared additive genetic factors could influence the manifestation of one phenotype while reducing that of the other, in the case of a negative genetic association. Results from multivariate twin analyses can explain common etiology and expand understanding of comorbid disorders. Under this model, studies using a twin design have researched the co-occurrence and comorbidity of substance use (SU), substance use disorder (SUD), and other substance- and non-substance-based phenotypes (e.g., psychiatric disorders, brain imaging) among other phenotypes.

Regarding the covariance between SU and SUDs and psychiatric disorders, population-based twin studies have repeatedly shown that comorbidity between major psychiatric disorders can be best explained by two correlated yet distinct Internalizing and Externalizing dimensions [61–66]. The latter consists of antisocial behaviors such as conduct disorder, antisocial personality disorder, as well as SU and SUDs, which are all significantly genetically correlated, thus providing the best explanation for the observed comorbidity [34, 67–69].

Prom-Wormley et al. [70] investigated the common genetic and environmental influences between average lifetime cigarette use (cigarettes-packs/year) and brain structure (i.e., subcortical and cortical volume, surface area, and thickness). The genetic covariance is derived from the within-twin cross-trait covariance, and the MZ and DZ cross-twin cross-trait covariances, and dividing the genetic covariance by the square root of the product of the two traits' genetic variances. Results indicated that the shared genetic and unique environmental factors generate negative phenotypic correlations of cigarette packs per year, which were seen for many subcortical and cortical volumes and cortical surface areas. These associations include genetic correlations of −0.28 to −0.40 (notably the lingual gyrus, caudal anterior cingulate cortex in the pars opercularis, precuneus, all in the right hemisphere; cuneus, cerebellar cortex, both in the left hemisphere) and environmental correlations of −0.19 to −0.31 (particularly the posterior cingulate cortex, pars orbitalis, accumbens, pallidum, all in the left hemisphere; rostral middle frontal gyrus, inferior temporal gyrus, both in the right hemisphere) with cigarette packs per year. Several of these regions are implicated in smoking-related behaviors such as reward, pleasure, and craving control. After correction for multiple testing, none of the areas remained significant, but it is worth noting the consistent direction of the correlations. Multivariate twin designs have been applied to study the associations of cannabis use with smaller subcortical gray matter volumes using US and Australian twin samples [71]. Similar to cigarette use and brain structures, magnetic resonance imaging (MRI) volumetric measures of putative regions of interest (ROIs; i.e., thalamus, caudate nucleus, putamen, pallidum, hippocampus, amygdala, and nucleus accumbens) were not associated with cannabis use after correcting for multiple testing. Nevertheless, lifetime maximum nicotine use was associated with significantly smaller volumes in the thalamus for middle-aged males. Similarly, in a study of adolescent drinking and brain morphometry using a co-twin control design, Wilson et al. [72] found that smaller volume in the right amygdala, cortical volume, and greater left cerebellar volume are associated with problematic alcohol use. Smaller cortical thickness in the left middle temporal gyrus appeared to be the result of alcohol exposure. Furthermore, smaller volumes in the left ventral diencephalon were associated with drinking alcohol.

Multivariate Analyses: Modelling the Genetic and Environmental Etiology of Between-Group Differences in SU and SUDs

Twin designs can also help to uncover between-group differences. From a heterogeneity point of view, studies using this type of modeling can assess if there are differences in the contributions of genetic and environmental factors between the groups. A particular case of heterogeneity models is the sex-limitation model. Depending on the types of twins in the data, the quantitative (i.e., magnitude of effects) and qualitative (i.e., nature of effects) differences can be estimated. There are two avenues to assess heterogeneity via the sex-limitation model. A design including same-sex monozygotic and dizygotic twins allows the estimation of quantitative sex differences. However, if opposite-sex dizygotic twins are included in the design, then qualitative differences can be estimated in addition to the quantitative.

Sheerin et al. [73] examined the genetic and environmental correlations between psychiatric resilience (PR) and alcohol resistance (AR), the quantitative and qualitative sex differences, and the variance attributable to additive genetic shared- and unique-environmental factors in these phenotypes. Based on interviews and measures of stressful life events, distress symptoms, alcohol use, and alcohol use disorder, they found that additive genetic factors influenced a higher proportion (albeit small difference) of PR

(M = 0.33, F = 0.29) and AR (M = 0.26, F = 0.25) in males than in females. Conversely, unique environmental factors explained more of the variance of PR (M = 0.67, F = 0.71) and AR (M = 0.74, F = 0.75) in females. Males and females shared an additive genetic correlation of 54% between the two phenotypes, with unique environmental factors correlating for PR and AR at 24% for males and 26% for females.

Using a common pathway model, Kendler et al. [74] investigated the latent liability to externalizing syndromes, including drug abuse (DA), criminal behavior (CB), and alcohol use disorders (AUD) from the Swedish twin registry. The heritability of the latent externalizing syndromes factor was higher in females (76%) than in males (62%). However, shared-environmental factors accounted for a higher proportion in males (23%) than in females (3%). The proportion of DA variance accounted for by additive genetic effects was the highest for both sexes (M = 48.9%; F = 68.6%), whereas the influence of shared-environmental factors on DA was stronger in males (32.5%) than in females (2.8%), potentially due to greater influences from peers and to conform with use of substances and with delinquency in males compared to females.

Future Directions

Much of the future of genetic research in substance use and other complex traits will no doubt involve molecular genetic markers, either an inexpensive microchip array with a sample of around 600,000 SNP markers or with whole-exome or whole-genome sequencing. There remain, however, several advantages to using data collected from relatives. First, in genomic studies, there is the constant concern that population stratification may adversely affect the results of studies seeking to associate SNP markers to complex trait outcomes. Usually, the effects of possible population stratification are controlled by using principal components of ancestry as covariates in SNP-outcome regression analyses. While useful as a better-safe-than-sorry measure, this approach risks missing some genuine association signals from regions with considerable allele frequency differences between populations. Such losses may partly contribute to the difference in heritability estimates between the genomic and the twin study approaches. Relatives reared in the same family, such as twins, have the advantage that they are from the same stratum of the population, so the effects of stratification are effectively removed from the association, and the relative impact of association vs. stratification can be measured by comparing the within-family effect of an allele substitution to that seen between families (e.g., [75]).

The use of twin data in discordant twin pair analyses or within SEM frameworks remains useful for causal modeling [76–79]. However, co-twin-control experimental studies – in which one twin is given a treatment while their co-twin is a control – are largely unsuitable for determining, e.g., how much of a drug is required to generate addiction. Ethical concerns rule out studies of this nature, and even if they did not, the experimental situation may not be a good representation of the realities of habit acquisition. Some potential still exists for the treatment of addiction, given a sufficient supply of twin pairs concordant for substance dependence. In naturalistic settings, direction of causation modeling can provide a valuable and different line of evidence with which to test specific hypotheses [79].

More recent and innovative approaches are now capable of jointly analyzing individual GWAS, and phenotypic data hold promise. By applying genomic relatedness-based restricted maximum-likelihood (GREML) [80] to structural equation modeling software packages [81], GWAS information can now be used to estimate cryptic relatedness in the form of kinship matrices, which are analogous to the expected MZ and DZ twin pair genetic correlations, except that the approach can be extended to much larger samples of related and unrelated individuals. In principle, causal inferences may be derived from unrelated genotyped persons, or simply DZ twin pairs who have been genotyped. In effect, the regression line drawn in Fig. 4.1 can be drawn around very little variation in genomic relatedness – sib pairs' resemblance has a standard deviation of approximately 0.02, so with large sample sizes it is realistic to expect relatedness to vary between 0.45 and 0.55. Although much larger sample sizes are required to obtain a precise regression, it should be noted that the number of pairs increases factorially with the sample size, since every participant can be matched with everyone else. This type of twin study, using measures of DZ twin pairs' genomic relatedness and excluding MZ twin pairs, is only one potential modification that genomic data may bring. We now briefly consider several of these options.

A recent special issue of the journal *Behavior Genetics* (Volume 51, Number 3) describes extensions to twin studies that have considerable potential for future research. First, and relevant to the assumptions discussed above, is the use of genotyped DZ twin pairs to estimate and control for the putative effects of failure of the equal environments assumption [82]. In essence, variance due to EEA failure is thought to be captured by the excess resemblance of MZ pairs once an estimate of heritability has been derived from the genotyped DZ pairs alone. Large samples (thousands of pairs of genotyped DZ pairs) are needed for sufficient statistical precision. Although initially very promising, it must be noted that epistatic interactions between loci would have the same type of effect, since the expected genomic sharing of DZ pairs is only 0.25 within a locus or for additive × additive genetic interactions. This sharing is even less when more than two loci interact. Research designs with different types of relatives may help to resolve this confound.

Second, adding polygenic risk scores or simple genotypes to the ACE model described above enables testing of the assumption that additive genetic and common environment sources do not covary [83]. Essentially, additive genetic variation is partitioned into that due to a polygenic score (typically one for the same trait that is under analysis) and a residual component not assayed by the SNP genetic markers. Covariance between A and C can be estimated between the polygenic score and the common environment because the former has been directly measured on the same individuals. The usual proviso that large sample sizes are needed for adequate statistical power applies to this design. For example, over 1000 pairs are required to detect A-C covariance with 80% power at the 0.05 alpha level when the polygenic score accounts for between 5 and 18% of phenotypic variance. For lower proportions of variance in this range, over 10,000 pairs may be required.

Third, there have been developments in multilevel modeling that have potential for further analyses of individual differences in substance use and abuse. An important potential confound in multi-site studies is that variation associated with study site, if not controlled, can inflate estimates of the familial (environmental and genetic) sources of variance. The application of multilevel modeling to Dutch data on height and geographical region [84] found approximately 2% of phenotypic variation to be due to region, but that this source of variance was no longer detectable when variation associated with measured genotype was controlled. This method likely will have valuable applications to substance use research in youth, such as the ABCD Study® which is collecting Magnetic Resonance Imaging, genomic, and phenotypic data from over 20 sites across the USA. Multivariate analyses of such data also hold considerable promise, albeit somewhat tempered by the need to control for multiple testing as neuroimaging data often feature very high dimensionality (320,000 voxels per brain is only the beginning of this problem). The multilevel analysis framework also holds potential for mega-analytic work, described by Maes et al. [85] in which statistical power is gained by establishing consortia of studies with relevant assessments.

Finally, it will also be interesting to see the results of substance use-focused applications of the combined Mendelian Randomization (MR) and direction-of-causation twin models. Minica et al. [86] describe the unification of these two research strategies to enable testing of the assumptions of MR methods. In particular, MR with unrelated persons tacitly assumes no reverse causation from hypothesized outcome to the putative risk factor, and no third variable involvement, but these assumptions can be tested in a design involving twins, measured genotypes, risk factors, and outcomes. Such hybrid research designs have their limitations, particularly the ascertainment of a sufficiently large sample of genotyped twins, but the meteoric reductions in costs for genotyping, combined with approximately 2% of the population who are twins, make them entirely practical for the future.

References

1. Polderman TJ, Benyamin B, de Leeuw CA, Sullivan PF, van Bochoven A, Visscher PM, et al. Meta-analysis of the heritability of human traits based on fifty years of twin studies. Nat Genet. 2015;47(7):702–9.
2. Jonsson H, Magnusdottir E, Eggertsson HP, Stefansson OA, Arnadottir GA, Eiriksson O, et al. Differences between germline genomes of monozygotic twins. Nat Genet. 2021;53(1):27–34.
3. Neale MC, Lubke G, Aggen SH, Dolan CV. Problems with using sum scores for estimating variance components: contamination and measurement non-invariance. Twin Res Hum Genet. 2005;8(6):553–68.
4. Neale MC, Eaves LJ. Estimating and controlling for the effects of volunteer bias with pairs of relatives. Behav Genet. 1993;23(3):271–7.
5. Fanelli D. Opinion: is science really facing a reproducibility crisis, and do we need it to? Proc Natl Acad Sci U S A. 2018;115(11):2628–31.
6. McArdle JJ, McDonald RP. Some algebraic properties of the reticular action model for moment structures. Br J Math Stat Psychol. 1984;37:234–51.
7. von Oertzen T, Brandmaier AM, Tsang S. Structural equation modeling with Ωnyx. Struct Equ Model Multidiscip J. 2015;22(1):148–61.
8. Verhulst B, Prom-Wormley E, Keller M, Medland S, Neale MC. Type I error rates and parameter bias in multivariate behavioral genetic models. Behav Genet. 2019;49(1):99–111.
9. Foley DL, Neale MC, Kendler KS. A longitudinal study of stressful life events assessed at interview with an epidemiological sample of adult twins: the basis of individual variation in event exposure. Psychol Med. 1996;26(6):1239–52.
10. Gillespie NA, Neale MC, Kendler KS. Pathways to cannabis abuse: a multi-stage model from cannabis availability, cannabis initiation and progression to abuse. Addiction. 2009;104(3):430–8.
11. Saccone SF, Hinrichs AL, Saccone NL, Chase GA, Konvicka K, Madden PA, et al. Cholinergic nicotinic receptor genes implicated in a nicotine dependence association study targeting 348 candidate genes with 3713 SNPs. Hum Mol Genet. 2007;16(1):36–49.
12. Kendler KS, Chen X, Dick D, Maes H, Gillespie N, Neale MC, et al. Recent advances in the genetic epidemiology and molecular genetics of substance use disorders. Nat Neurosci. 2012;15(2):181–9.
13. Heath AC, Kessler RC, Neale MC, Hewitt JK, Eaves LJ, Kendler KS. Testing hypotheses about direction of causation using cross-sectional family data. Behav Genet. 1993;23(1):29–50.
14. Heath AC, Martin NG. Genetic models for the natural history of smoking: evidence for a genetic influence on smoking persistence. Addict Behav. 1993;18(1):19–34.
15. Kendler KS, Neale MC, Sullivan P, Corey LA, Gardner CO, Prescott CA. A population-based twin study in women of smoking initiation and nicotine dependence. Psychol Med. 1999;29(2):299–308.
16. Neale MC, Harvey E, Maes HH, Sullivan PF, Kendler KS. Extensions to the modeling of initiation and progression: applications to substance use and abuse. Behav Genet. 2006;36(4):507–24.
17. Boker S, Neale M, Maes H, Wilde M, Spiegel M, Brick T, et al. OpenMx: an open source extended structural equation modeling framework. Psychometrika. 2011;76(2):306–17.
18. Neale MC, Hunter MD, Pritikin JN, Zahery M, Brick TR, Kirkpatrick RM, et al. OpenMx 2.0: extended structural equation and statistical modeling. Psychometrika. 2016;81(2):535–49.
19. Steiger JH, Shapiro A, Browne MW. On the multivariate asymptotic distribution of sequential chi-square statistics. Psychometrika. 1985;50:253–64.
20. Treur JL, Verweij KJH, Abdellaoui A, Fedko IO, de Zeeuw EL, Ehli EA, et al. Testing familial transmission of smoking with two different research designs. Nicotine Tob Res. 2018;20(7):836–42.
21. Maes HH, Prom-Wormley E, Eaves LJ, Rhee SH, Hewitt JK, Young S, et al. A genetic epidemiological mega analysis of smoking initiation in adolescents. Nicotine Tob Res. 2017;19(4):401–9.
22. Verweij KJ, Zietsch BP, Lynskey MT, Medland SE, Neale MC, Martin NG, et al. Genetic and environmental influences on cannabis use initiation and problematic use: a meta-analysis of twin studies. Addiction. 2010;105(3):417–30.
23. Bergen SE, Gardner CO, Kendler KS. Age-related changes in heritability of behavioral phenotypes over adolescence and young adulthood: a meta-analysis. Twin Res Hum Genet. 2007;10(3):423–33.
24. Goldman D, Oroszi G, Ducci F. The genetics of addictions: uncovering the genes. Nat Rev Genet. 2005;6(7):521–32.
25. Bienvenu OJ, Davydow DS, Kendler KS. Psychiatric 'diseases' versus behavioral disorders and degree of genetic influence. Psychol Med. 2011;41(1):33–40.
26. Dash GF, Martin NG, Agrawal A, Lynskey MT, Slutske WS. Are prescription misuse and illicit drug use etiologically distinct? A genetically-informed analysis of opioids and stimulants. Psychol Med. 2021:1–8.
27. Gillespie NA, Bates TC, Hickie IB, Medland SE, Verhulst B, Kirkpatrick RM, et al. Genetic and environmental risk factors in the non-medical use of over-the-counter or prescribed analgesics, and their relationship to major classes of licit and illicit sub-

stance use and misuse in a population-based sample of young adult twins. Addiction. 2019;114(12):2229–40.
28. Kendler KS, Prescott CA. Genes, environment, and psychopathology: understanding the causes of psychiatric and substance use disorders. 1st ed. New York: The Guilford Press; 2006. 412 pp.
29. Kendler KS, Myers J, Prescott CA. Specificity of genetic and environmental risk factors for symptoms of cannabis, cocaine, alcohol, caffeine, and nicotine dependence. Arch Gen Psychiatry. 2007;64(11):1313–20.
30. Kendler KS, Prescott CA, Jacobson K, Myers J, Neale MC. The joint analysis of personal interview and family history diagnoses: evidence for validity of diagnosis and increased heritability estimates. Psychol Med. 2002;32(5):829–42.
31. Kendler KS, Schmitt E, Aggen SH, Prescott CA. Genetic and environmental influences on alcohol, caffeine, cannabis, and nicotine use from early adolescence to middle adulthood. Arch Gen Psychiatry. 2008;65(6):674–82.
32. Dick DM, Meyers JL, Rose RJ, Kaprio J, Kendler KS. Measures of current alcohol consumption and problems: two independent twin studies suggest a complex genetic architecture. Alcohol Clin Exp Res. 2011;35(12):2152–61.
33. Kendler KS, Jacobson KC, Prescott CA, Neale MC. Specificity of genetic and environmental risk factors for use and abuse/dependence of cannabis, cocaine, hallucinogens, sedatives, stimulants, and opiates in male twins. Am J Psychiatry. 2003;160(4):687–95.
34. Tsuang MT, Lyons MJ, Meyer JM, Doyle T, Eisen SA, Goldberg J, et al. Co-occurrence of abuse of different drugs in men: the role of drug-specific and shared vulnerabilities. Arch Gen Psychiatry. 1998;55(11):967–72.
35. Liu QR, Drgon T, Johnson C, Walther D, Hess J, Uhl GR. Addiction molecular genetics: 639,401 SNP whole genome association identifies many "cell adhesion" genes. Am J Med Genet B Neuropsychiatr Genet. 2006;141B(8):918–25.
36. Walters RK, Polimanti R, Johnson EC, McClintick JN, Adams MJ, Adkins AE, et al. Transancestral GWAS of alcohol dependence reveals common genetic underpinnings with psychiatric disorders. Nat Neurosci. 2018;21(12):1656–69.
37. Pasman JA, Verweij KJH, Gerring Z, Stringer S, Sanchez-Roige S, Treur JL, et al. GWAS of lifetime cannabis use reveals new risk loci, genetic overlap with psychiatric traits, and a causal influence of schizophrenia. Nat Neurosci. 2018;21(9):1161–70.
38. Liu M, Jiang Y, Wedow R, Li Y, Brazel DM, Chen F, et al. Association studies of up to 1.2 million individuals yield new insights into the genetic etiology of tobacco and alcohol use. Nat Genet. 2019;51(2):237–44.
39. Kendler KS, Lonn SL, Salvatore J, Sundquist J, Sundquist K. Divorce and the onset of alcohol use disorder: a Swedish population-based longitudinal cohort and co-relative study. Am J Psychiatry. 2017;174(5):451–8.
40. Waldron M, Heath AC, Lynskey MT, Bucholz KK, Madden PA, Martin NG. Alcoholic marriage: later start, sooner end. Alcohol Clin Exp Res. 2011;35(4):632–42.
41. Wichers M, Gillespie NA, Kendler KS. Genetic and environmental predictors of latent trajectories of alcohol use from adolescence to adulthood: a male twin study. Alcohol Clin Exp Res. 2013;37(3):498–506.
42. Olivares EL, Kendler KS, Neale MC, Gillespie NA. The genetic and environmental association between parental monitoring and risk of cannabis, stimulants, and cocaine initiation in a sample of male twins: does parenting matter? Twin Res Hum Genet. 2016;19(4):297–305.
43. Gillespie NA, Zhu G, Neale MC, Heath AC, Martin NG. Direction of causation modeling between cross-sectional measures of parenting and psychological distress in female twins. Behav Genet. 2003;33(4):383–96.
44. den Hoed M, Brage S, Zhao JH, Westgate K, Nessa A, Ekelund U, et al. Heritability of objectively assessed daily physical activity and sedentary behavior. Am J Clin Nutr. 2013;98(5):1317–25.
45. Kendler KS, Myers J. A developmental twin study of church attendance and alcohol and nicotine consumption: a model for analyzing the changing impact of genes and environment. Am J Psychiatry. 2009;166(10):1150–5.
46. Button TM, Stallings MC, Rhee SH, Corley RP, Hewitt JK. The etiology of stability and change in religious values and religious attendance. Behav Genet. 2011;41(2):201–10.
47. Kendler KS, Baker JH. Genetic influences on measures of the environment: a systematic review. Psychol Med. 2007;37(5):615–26.
48. Kendler KS, Jacobson KC, Gardner CO, Gillespie N, Aggen SA, Prescott CA. Creating a social world: a developmental twin study of peer-group deviance. Arch Gen Psychiatry. 2007;64(8):958–65.
49. Gillespie NA, Neale MC, Jacobson K, Kendler KS. Modeling the genetic and environmental association between peer group deviance and cannabis use in male twins. Addiction. 2009;104(3):420–9.
50. Mann FD, Patterson MW, Grotzinger AD, Kretsch N, Tackett JL, Tucker-Drob EM, et al. Sensation seeking, peer deviance, and genetic influences on adolescent delinquency: evidence for person-environment correlation and interaction. J Abnorm Psychol. 2016;125(5):679–91.
51. Vinkhuyzen AA, van der Sluis S, de Geus EJ, Boomsma DI, Posthuma D. Genetic influences on 'environmental' factors. Genes Brain Behav. 2010;9(3):276–87.
52. Dolan CV, de Kort JM, van Beijsterveldt TC, Bartels M, Boomsma DI. GE covariance through phenotype to environment transmission: an assessment in longitudinal twin data and application to childhood anxiety. Behav Genet. 2014;44(3):240–53.

53. Maes HH, Sullivan PF, Bulik CM, Neale MC, Prescott CA, Eaves LJ, et al. A twin study of genetic and environmental influences on tobacco initiation, regular tobacco use and nicotine dependence. Psychol Med. 2004;34(7):1251–61.
54. Kendler KS, Gardner CO Jr. Twin studies of adult psychiatric and substance dependence disorders: are they biased by differences in the environmental experiences of monozygotic and dizygotic twins in childhood and adolescence? Psychol Med. 1998;28(3):625–33.
55. Miles DR, van den Bree MB, Gupman AE, Newlin DB, Glantz MD, Pickens RW. A twin study on sensation seeking, risk taking behavior and marijuana use. Drug Alcohol Depend. 2001;62(1):57–68.
56. van den Bree MB, Johnson EO, Neale MC, Pickens RW. Genetic and environmental influences on drug use and abuse/dependence in male and female twins. Drug Alcohol Depend. 1998;52(3):231–41.
57. Rhee SH, Hewitt JK, Young SE, Corley RP, Crowley TJ, Stallings MC. Genetic and environmental influences on substance initiation, use, and problem use in adolescents. Arch Gen Psychiatry. 2003;60(12):1256–64.
58. Kendler KS, Karkowski LM, Neale MC, Prescott CA. Illicit psychoactive substance use, heavy use, abuse, and dependence in a US population-based sample of male twins. Arch Gen Psychiatry. 2000;57(3):261–9.
59. McGue M, Elkins I, Iacono WG. Genetic and environmental influences on adolescent substance use and abuse. Am J Med Genet. 2000;96(5):671–7.
60. Agrawal A, Neale MC, Jacobson KC, Prescott CA, Kendler KS. Illicit drug use and abuse/dependence: modeling of two-stage variables using the CCC approach. Addict Behav. 2005;30(5):1043–8.
61. Krueger RF, Caspi A, Moffitt TE, Silva PA. The structure and stability of common mental disorders (DSM-III-R): a longitudinal-epidemiological study. J Abnorm Psychol. 1998;107(2):216–27.
62. Krueger RF. The structure of common mental disorders. Arch Gen Psychiatry. 1999;56(10):921–6.
63. Vollebergh WA, Iedema J, Bijl RV, de Graaf R, Smit F, Ormel J. The structure and stability of common mental disorders: the NEMESIS study. Arch Gen Psychiatry. 2001;58(6):597–603.
64. Krueger RF, Tackett JL. Personality and psychopathology: working toward the bigger picture. J Personal Disord. 2003;17(2):109–28.
65. Eaton NR, Krueger RF, Keyes KM, Skodol AE, Markon KE, Grant BF, et al. Borderline personality disorder co-morbidity: relationship to the internalizing-externalizing structure of common mental disorders. Psychol Med. 2011;41(5):1041–50.
66. Kendler K, Aggen SH, Knudsen GP, Roysamb E, Neale MC, Reichborn-Kjennerud T. The structure of genetic and environmental risk factors for syndromal and subsyndromal common DSM-IV axis I and all axis II disorders. Am J Psychiatry. 2011;168(1):29–39.
67. Grove WM, Eckert ED, Heston L, Bouchard TJ Jr, Segal N, Lykken DT. Heritability of substance abuse and antisocial behavior: a study of monozygotic twins reared apart. Biol Psychiatry. 1990;27(12):1293–304.
68. Lyons MJ, True WR, Eisen SA, Goldberg J, Meyer JM, Faraone SV, et al. Differential heritability of adult and juvenile antisocial traits. Arch Gen Psychiatry. 1995;52(11):906–15.
69. True WR, Heath AC, Scherrer JF, Xian H, Lin N, Eisen SA, et al. Interrelationship of genetic and environmental influences on conduct disorder and alcohol and marijuana dependence symptoms. Am J Med Genet. 1999;88(4):391–7.
70. Prom-Wormley E, Maes HHM, Schmitt JE, Panizzon MS, Xian H, Eyler LT, Franz CE, et al. Genetic and environmental contributions to the relationships between brain structure and average lifetime cigarette use. Behav Genet. 2015;45(2):157–70. (1573–3297 (Electronic)).
71. Gillespie NA, Neale MC, Bates TC, Eyler LT, Fennema-Notestine C, Vassileva J, et al. Testing associations between cannabis use and subcortical volumes in two large population-based samples. Addiction. 2018;
72. Wilson S, Malone SM, Thomas KM, Iacono WG. Adolescent drinking and brain morphometry: a co-twin control analysis. Dev Cogn Neurosci. 2015;16:130–8.
73. Sheerin CA-OX, Bustamante D, Bountress KE, Cusack SE, Aggen SH, Kendler KS, et al. Psychiatric resilience and alcohol resistance: a twin study of genetic correlation and sex differences. https://doi.org/10.1007/s10519-021-10059-7. (1573–3297 (Electronic)).
74. Kendler KS, Lonn SL, Maes HH, Lichtenstein P, Sundquist J, Sundquist K. A Swedish population-based multivariate twin study of externalizing disorders. Behav Genet. 2016;46(2):183–92.
75. Neale MC, Cherny SS, Sham PC, Whitfield JB, Heath AC, Birley AC, et al. Distinguishing population stratification from genuine allelic effects with Mx: association of ADH2 with alcohol consumption. Behav Genet. 1999;29:233–44.
76. Kendler KS, Bulik CM, Silberg J, Hettema JM, Myers J, Prescott CA. Childhood sexual abuse and adult psychiatric and substance use disorders in women - an epidemiological and Cotwin control analysis. Arch Gen Psychiatry. 2000;57(10):953–9.
77. Kendler KS, Neale MC, MacLean CJ, Heath AC, Eaves LJ, Kessler RC. Smoking and major depression. A causal analysis. Arch Gen Psychiatry. 1993;50(1):36–43.
78. Gillespie NA, Kendler KS. Use of genetically informed methods to clarify the nature of the association between cannabis use and risk for schizophrenia. JAMA Psychiat. 2021;78(5):467–8.
79. Gillespie NA, Martin NG. Modeling direction of causation. In: Everitt N, Howell DC, editors.

Encyclopedia of statistics in behavioral science. Chichester: Wiley; 2005. p. 496–9.
80. Yang J, Lee SH, Goddard ME, Visscher PM. GCTA: a tool for genome-wide complex trait analysis. Am J Hum Genet. 2011;88(1):76–82.
81. Kirkpatrick RM, Pritikin JN, Hunter MD, Neale MC. Combining structural-equation modeling with genomic-relatedness-matrix restricted maximum likelihood in OpenMx. Behav Genet. 2021;51(3):331–42.
82. Hwang LD, Mitchell BL, Medland SE, Martin NG, Neale MC, Evans DA-O. The augmented classical twin design: incorporating genome-wide identity by descent sharing into twin studies in order to model violations of the equal environments assumption. Behav Genet. 2021;51(3):223–36. (1573–3297 (Electronic)).
83. Dolan CV, Huijskens RCA, Minică CC, Neale MC, Boomsma DI. Incorporating polygenic risk scores in the ACE twin model to estimate A-C covariance. Behav Genet. 2021;51(3):237–49. (1573–3297 (Electronic)).
84. Tamimy ZA-O, Kevenaar SA-O, Hottenga JA-O, Hunter MA-O, de Zeeuw EA-O, Neale MA-OX, et al. Multilevel twin models: geographical region as a third level variable. Behav Genet. 2021;51(3):319–30. (1573–3297 (Electronic)).
85. Maes HH, Prom-Wormley E, Eaves LJ, Rhee SH, Hewitt JK, Young S, et al. A genetic epidemiological mega analysis of smoking initiation in adolescents. Nicotine Tob Res. 2017;19(4):401–9. (1469–994X (Electronic)).
86. Minica CC, Dolan CV, Boomsma DI, de Geus E, Neale MC. Extending causality tests with genetic instruments: an integration of Mendelian randomization with the classical twin design. Behav Genet. 2018;48(4):337–49.

5 Family and Adoption Studies of Substance Use

Michael C. Stallings, Kyle R. Kent, and Maia J. Frieser

Family Studies

Introduction

Family studies have taken many forms, utilizing a variety of analytical approaches from proband family history reports and case/control studies, to dyadic comparisons of parent-offspring and sibling risk factors, to family transmission models that consider the family/pedigree as the unit of analysis. A specific variety of family studies, discussed in a separate chapter of this monograph, is analysis of twins, which has been the most common biometric genetic design for investigating the sources of individual variation in *substance* use and misuse and liability[1] to addiction. Nonetheless, family and adoption studies provide important complementary data about those sources. Here we review findings from family studies of substance-related behavior over the past several decades. This research, as most of substance use-related studies, has been largely focused on the risk for substance use disorders, although negative consequences of substance use are not limited to those stemming from a diagnosable disorder.

Generally, because the behavior of family members is influenced by both shared genetic and environmental factors, family studies cannot disentangle the underlying sources of familial resemblance (e.g., parent-offspring or sibling resemblance). However, they have made major contributions to the identification of important intra- and extra-familial risk factors, the extent to which risk (both genetic and environmental) is transmitted in families, how familial influences change over time/development, and the extent to which family environments/contexts moderate transmissible risk. Early family studies often compared the incidence or prevalence of substance-related behaviors in the relatives of probands with and without substance use diagnoses. A landmark review of 39 such studies inves-

M. C. Stallings (✉) · M. J. Frieser
Department of Psychology and Neuroscience, University of Colorado, Boulder, Boulder, CO, USA

Institute for Behavioral Genetics, University of Colorado, Boulder, Boulder, CO, USA
e-mail: Michael.Stallings@Colorado.Edu; Maia.Frieser@Colorado.Edu

K. R. Kent
Department of Psychology and Neuroscience, University of Colorado, Boulder, Boulder, CO, USA
e-mail: Kyle.Kent@Colorado.Edu

[1] Liability (Falconer, 1965) is a latent (unobserved) trait subsuming the effects of all factors influencing variation in the risk for a disorder. Below a certain point on its scale, termed the threshold, the phenotypes are generally unaffected, and above, affected.

M. M. Vanyukov (ed.), *Genetics of Substance Use*, https://doi.org/10.1007/978-3-030-95350-8_5

tigating the incidence of alcoholism in families [1] convincingly demonstrated that rates of alcoholism are substantially higher in the relatives of alcoholics than in the relatives of non-alcoholics. Approximately one-third of any sample of alcoholics had at least one parent who was also an alcoholic. A review of smoking behavior [2] also demonstrated familial resemblance, but showed weaker evidence for associations between parental and adolescent offspring smoking than for sibling and peer smoking. Merikangas et al. [3] examined the adult first-degree relatives of 231 probands with dependence on opioids, cocaine, cannabis, and alcohol and the relatives of 61 control probands and found an eightfold increased odds of substance use disorders across the range of substances studied. Although these early studies demonstrate the familial aggregation of substance-related behaviors and disorders, they provide limited information regarding specific risk factors and how those risks are transmitted within families.

Family Risk Factors

Substance use disorders are among the most strongly familial psychiatric disorders [4]. However, because family studies cannot resolve the extent to which genetic influences confound these risk factors, the etiology of familial risks is difficult to determine. For example, numerous family studies have shown that parental substance use is an important predictor of child substance use [e.g., 3, 5–12]. However, this association may be due to direct genetic or environmental transmission of risk from parents to children, or both, as well as other complex influences including gene-environment interplay. Gene-environment correlation (rGE) occurs when genetic factors influence exposure to different environments (e.g., parents provide environments for their children that are correlated with their genetic predispositions, and individuals create or select into environments that are correlated with their own genetic predisposition). Gene-environment interaction (G×E) occurs when genetic factors influence sensitivity to environments (e.g., when genetic vulnerability to addiction is influenced by the availability of drugs). Nevertheless, family studies have identified numerous family characteristics associated with substance use that are important targets for further investigation.

Parental separation and divorce have been associated with increased substance use risk. Conway and colleagues [13] showed that the prevalence of substance use is greater among adolescents living with a single parent or one or more step-parents, than for those living with both biological parents. Using data from a large Danish population registry, Holst et al. [14] also found that the prevalence of non-intact family structure was greater among families with parental alcohol use disorder (AUD). However, parental separation may be influenced, in part, by substance abuse in one or both parents. McCutcheon and colleagues [15], using high-risk family data (selected for high levels of parental AUD) from the Collaborative Studies on the Genetics of Alcoholism (COGA), examined the influence of both parental AUD and parental separation on substance use in their children. They found that both risk factors were independent predictors of increased risk for early alcohol, tobacco, and cannabis use in offspring. In fact, parental separation had a stronger association with the timing of first use of alcohol relative to having one parent with an AUD (hazard ratios, HR, 2.16 vs. 1.28) but not two affected parents (HR = 1.59). Using a sample of children of twins, Waldron et al. [16] also found that parental separation was an independent risk factor for early substance involvement, over and above genetic and environmental influences specific to parental alcohol and cannabis dependence.

Although these studies controlled for a number of potential confounding variables, the relationship between parental separation and child substance use is likely complex. Separation may be preceded by substantial parental conflict that is likely to affect parenting behaviors [17] as well as parent-child attachment, support, and communication. In some cases, separation may actually resolve some of these issues; in other cases the effects may be long-lasting. Many studies have examined how parental separation influences early substance use in adolescence, but few studies have examined long-term effects. Further, the age and sex of children may moderate the effects of parental separation [e.g., 18]. Newer studies are addressing the complexities of this relationship and are beginning to disentangle the mechanisms underlying the association between parental separation and substance use risk, but more work needs to be done.

How do parenting behaviors influence substance abuse risk? One hypothesis is that parenting skills suffer when parents are substance users [11]. Hill and colleagues [19] suggest that the influence of parental cannabis use on offspring cannabis use is, in part, mediated by substance-related impaired parenting. A number of studies have shown associations between substance abuse and poor parental monitoring [20–24], poor parent-child communication [25], and ineffective discipline strategies [11, 17, 26, 27]. Other family-level predictors of substance use include family closeness and attachment [27, 28] and opportunities and rewards for prosocial involvement [29]. Ryan et al. [30] reviewed the literature for eight parenting factors associated with adolescent drinking or age of onset of alcohol use: parental modeling, parental provision and alcohol accessibility (allowing alcohol use at home), parental disapproval of adolescent drinking, discipline practices, parental monitoring, parent-child relationship quality, parental involvement (sharing activities together), and general communication. Although the findings across the 77 studies they reviewed were mixed, a preponderance of evidence suggests that these family factors were associated with age of initiation and adolescent drinking. Conversely, they found little evidence to support that alcohol-specific communication (discussions between parents and adolescents specifically about alcohol), rules prohibiting adolescent drinking, family conflict (family arguments and hostility), or parental support (help, guidance, and parental acceptance) was strongly associated with early initiation or later drinking behavior. Parental influences are likely to be moderated by different contextual variables. A review and meta-analysis of 81 studies [31] found that parental influences varied by type of substance and offspring age. Dever and colleagues [21], utilizing 36,514 eighth and tenth grade participants in the nationally representative *Monitoring the Future* study, found that parental monitoring was associated with lower alcohol and cannabis use and that these effects were strongest among high-risk takers and females. Parental monitoring had a greater impact on substance use than either school bonding or sports participation. Hill et al. [23] also found that the quality of family management (which included measures of parental monitoring) moderated the relationship between behavioral disinhibition (e.g., ability to inhibit inappropriate behavior) in adolescence and adult alcohol use and dependence. Hill and colleagues found that adolescents high in behavioral disinhibition were at increased risk for later substance abuse problems if they were reared in poorly managed family environments during adolescence. In well-managed families, the increased risk due to high levels of behavioral disinhibition was minimized. In a meta-analysis of 161 studies exploring the relationship between parenting behaviors and delinquency, Hoeve and colleagues [24] found that the strongest associations were with parental monitoring, psychological control (e.g., authoritative versus authoritarian control), and negative support (e.g., rejection and hostility). However, few of these studies consider genetic risk transmitted from parents to offspring, which remains an important potential confounder when interpreting these findings.

Parental psychopathology has also been associated with both parental substance use and substance use in their children. Although both parental externalizing and internalizing psychopathology have been associated with offspring substance use, parental externalizing has perhaps been given the most attention. Numerous studies have shown that parental antisocial behavior is predictive of substance use behaviors in their children. For example, parental histories of cannabis use disorder, antisocial behavior, and rule-breaking behavior were predictive of cannabis use in adolescent and young adult offspring [32]. However, the fact that parental antisocial behavior is often concurrent with parental substance use makes it difficult to determine how parental psychopathology contributes specifically to offspring substance use risk. In fact, the latter may be a facet of externalizing behavior, one of its possible manifestations. Hicks et al. [33] investigated the extent to which the family transmission of risks for externalizing disorders, including conduct disorder, adult antisocial behavior, alcohol dependence, and drug dependence, was due to general (common) or disorder-specific liabilities. Although some evidence for specific transmission was found, most of the familial resemblance could be accounted for through the transmission of generalized risk. Kendler and colleagues [7], using a large cohort of Swedish men, found that the strongest predictors of AUD were externalizing and criminal behavior. In addition to pathways to AUD via father's alcohol consumption, they found strong evidence for a general externalizing pathway. They note, however, that these pathways are complex, interact over development, and include multiple mediational processes. Although genetic studies suggest common genetic mechanisms underlie the association between substance use and externalizing psychopathology [34, 35], the underlying mechanisms have not been determined. For example, deficits in inhibitory control are associated with antisocial and aggressive behavior [34, 36, 37]. Thus, one hypothesis is that parents with poor inhibitory control are unlikely to be able to form healthy attachments with their children and utilize effective discipline strategies [11, 17, 38]. However, because paternal substance use disorder (SUD) is often comorbid with other forms of psychopathology, it is difficult to disentangle whether cognitive deficits that interfere with effective parenting are due to psychopathology or chronic substance use [38].

The evidence for the role of internalizing psychopathology in the intergenerational transmission of substance use and addiction risks is perhaps weaker. However, several studies have shown that internalizing disorders are also associated with substance-related behavior [13, 39–44]. In a nationally representative sample of tenth graders, Conway and colleagues (2013) found that polysubstance use was strongly associated with depressive and somatic symptoms. Acheson et al. [39] used principal component analyses to differentiate young adults with a positive family history of alcohol or other drug use disorder from individuals without a positive family history. Three principal components significantly predicted positive family history. The first principal component consisted of measures indexing internalizing traits, with high scores indicating greater depression, anxiety, and emotional instability. The second principal component consisted of measures of externalizing traits, while the third consisted of cognitive measures (IQ and delayed discounting), SES, and education. Rothenberg and colleagues [45] found evidence for a depressive pathway to adolescent substance use after controlling for opportunities for use and externalizing symptoms. The authors propose that childhood internalizing symptoms may lead to later externalizing behavior, affiliations with deviant peers, and substance use in adolescence. Although there is evidence that internalizing behaviors are associated with substance misuse, less is known regarding the impact of the transmissible risk for internalizing disorders in parents on substance abuse risk in their children. Buu et al. [46] showed that after controlling for the effect of parental nicotine dependence symptoms, parental lifetime major depressive disorder (MDD) still predicted adolescent nicotine dependence symptoms. Kerr and colleagues [47] also showed that parental MDD and bipolar disorder symptoms increased the risk of MDD and SUDs in their offspring. Other studies have found no independent relationship between inhibitory traits in parents and substance use disorder in offspring [23, 32, 48], but the age at which offspring are assessed may be a factor. With some exceptions, most family studies focused on offspring in childhood and adolescence. Cloninger and colleagues [49, 50] have hypothesized that substance abuse onset after age 25 is characterized by internalizing behavior while early onset use is associated with disinhibitory externalizing behavior.

Sibling Resemblance

Family studies have consistently shown that sibling similarity is greater than parent-offspring similarity. This has been found in studies of smoking [6, 51], drinking [52–54], and cannabis use behavior [55]. Although the greater sibling similarity relative to parent-offspring similarity may be due to genetic differences (e.g., siblings share nonadditive genetic influences that parents and children do not), evidence suggests that siblings share more environmental influences than they share with their parents. Within families sibling interaction and direct behavioral modeling (contagion) have been proposed as important influences. Older siblings may facilitate access to substances for younger siblings or influence attitudes toward use. Several studies have shown that having an older sibling involved with smoking or other drug use is a strong predictor of smoking in younger siblings [27, 56]. The age difference between siblings and whether siblings are same-sex or opposite-sex may also be important moderators of sibling influence [57, 58]. In a recent review of twin studies of tobacco, alcohol, and cannabis use and dependence, Stallings et al. [59] showed that opposite-sex twin correlations were consistently lower than same-sex twin correlations. Although this could be genetic in origin (i.e., different genetic influences could be operating in males and females), it is equally or perhaps more likely that environmental factors operate differently in males and females, increasing the similarity of same-sex siblings relative to opposite-sex siblings.

The greater resemblance of siblings may also be the result of shared influences outside the family. The importance of extra-familial influences, particularly peer influences, both as main effects and as potential moderators of familial risk, has been investigated extensively [e.g., 29, 60–66]. Peer relationships play an important role in adolescent development, and affiliation with substance using peers is one of the strongest predictors of substance use in adolescence [31, 63, 65, 67]. Scherrer and colleagues [27] found that having a friend who was a smoker was the greatest predictor of offspring smoking—after accounting for familial liability (paternal and maternal nicotine dependence and heavy smoking status) and numerous parent and sibling level effects (e.g., parental discipline style, consistency of rules, parent-offspring closeness, and perceived parental and sibling other substance use). Further the prevalence of ever smoking, regular smoking, and nicotine dependence increased as the number of perceived friends who smoked increased.

Whether peer influences play a direct causal role in the development of substance use remains uncertain. Direct causality may arise from peers' serving as role models, influencing attitudes towards substance use, and facilitating access to substances. Alternatively, adolescents may select friends with similar substance use habits [62, 63], termed homophily. Individuals do not choose friends randomly, and there is evidence that genetic factors influence exposure to substance-using peers [62, 68]. Because of this selection process, genetic factors that increase one's risk for use may also explain, in part, resemblance of use with one's peers—a form of gene-environment correlation. It is likely that both peer selection and peer socialization (contagion influences) underlie peer resemblance for substance-related behavior. Fowler and colleagues [62] found evidence that active or reactive gene-environment correlation (rGE) contributes to peer selection effects, although passive rGE could have played some role as well. Active rGE occurs when an individual's genetic predisposition influences the selection and modification of their environment, while reactive rGE occurs when one's genetic predisposition influences the extent to which they are selected by others. Using genetically informative same-sex sibling pairs and their best friends from the National Longitudinal Study on Adolescent Health, Harden et al. [63] also found evidence for gene-environment correlation (i.e., friends' resemblance was influenced by the same genetic factors that contribute directly to substance use), but they found evidence for causal/socialization influences as well.

The relative importance of peer selection and socialization (contagion) influences in substance-related behavior likely depends on developmental phase. For example, Burk et al. [69] reported that both peer selection and socialization effects were present in early to late adolescence, with peer socialization influences becoming especially prominent in middle and later adolescence. Kirillova et al. [70] showed that sexual maturation in adolescent girls was predictive of peer deviance and that the relationship between sexual maturation and SUD risk was mediated by peer deviance. Alternatively, selection effects have been found to be more prominent in young adulthood [71, 72]. However, more well-designed longitudinal studies will be necessary to better disentangle the impact of peer socialization and selection processes [73]. Further, important moderators of peer influences need to be identified. For example, Harden and colleagues [63], using data from twins, non-twin siblings, and closest friends from the Add Health Study [74], found that the effects of friends' substance use were found to be strongest for adolescents with the highest genetic liability for use. Allen et al. [75] found that the influence of peers may vary as a function of internal factors (e.g., level of autonomy and parental support) and external factors (social status and acceptance of friends). They found that adolescents susceptible to peer influence (having low autonomy and poor deviance refusal skills) were very similar to their peers for drug and alcohol use, whereas more dominant (autonomous) adolescents were less similar to their peers. The findings suggest that peer pressure or peer influence is more likely a transactional (versus unidirectional) process that depends on characteristics of the peers involved in the relationship. Nearly all of this work has primarily examined dyadic relationships (e.g., target and best friend). It is likely that investigating larger peer networks will be necessary to better understand the extent of peer influences on substance-related behavior.

Family Transmission Models

An important strength of many of the family studies reviewed above is the use of multivariate structural equation models to test hypotheses underlying familial resemblance. However, dyadic approaches that focus on parent-offspring resemblance, siblings, or peer influences separately are also quite common. Unfortunately, when dyadic family relationships are examined separately, the presence of higher-order familial covariances can lead to biased parameter estimates. For example, interpreting parent-offspring or sibling correlations without taking spouse/mate correlations into account can lead to misinterpretations of the data. On the other hand, a substantial problem when conducting family analyses is that families come in all sizes and configurations. To accommodate this, sibling studies often study closest-in-age siblings, and parent-offspring studies focus on first-born children.

Although new approaches to family analysis are being developed, the work of Eaves et al. [76, 77] and Rice and Cloninger and colleagues in the late 1970s [62, 78, 79] paved the way for the development of analytical methods that treated the family as the unit of analysis. Their early work demonstrated how hypotheses about assortative mating, vertical parent-offspring transmission, and horizontal sibling influences could be modelled and tested simultaneously. They accommodated the unique family configurations encountered in studying families as a special case of missing data, and they showed how multivariate extensions of their models were straightforward generalizations. Their work, and the work of others, paved the way for current family study designs, including parents of twins, children of twins, and multivariate family designs.

Figure 5.1 shows the family transmission model used by Hopfer and colleagues (2003). The basic model allows one to simultaneously determine the extent to which familial resemblance for a given measured phenotype can be explained by vertical parent-offspring transmission of genetic and environmental influences (t), residual horizontal influences shared by siblings (H) that are not transmitted from parents to children, the effects of marital assortment (D), and non-transmissible influences (u) unique to individuals. The model demonstrates how expected parent-offspring and sibling correlations depend

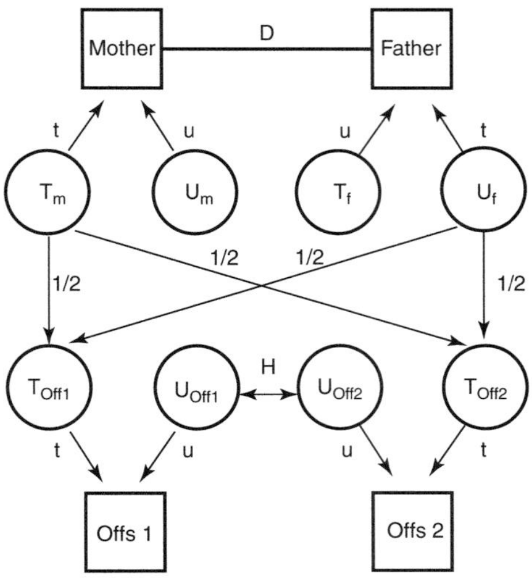

Fig. 5.1 Family transmission model

on higher-order correlations in the pedigree—specifically, assumptions about parental correlations for a given trait/behavior. If there is no assortative mating ($D = 0$), the expected correlation between an offspring and one parent is $1/2\ t^2$. However, if $D > 0$, then the expected parent-offspring correlation is $1/2\ t^2 + 1/2\ Dt^2$, the second term resulting from the magnitude of the correlation among parents. Note that the expected sibling correlation also depends on whether or not $D > 0$. Another feature of family transmission models (and structural equation models in general) is that they make assumptions explicit. In this model, t, the transmission parameter is the same in both generations. This assumption of intergenerational equilibrium, which is unlikely to hold for substance-related traits generally, is an assumption of all multigenerational parent-offspring designs. It assumes that genetic and environmental influences transmitted from parents to children have the same effect on both parental and offspring traits—despite the fact that they are usually assessed at quite different ages/developmental stages. Given generational differences in availability, substance use trends, and other factors, this is a strong assumption.

The basic model can be readily extended to the multivariate case in a straightforward manner [80, 81]. The variables and paths in the model become matrices of various forms (e.g., diagonal or full matrices). Further, it is not necessary that paternal and maternal transmission parameters are equal, and differences in parental resemblance with same-sex versus opposite-sex offspring can also be examined. Similarly, differential sibling effects for same-sex versus opposite-sex siblings can also be modelled.

This brief summary of family transmission models serves two purposes: (1) to recognize the pioneering work of Eaves et al. and Rice and colleagues and the tremendous influence this early work has had on the field [see 58, 62, 82–86]; and many others for extensions of this work] and (2) to note some of the assumptions that should be considered when interpreting parent-offspring and sibling correlations or predictions from family studies.

A number of family studies using variations or extensions of this model have been conducted. Observed spousal/mate, parent-offspring, and sibling correlations (or model-based estimates) for different substance-related behaviors are shown in the top portion of Table 5.1. For comparisons with estimates of sibling correlations from twin studies, the bottom portion of the Table includes weighted averages of same-sex dizygotic twin correlations (same-age siblings) from a recent review of twin studies of tobacco, alcohol, and cannabis behaviors [59]. The first notable finding in Table 5.1 is that spouse/mate correlations are not zero. In fact, they are frequently as great as, or greater than, the sibling correlations. First, this suggests that the assumption of random mating in the classic twin design is not supported. Second, it suggests that the interpretation of parent-offspring and sibling correlations from family studies of substance-related behavior should take spouse/mate correlations into account. Unfortunately, there is often insufficient information to determine the source of spouse/mate correlations. Mate/spousal similarity (homogamy) is likely due to a number of factors [87–89], including direct phenotypic assortment (selection of mates based on similar-

Table 5.1 Family correlations for substance-related behaviors

Reference	Year	Sample	Phenotype	R_{SP}	R_{PO}	R_{SIB}	R_{DZ}
Stallings et al.[a]	1997 [92]	CO Adolescent Substance Abuse study	Alcohol				
			DSM-IV criterion count (Alcohol Abuse plus Dependence)	0.31[d]	0.24[d]	0.26[d]	---
Hopfer et al. [a]	2003 [55]	CO Center on Antisocial Drug Dependence	Cannabis				
			Ever Use	0.70[d]	0.30[d]	0.39[d]	---
			Abuse	0.33[d]	0.28[d]	0.44[d]	
			Dependence	0.40[d]	0.17[d]	0.34[d]	
Hartman et al. [a]	2006 [53]	CO Center on Antisocial Drug Dependence	Alcohol Abuse	0.37[d]	0.19[d]	0.29[d]	
			Alcohol Dependence	0.14[d]	0.24[d]	0.34[d]	---
Agrawal et al.	2006 [90]	Australian Twin Sample	Regular Smoking	0.30	---	---	---
			Nicotine Dependence	0.31			
			Regular Alcohol Use	0.38			
			Alcohol Dependence	0.15			
Reynolds et al.	2006 [86]	Swedish Twin Registries	Tobacco Use	0.33			
			Tobacco Freq/Quant.	0.27			
			Alcohol Freq/Quant.	0.58			
Hicks et al.[b]	2013 [82]	Minnesota Twin and Family Study and Sibling Interaction and Behavior Study					
			Latent Externalizing	0.45		0.45	---
			Mother-Offspring		0.27		
			Father-Offspring		0.30		
Kendler et al.	2015 [85]	Swedish National Cohort Triparental Families	Drug Abuse				
			Mother-Father	0.18	---	---	---
			Mother-Stepfather	0.37			
			Alcohol Use Disorder				
			Mother-Father	0.05			
			Mother-Stepfather	0.25			
Samek et al.[b]	2015 [58]	Sibling Interaction and Behavior Study	Alcohol				
			Comp. Alcohol Use	0.45[d]		0.29[d]	---
			Older Sibling		0.10[d]		
			Younger Sibling		0.14[d]		
Saunders et al.[b]	2016 [93]	Minnesota Center For Twin and Family Research	Alcohol				
			Comp. Alcohol Use	---	0.21[c]	---	---
			Problem Use (sum of DSM-IIIR criteria)		0.15[c]		
Stallings et al.	2016 [59]	Review of Twin Studies	Tobacco	---	---	---	
			Use Adolescence				0.64
			Use Adulthood				0.40
			Freq/Quant Adoles.				0.55
			Freq/Quant Adult				0.54
			ND/HS Adolescence				0.60
			ND/HS Adult				0.29
Stallings et al.	2016 [59]	Review of Twin Studies	Alcohol	---	---	---	
			Use Adolescence				0.77
			Use Adulthood				0.58
			Freq/Quant Adoles.				0.42
			Freq/Quant Adult				0.35
			PRB Use Adoles.				0.59
			PRB Use Adult				0.27

Table 5.1 (continued)

Reference	Year	Sample	Phenotype	R_{SP}	R_{PO}	R_{SIB}	R_{DZ}
Stallings et al.	2016 [59]	Review of Twin Studies	Cannabis	---	---	---	
			Use Adolescence				0.68
			Use Adulthood				0.46
			Freq/Quant Adoles.				0.13
			Freq/Quant Adult				0.49
			PRB Use Adoles.				0.62
			PRB Use Adult				0.37

[a, b]indicates some sample overlap
[c]indicates mid-parent correlations averaged over offspring ages 14 to 29 use, 17–29 problem use
[d]correlations estimated from model parameters
ND/HS nicotine dependence or persistent/heavy smoking, *PRB Use* problem drinking or alcohol use disorder

ity in heritable traits), cohabitation effects (contagion, where mates influence one another to become more similar in behavior over time), and social homogamy (similarity due to environmental factors such as geographic location or SES). Phenotypic assortment leads to increased genetic resemblance among nonrelated mates, while cohabitation effects and social homogamy do not [86]. Reynolds and colleagues used a spouses-of-twins design to test phenotypic assortment and social homogamy processes underlying mate similarity for tobacco, alcohol, and caffeine use in participants from two Swedish studies. They found evidence for both phenotypic assortment and social homogamy underlying mate similarity for alcohol use, but only phenotypic assortment for tobacco and caffeine use. Agrawal et al. [90], also using a spouses-of-twins design, found evidence for assortative mating for regular cigarette smoking, nicotine dependence, regular alcohol use, and alcohol dependence in female twins and their partners from the Australian Twin Sample. They found no evidence for marital interaction (e.g., cohabitation effects) on regular smoking but mixed results for alcohol-related traits. Kendler and colleagues [91] found evidence for cohabitation effects for alcohol use disorder. Using a large sample of spouses from population-wide Swedish registries, they concluded that "a married individual's risk for alcohol use disorder is likely directly and causally affected by the presence of alcohol use disorder in his or her spouse." Studies that improve our understanding of the etiological origins of spouse/mate correlations and the implications of different mechanisms on parent-offspring and sibling resemblance for substance-related traits are clearly important.

Another notable finding from Table 5.1 is that sibling correlations tend to be larger than parent-offspring correlations. Sibling similarity has also been found to be greater than parent-offspring similarity in other studies reporting odds ratios and other statistics as well [6, 51, 52, 54]. Genetically, the expected genetic resemblance between parents and offspring and among siblings is similar [94]. Although siblings share non-additive genetic effects that parents and children do not, so genetic factors cannot be ruled out, the greater sibling versus parent-offspring resemblance may also suggest that the environment that siblings share may play a greater role in sibling similarity for substance-related behavior than the family environment influenced by parents. The comparison of non-twin sibling correlations with dizygotic (DZ) twin correlations also provides an important comparison. DZ twins and non-twin siblings have the same expected genetic covariance. Any differences between DZ twin and non-twin sibling correlations cannot be explained by direct genetic influences. This suggests that environmental differences between same-age twins and discordant-age siblings are responsible for the greater DZ twin correlations.

In the bottom portion of Table 5.1 are weighted averages of DZ twin correlations from twin studies reviewed by Stallings et al. [59]. The average DZ (same-age) twin correlations are consistently, and substantially, greater than the discordant-age sibling correlations from the family studies in Table 5.1. This is consistent with the hypothesis that sibling and peer influences, as well as peer selection effects, may make a larger contribution to the resemblance among same-age siblings than discordant-age siblings.

General (Common) Liability

Substance use is rarely limited to one drug. Individuals who abuse one substance are more likely to abuse others [4, 95–98]. Indeed, polysubstance use appears to be the norm—particularly in adolescence and young adulthood [13, 99–101]. Consistent with findings from twin studies, family studies have also found evidence for both common and specific risks for substance-related behaviors. For example, Obot et al. [102] found that the offspring of alcohol-dependent parents were also more likely to smoke tobacco and marijuana, and Merikangas et al. [3] found higher rates of nicotine dependence in the relatives of probands with alcohol and cannabis use disorders than in relatives of controls. Young et al. [101] examined use and problem use (defined as meeting one or more DSM-IV dependence criteria) of tobacco, alcohol, and cannabis in a sample of 3744 adolescents (ages 12–18), including 1347 twin pairs, 429 non-twin sibling pairs, and 96 adoptive sibling pairs. Heritability estimates for tobacco, alcohol, and cannabis use were relatively modest, ranging from 5% to 46%, and genetic correlations among use measures were also modest, ranging from 0.14 to 0.31. Sibling resemblance for substance use was primarily explained by shared environmental influences, with a substantial proportion due to shared environmental factors shared by twins or same-age siblings. For problem use of tobacco, alcohol, and cannabis, respectively, heritability estimates increased to 60%, 54%, and 70%. Genetic correlations also increased substantially, ranging from 0.56 to 0.62, whereas correlations among shared environmental factors were negligible. These findings suggest that genetic factors play a greater role in variation in liability to problem use than to substance use initiation, and the extent to which common genetic factors contribute to comorbidity increases for more severe patterns of use. Other family studies have stressed the importance of both common and specific familial risks [e.g., 103], and Volk et al. [104], using a children-of-twins design, found evidence for the specificity of genetic influences on nicotine dependence and alcohol dependence.

Substance use also frequently co-occurs with conduct problems and other disruptive antisocial behavior [105–109]. Conduct problems usually precede substance involvement [110, 111], and clear trajectories have been noted from early externalizing behavior to a range of problems during adolescence and adulthood, including delinquency, substance abuse, and antisocial behavior [112–115]. Family studies have made important contributions to our understanding of the comorbidity of antisocial behavior and substance use. For example, Lynskey et al. [116] showed that 15-year-old offspring of parents with alcohol problems were three times as likely to receive a diagnosis of conduct disorder or oppositional defiant disorder than were offspring of parents with no history of alcohol problems. Kendler et al. [117] reported that offspring of parents with alcohol dependence or antisocial personality disorder were twice as likely to develop these disorders, and Markon et al. [118] showed that alcohol dependence, drug dependence, and antisocial personality disorder could be modeled as a single externalizing factor. Hicks and colleagues have suggested that "what parents transmit to their offspring is a non-specific, genetic liability to multiple externalizing disorders" [82]. Franco and colleagues [119] also provide evidence that substance use disorders (SUDs) increase the risk of adverse adult outcomes primarily through a general predisposition, or mechanisms shared across substance use disorders, rather than substance-specific outcomes.

What underlies this general liability remains an important question of study. However, one hypothesis that has received considerable empirical support is the notion that SUDs, in particular early-onset SUD, are one facet of a syndrome of externalizing behaviors characterized by disinhibitory psychopathology related to pursuit of reward and the diminished ability to inhibit inappropriate behavior in the face of negative consequences [33–35, 37, 50, 109, 112, 120–127]. This hypothesis is not new. Jessor and Jessor [107] proposed their generalized problem behavior theory in the 1970s, and Gorenstein and Newman [128] hypothesized "that [antisocial behavior] and [alcohol dependence] co-occur because, like other related problems, they are indicators of a common, genetically influenced latent factor of general disinhibition or impulsivity." What is new is that evidence is converging in support of this hypothesis. Consistent with the notion that disinhibitory psychopathology is a common feature of externalizing disorders, findings from neurophysiological studies [34, 129–132] provide evidence related to prefrontal cortex dysfunction. The prefrontal cortex has been implicated in inhibiting inappropriate responses and regulating behavior in relation to future reward [132]. Attenuated amplitude of the P300 component of the electrocortical event-related potential has also been associated with youth at risk for SUD [34, 133, 134], as well as with other externalizing disorders such as conduct problems [129], attention-deficit hyperactivity disorder (ADHD) [135, 136], and impulsivity [137]. Iacono and colleagues [130, 131] have shown that reduced P3 amplitude at age 17 predicts SUDs in general 3 years later at age 20. Moreover, reduced P3 amplitude was associated with the full spectrum of externalizing disorders, including ADHD, conduct disorder, oppositional defiant disorder, antisocial personality disorder, and SUDs. Although the biological relationship between P3 amplitude and executive cognitive function remains unknown, Begleiter and Porjesz [138] have proposed that P3 amplitude most strongly reflects frontal-parietal cortical activity, and reduced P3 amplitude may be a marker of impaired inhibitory regulation. Although there are likely to be multiple pathways to SUD, there is now accumulating evidence that SUDs share common etiological features with each other and with other disinhibitory or externalizing behaviors and disorders [for a review, see 132].

Studies have found evidence for substance-specific transmission as well [85, 103, 104, 139, 140]. Although Bornovalova et al. [139] found that parent-child resemblance was accounted for by the transmission of a general liability to externalizing disorders, specific effects were also detected, but specific influences primarily contributed to sibling resemblance. Farmer and colleagues [140] found support for both general and specific risk associated with abuse of or dependence on specific substances and found that within families sibling influences on a proband were generally stronger than maternal and paternal influences. Long et al. [141] have also reported some evidence for specificity. They showed that the offspring of parents with AUD showed a two- to threefold increased risk for AUD, but also drug abuse, criminal behavior, and ADHD. Maternal AUD was associated with a greater risk than paternal AUD for both sons and daughters, and having two parents with AUD increased risk more than only having one. For drug abuse and criminal behavior, they found sex differences (in both parents and children) that moderated parent-offspring risk. Nadel and Thornberry [9] suggest that evidence for familial transmission depends on when in the parent's life course substance use occurs or is assessed, and Saunders et al. [93] have shown that parent-offspring correlations vary as a function of age. Vrieze et al. [142] have shown that adolescent substance abuse and dependence are largely due to common or generalized risk. However, as young people age, factors contributing to liability variation become more substance-specific. This emphasizes the need for more long-term longitudinal family studies that follow offspring well into adulthood.

In summary, research on substance use and SUDs has tended to focus on single substances or a single class of substances. Although much insight into the addiction process has been gained through this strategy, polysubstance use is normative and characteristic of most individuals with SUD. Furthermore, substance use is frequently comorbid with a spectrum of other externalizing traits and behaviors. Indeed, it is becoming clear that a complete understanding of the addiction process will likely require the investigation of substance use within this comorbid context, rather than in isolation. Multivariate family and adoption studies have provided compelling evidence that common genetic risk and protective factors influence substance use and vulnerability to addiction to all classes of addictive drugs. Furthermore, there is substantial evidence that the same genetic factors contribute to variation in liability to a broad spectrum of externalizing disorders and disinhibitory traits. Although many of the studies reviewed have reported evidence for generalized risk, substance-specific effects are found as well. Understanding both will be important for improving our understanding of the familial aggregation of substance-related behaviors.

Developmental Studies

Substance use disorders and comorbid psychopathology develop over time. While some factors may influence multiple developmental stages, there is evidence to suggest that different risk and protective factors are uniquely associated with the onset, progression, and persistence of substance use. To be fully understood, prospective longitudinal assessment is imperative. However, many family studies are cross-sectional and use lifetime or single-point assessments of substance use in parents and offspring. Longitudinal family studies are providing important insights about familial resemblance not possible from cross-sectional studies. For example, Vuolo and Staff [51] showed that the length of time a parent smokes may have important implications for offspring risk. They made use of 19 assessments of parent and offspring smoking over a 23-year period to show that the risk of smoking in offspring was greater for parents who were persistent heavy smokers than for lighter smokers and smokers that quit later in adulthood. The observed differences were modest, however, and having an older sibling who smoked mediated the effect of parent use in heavy smoking households. Sibling and peer influences on drinking behavior have also been shown to decrease with age. Saunders et al. [93] examined parent-offspring correlations across multiple assessments spanning offspring age 14 to age 29. They found evidence that parent-offspring correlations for alcohol use and problem use tended to peak at age 17 and then decrease over time to age 29. This pattern was more notable for problem alcohol use than for a composite drinking index. On the other hand, O'Loughlin and colleagues [10] found that the odds of offspring using cannabis in high school and young adulthood given their parents reported past-year cannabis use were essentially the same.

In family studies parent-offspring resemblance confounds genetic and environmental effects. The same is true for peer influences. As noted above, peer influences likely include direct influences (e.g., imitation, facilitating access to drugs) as well as the effects of peer selection. Genetic predisposition likely plays an important role in the selection of peers and maintenance of friendships. The following studies examine an important issue: the extent to which parental and peer influences may change over development. However, it is important to keep these confounds in mind when interpreting these findings. Several studies have shown a decrease in the effect of putative family environmental influences and an increase in the influence of peers over time—presumably as adolescents mature and gain more autonomy [29, 64, 65]. Van Ryzin and colleagues [65] found that parental monitoring, quality of family relationships, and affiliation with deviant peers were predictive of substance use in adolescence, but peer deviance was the only significant predictor of use in early adulthood. In adulthood, the influence of parental monitoring and family relationship quality (family context) on substance use risk was mediated by peer deviance (peer group affiliation). Kirillova et al. [70] also found that peer deviance developmentally mediated the effect of parental SUD load (number of affected parents) on children's SUD risk. In contrast, Scholte et al. (2007) found that the relative risk of alcohol use given regular drinking friends decreased from 4.79 at ages 12–15, to 2.19 at ages 16–20, to 1.76 by ages 21–25. Epstein and colleagues [143] investigated the influence of family monitoring and antisocial peers as time-varying effects on cannabis use in a longitudinal study of youth ages 11 to 19. They found that these influences remained steady over this age range and were stronger for girls than boys. Although this is a fairly narrow age range, these data are inconsistent with the hypothesis that family environmental influences (direct environmental effects) become less important across adolescence while peer influences increase. Some evidence suggests developmental patterns may vary as a function of substance used. For example, Kendler et al. [144] showed that substantial shared environmental influences on cannabis use (including both familial and extra-familial influences) may extend further into young adulthood than for smoking and drinking. Although it is clear that family factors contribute to substance abuse risk, newer longitudinal family studies are beginning to shine a light on the complex nature of these processes. These findings have highlighted important changes in parent-offspring and sibling resemblance across development that need further investigation.

Adoption Studies

Unlike studies of biological families, adoption studies provide researchers a tool for separating the relative contributions of genetic and environmental influences on liability variation. In a typical adoption study design, data are available from adoptive children (adoptees), their biological parents (from whom they were separated early in life), and their adoptive parents (to whom they are biologically unrelated). The degree of resemblance between adoptive children and their biological parents ("genetic parents"), with whom they share genetic factors but not (or limited) environmental factors, provides an estimate of the contribution of genetic influences. The degree of resemblance between adoptive children and their genetically unrelated adoptive parents ("environmental parents") provides an estimate of the importance of environmental influences that contribute to parent-offspring resemblance. In extended adoption designs that include adoptive siblings, the degree of resemblance among genetically unrelated siblings provides an estimate of the importance of shared environmental influences that contribute to the resemblance of siblings raised together in the same family [for more details, see 145–147].

Figure 5.2 shows a full adoption design that includes nonadoptive control families (both genetic and environmental transmission; top portion of the Figure) and adoptive families (environmental transmission only; lower portion). Like in family studies, a number of assumptions must be made in interpreting findings from adoption studies. First, as noted previously, a limitation of any intergenerational family design is the potential for generational differences in substance availability, use patterns, or other factors that differ between parents and children. When genetic and environmental influences differ between generations, the interpretation of parent-offspring resemblance is not straightforward [147]. The inclusion of adoptive and nonadoptive siblings into the adoptive family design can provide a means for addressing this limitation. Although age and cohort effects may still apply to siblings (e.g., siblings may differ in age by several years), these influences would be expected to be less substantial compared to generational differences. Adoption designs also assume the absence of "selective placement." Selective (nonrandom) placement of adoptive children with adoptive parents can occur when adoptees are placed with relatives or when there is some direct or indirect matching of biological and adoptive family characteristics during placement. The influence of selective placement can be tested by assessing the resemblance between biological and adoptive parents for the trait or behavior of interest; significant parental correlations would suggest selective placement effects.

Another assumption of the adoption design is that *only* genetic factors contribute to the resemblance between biological parents and their

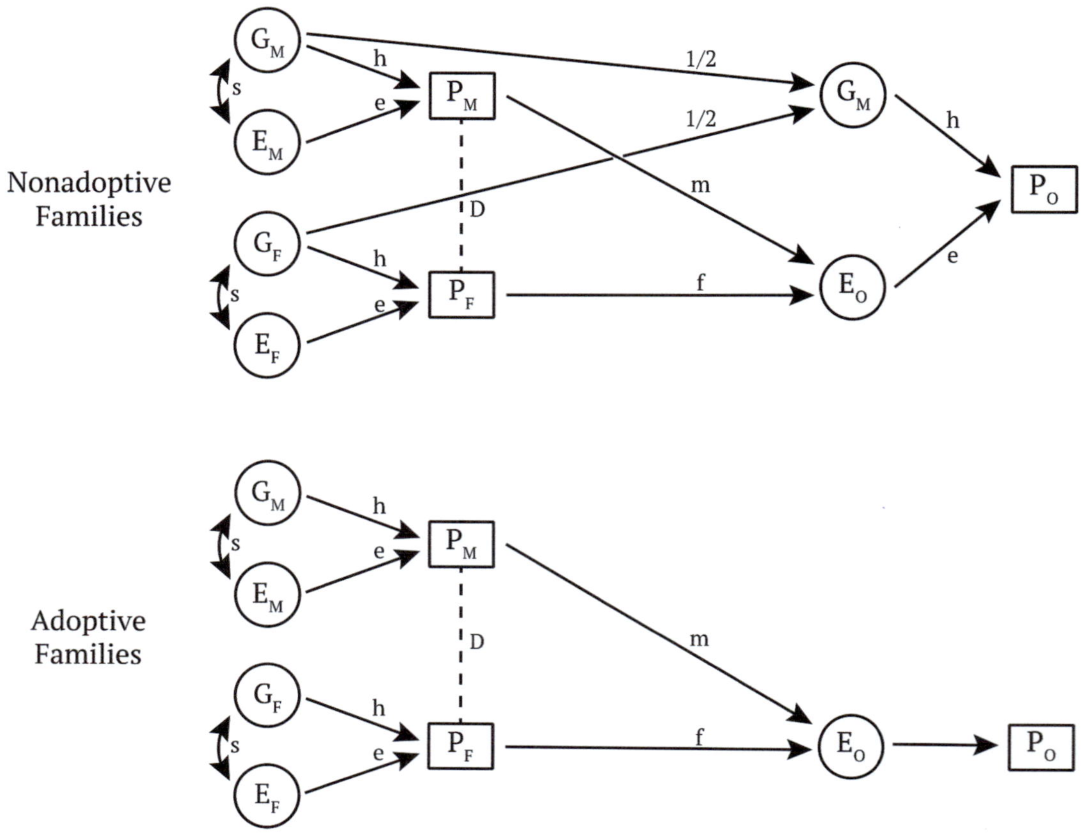

Fig. 5.2 Genetic and environmental resemblance in adoptive and nonadoptive families

adopted-away offspring. However, the extent to which prenatal and pre-adoption postnatal environmental influences may also contribute should be addressed. Although early placement of adoptees in adoptive homes is assumed in adoption designs (and presumed to minimize such influences), prenatal environmental effects and early maternal effects may still contribute to the resemblance between adopted-away children and their biological mothers. Greater similarity between adopted-away children and their mothers, compared to their fathers, may indicate early maternal environmental effects. Adoption designs have also been criticized for potential environmental range restriction in adoptive families [148]. That is, given that most adoption agencies engage in some screening of adoptive parents, it has been argued that extreme behaviors (e.g., serious substance abuse or psychopathology) have been selected against, resulting in a population of adoptive parents that is not representative of parents in general. However, McGue et al. [149] have reported only limited evidence for range restriction on a number of environmental dimensions that would be expected to be associated with substance use in the Minnesota Sibling Interaction and Behavior Study. Moreover, although they did find some evidence for restricted range in adoptive parents, they found no evidence that range restriction on these dimensions affected estimates of adoptive-sibling correlations for measures of substance use, delinquency, or IQ.

Early adoption studies of adult alcohol-related behavior [49, 150–152] have reported significant associations between family history of alcoholism in biological relatives and adoptee drinking behavior. In a follow-up of the Iowa adoption studies [150, 151], Yates et al. [153] reported further evidence for genetic influences and found the magnitude of genetic effects was dependent on the severity of problem alcohol use in the adoptees. In contrast, findings regarding associations with adoptive relative histories have been mixed. McGue et al. [57] specifically examined the differential effects of parent and sibling influences in a US adolescent adoption cohort (aged 12–18), drawn from adoption agencies in Colorado, Illinois, Minnesota, and Wisconsin. The 653 adoptive families included 68 families with a second adolescent offspring biologically related to the adoptive parents (birth offspring) and 187 families with a second adopted child. They found that parental problem drinking was significantly correlated with adolescent alcohol involvement in the smaller birth offspring sample but not in the much larger adopted offspring sample. Correlations were highest between mothers and their birth daughters ($r = 0.33$) and between fathers and birth sons ($r = 0.64$). Correlations between adoptive parents and their adoptive offspring ranged from $r = 0.00$ to 0.07. Measures of family functioning characteristics (e.g., religious, cohesive, authoritarian, intellectual, organized) were highly predictive of alcohol involvement in birth offspring ($r^2 = 0.23$), but only modestly predictive ($r^2 = 0.04$) for adoptive offspring. This differential prediction suggests that these measures of family function are not simply indices of the family environment. The findings are more consistent with the notion that genetic factors, at least in part, are a source of the relationship between parental drinking, family functioning, and adolescent alcohol involvement. Conversely, this study also reported an adoptive sibling correlation for alcohol involvement of $r = 0.24$, which provides a direct estimate of shared environmental influences on sibling resemblance. That is, approximately 24% of the variance in alcohol involvement in this study of adolescents could be explained by environmental factors shared by siblings. The adoptive sibling correlation was also increased for same-sex siblings ($r = 0.36$) and for siblings closer in age ($r = 0.35$), which is consistent with the hypothesis that sibling modeling/imitation and overlapping peer influences underlie adoptive sibling resemblance. Consistent with some of the family studies above, these findings suggested that adolescent drinking is substantially influenced by shared environmental effects specific to siblings but only minimally by the environmental consequences of family functioning and parental drinking behavior. Using longitudinal data from ages 14 to 18 from the Colorado Adoption Project, Huibregtse et al. [154] found evidence for increasing genetic influences on variation in tobacco and alcohol use across adolescence. Kendler et al. [155] made use of three-generation family data from a large Swedish cohort to show that the familial transmission of AUD risk was remarkably stable over three generations. They found that males and females transmit risk for AUD equally to their descendants, but found that parents transmit higher liability to their same-sex descendants than to their opposite-sex descendants (e.g., mother-daughter resemblance was greater than mother-son resemblance).

Findings from adoption studies also provide evidence for a pathway to SUD through disinhibitory behavior. Cadoret and colleagues [150, 151, 156] reported two independent genetic pathways to drug abuse/dependence. The first pathway involved the direct transmission of substance-related risk factors from biological parents to their children. A second pathway started with antisocial personality disorder in the parents leading to antisocial behavior and then, ultimately, drug abuse/dependency in their children [156]. A reanalysis of updated data [157] confirmed these pathways but also suggested that the combination of antisocial behavior and substance problems may represent another distinct pathway. Findings from the Minnesota Adoption Study [158] provided evidence for generalized genetic risk, as well as a non-specific environmentally mediated pathway. In adoptive families, exposure to parental smoking was found to be an environmental risk for substance use in adolescent offspring. However, exposure to parental smoking in nonadoptive families had both stronger and more diverse influences. Smoking in biological parents was associated with greater substance use, disruptive behavior disorders, delinquency, deviant peer affiliations, aggressive attitudes, and preference for risk taking. King et al. [159] found similar results for alcohol-related traits. They compared adopted and non-adopted adolescents reared in families where at least one parent was diagnosed with alcohol dependence (ever or currently) to those reared in families where neither parent met criteria for a lifetime diagnosis of alcohol abuse or dependence. A history of parental alcohol dependence was associated with higher levels of disinhibition only when adolescents were biologically related to their rearing parents. This suggests that the effects of parental alcohol dependence on offspring behavioral disinhibition were largely attributable to genetic rather than environmental transmission. Further, parental alcohol dependence was associated with elevated levels on a variety of indicators of behavioral disinhibition, and not just on alcohol or other substance use. Hicks et al. (2013) [82] found strong evidence for the transmission of general liability to addiction rather than substance-specific transmission. Parent-offspring correlations for a general externalizing factor for biological parents were $r = 0.27$ and $r = 0.30$ for mothers and fathers, respectively, but were not significant for adoptive parents ($r = 0.03$ and 0.07, for adoptive mothers and fathers). In contrast, adoptive siblings showed significant correlations on the general externalizing liability ($r = 0.21$). Findings indicated that the general externalizing liability was highly heritable, but they also found significant shared environmental influences specific to siblings. Fewer adoption studies have investigated pathways to SUD through internalizing disorders. Marmorstein et al. (2012) [48] found no evidence that parental major depressive disorder (MDD) increased the risk of SUDs in either adoptive or non-adoptive families. However, parental nicotine dependence and cannabis use disorder predicted increased risk for MDD in non-adopted, but not adopted adolescents, indicating a genetic origin for the association between parental SUD and offspring MDD.

Alternative Family Designs

Of the methods available to behavioral geneticists, adoption studies provide the most convincing evidence for genetic and environmental influences on variation in complex human traits [145]. However, adoption data can be more difficult to acquire due to legal and confidentiality issues and often require comparisons between adoptive and non-adoptive families that may differ on characteristics that are unknown. Kendler et al. [85] took advantage of more common step-parent families in a large Swedish national sample to examine parent-offspring resemblance for AUD, drug abuse, and criminal behavior in "tri-parental families." In these families every offspring had one biological parent who reared them (shared genes plus rearing effects), one "not-lived-with" biological parent with whom they had minimal contact (shared genes only), and one step-parent (rearing influences only). The design allows for tests of some of the same hypotheses as adoption studies, but utilizes within-family data that is more readily available than in traditional adoption studies. Kendler and colleagues [85] found that parent-offspring resemblance was greatest for offspring and their "reared-with" biological mother (influenced by both shared genetic and shared environmental factors), intermediate with "not-lived-with" biological fathers (genetic influences only), and least for offspring and step-fathers (shared environmental influences only) for drug abuse, AUD, and criminal behavior. Given the lower but significant resemblance to step-fathers, the findings suggest that both shared genetic and shared environmental influences underlie parent-offspring similarity, with genetic influences playing a greater role. Kendler et al. [160] developed a similar sibling design that utilizes differences in the expected genetic and environmental contributions to the similarity of full-siblings, half-siblings, and step-siblings, taking cohabitation history into account. Heritability estimates based on non-twin siblings were comparable to twin estimates for alcohol and drug use behavior. In general, findings from adoptive families have been very consistent with family studies. Because adoptive families allow estimation of genetic and environmental contributions to familial correlations, they can provide important insights into the potential mechanisms underlying the familial aggregation of substance-related behaviors that traditional family studies cannot. Unfortunately, due to ethical issues, confidentiality, and other pragmatic concerns, adoption studies are much less common than family studies. However, recent studies by Kendler and colleagues [85, 160] suggest promising methods for investigating genetic and environmental hypotheses regarding familial resemblance using family data.

Summary and Future Directions

The findings reviewed in this chapter clearly demonstrate that substance use and substance use disorders aggregate in families. Consistent with the twin literature, family and adoption studies also provide evidence that both general and specific familial risk factors are transmitted from parents to offspring. There is compelling evidence for a pathway to SUD through generalized liability to a broad spectrum of externalizing disorders and disinhibitory traits, but some studies have suggested internalizing behavior pathways as well. Important intra- and extra-familial predictors of substance use have been identified, and similar moderators of parent-offspring and sibling resemblance for substance-related behaviors have been reported. More longitudinal family and adoption studies that allow for the investigation of developmental changes in familial influences are essential. Importantly, family and adoption studies, which make different assumptions than twin studies, have provided very similar findings to those from twin studies. This contradicts the possibility that the overestimation of heritability from twin studies is a major contributor to the "missing heritability" problem (i.e., that known associations with genetic polymorphisms do not account for those heritability estimates).

This chapter also highlights some of the shortcomings of available data and challenges future studies will need to address. The family and adoption studies reviewed here primarily include participants of European ancestry. Studies that do include participants from understudied populations often lack the power to investigate group differences or moderating influences. This may limit the generalizability of findings if important, but undetected, differences in familial risk are not accommodated. Although numerous studies have investigated substance-related behaviors in different cultures and racial/ethnic groups at the individual level [e.g., 161–165], there are few family and adoption studies with adequate representation of diverse populations. Efforts to increase diversity in genetically informative studies are underway, but concerns regarding generalizability are a shortcoming of the currently available data.

Although longitudinal family and adoption data are becoming available, it is clear that more prospective family studies that assess offspring from childhood into adulthood are needed. Moreover, when and how parental substance use is assessed is also important. Many of the family and adoption studies reviewed here are cross-sectional, and most have focused on offspring substance use during the adolescent years. Parental substance use is often assessed with lifetime indices of substance use or disorder that do not consider age of onset, current use, or chronicity of use. These cross-sectional studies have made important contributions to the field, but they offer just a snapshot of familial influences at a specific point in development. It is quite possible that some of the inconsistency in findings across studies is due to developmental differences in assessment and study design. Studies that did assess parents or offspring on multiple occasions tended to find evidence for developmental changes in parental, sibling, and peer influences, as well as changes in the moderation of effects across development [e.g., 9, 51, 65, 166]. Substance use and substance use disorders develop over time. To fully understand the etiological sources of familial risk, and how those risks are transmitted in families and shared among siblings and peers, longitudinal analyses are imperative.

Family and adoption studies have identified important family processes and pathways that contribute to substance abuse risk, and these study designs will continue to provide important insights into the future. However, efforts to identify the specific genetic variants that contribute to transmissible genetic risk have only recently begun. Although very large genome-wide association studies (GWAS) have identified some replicated individual variants associated with substance-related traits [e.g., 167], polygenic scores [168] that essentially sum the allelic effects of single nucleotide polymorphisms (SNPs) across the entire genome have become an important tool for substance abuse researchers. As polygenic scores (PGSs) derived from larger and larger discovery samples show increased prediction utility, the innovative use of polygenic scores in family studies will enable investigations to disentangle genetic risks that are directly transmitted from parents to children from gene-environment correlational mechanisms including "genetic nurturing" (where parental genetic predispositions shape the environment they provide for their children). Kong et al. [169] have shown that prediction using a typical PGS from the alleles transmitted from father and mother (T_P and T_M in Fig. 5.3) also includes any indirect effects of parental genotypes on environmental variables (Y_P and Y_M). Although Kong et al. investigated a PGS for educational attainment, the same process applies to substance-related behavior. For example, suppose X_0 in Fig. 5.3 represents a substance use behavior in offspring. Parental genotypes (paternal genotypes in the rectangle and maternal genotypes in the circle) influence the offspring trait (X_0) through direct genetic transmission (the direct effect of transmitted alleles T_P and T_m on X_0) but also an indirect path through their genetic effects on the environment they provide for their children. By creating PGS using both transmitted alleles (T_P, T_M) and non-transmitted alleles (NT_P, NT_M), the

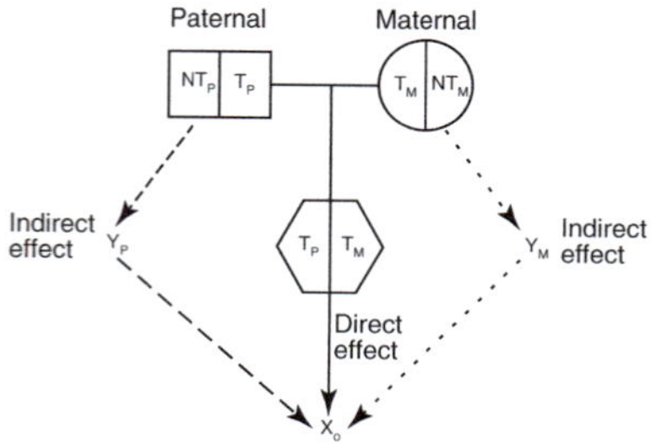

Fig. 5.3 Distinguishing direct and indirect genetic influences using polygenic scores based on transmitted and non-transmitted alleles; adapted from Kong et al. [169]

effects of these two paths can be estimated. Similarly, PGS can be used to investigate peer socialization versus peer selection processes. If peers influence each other via environmental mechanisms, their PGS should not correlate. If, however, individuals select peers who are similar to them (peer selection; homophily), then one may see correlations among their PGS. Family and adoption studies continue to make important contributions to our understanding of how genetic and environmental components of variation in risk for substance-related behaviors are transmitted and shared among family members. The progress in molecular genetic studies of substance abuse will not make family studies obsolete. On the contrary, the incorporation of genomic variables into family studies has considerable promise for the future.

References

1. Cotton NS. The familial incidence of alcoholism: a review. J Stud Alcohol. 1979;40:89–116.
2. Avenevoli S, Merikangas KR. Familial influences on adolescent smoking. Addiction. 2003;98:1–20.
3. Merikangas KR, Stolar M, Stevens DE, Goulet J, Preisig MA, Fenton B, et al. Familial transmission of substance use disorders. Arch Gen Psychiatry. American Medical Association. 1998;55:973–9.
4. Kessler RC, McGonagle KA, Zhao S, Nelson CB, Hughes M, Eshleman S, et al. Lifetime and 12-month prevalence of DSM-III-R psychiatric disorders in the United States: results from the National Comorbidity Survey. Arch Gen Psychiatry. American Medical Association. 1994;51:8–19.
5. Homel J, Warren D. The relationship between parent drinking and adolescent drinking: differences for mothers and fathers and boys and girls. Substance Use & Misuse. Taylor & Francis. 2019;54:661–9.
6. Leonardi-Bee J, Jere ML, Britton J. Exposure to parental and sibling smoking and the risk of smoking uptake in childhood and adolescence: a systematic review and meta-analysis. Thorax. BMJ Publishing Group Ltd. 2011;66:847–55.
7. Kendler KS, Ohlsson H, Edwards AC, Sundquist J, Sundquist K. A developmental model for alcohol use disorders in Swedish men. Psychol Med. 2016;46:2759–70.
8. Kosty DB, Farmer RF, Seeley JR, Merikangas KR, Klein DN, Gau JM, et al. The number of biological parents with alcohol use disorder histories and risk to offspring through age 30. Addict Behav. 2020;102:106196.

9. Nadel EL, Thornberry TP. Intergenerational consequences of adolescent substance use: patterns of homotypic and heterotypic continuity. Psychol Addict Behav. US: American Psychological Association. 2017;31:200–11.
10. O'Loughlin JL, Dugas EN, O'Loughlin EK, Winickoff JP, Montreuil A, Wellman RJ, et al. Parental cannabis use is associated with cannabis initiation and use in offspring. J Pediatr. 2019;206:142–147.e1.
11. Pears K, Capaldi DM, Owen LD. Substance use risk across three generations: the roles of parent discipline practices and inhibitory control. Psychol Addict Behav US: American Psychological Association. 2007;21:373–86.
12. Sher KJ, Walitzer KS, Wood PK, Brent EE. Characteristics of children of alcoholics: putative risk factors, substance use and abuse, and psychopathology. J Abnorm Psychol. US: American Psychological Association. 1991;100:427–48.
13. Conway KP, Vullo GC, Nichter B, Wang J, Compton WM, Iannotti RJ, et al. Prevalence and patterns of polysubstance use in a nationally representative sample of 10th graders in the United States. J Adolesc Health. 2013;52:716–23.
14. Holst C, Tolstrup JS, Sørensen HJ, Becker U. Family structure and alcohol use disorder: a register-based cohort study among offspring with and without parental alcohol use disorder. Addiction. 2020;115:1440–9.
15. McCutcheon VV, Agrawal A, Kuo SI-C, Su J, Dick DM, Meyers JL, et al. Associations of parental alcohol use disorders and parental separation with offspring initiation of alcohol, cigarette and cannabis use and sexual debut in high-risk families. Addiction. 2018;113:336–45.
16. Waldron M, Grant JD, Bucholz KK, Lynskey MT, Slutske WS, Glowinski AL, et al. Parental separation and early substance involvement: results from children of alcoholic and cannabis dependent twins. Drug Alcohol Depend. 2014;134:78–84.
17. Martin MJ, Conger RD, Robins RW. Family stress processes and drug and alcohol use by Mexican American adolescents. Dev Psychol. American Psychological Association. 2019;55:170–83.
18. Windle M, Windle RC. Parental divorce and family history of alcohol disorder: associations with Young adults' alcohol problems, marijuana use, and interpersonal relations. Alcohol Clin Exp Res. 2018;42:1084–95.
19. Hill M, Sternberg A, Suk HW, Meier MH, Chassin L. The intergenerational transmission of cannabis use: associations between parental history of cannabis use and cannabis use disorder, low positive parenting, and offspring cannabis use. Psychol Addict. Behav US: American Psychological Association. 2018;32:93–103.
20. Dishion TJ, Capaldi DM, Yoerger K. Middle childhood antecedents to progressions in male adolescent substance use: an ecological analysis of risk and protection. J Adolescent Res. SAGE Publications Inc. 1999;14:175–205.
21. Dever BV, Schulenberg JE, Dworkin JB, O'Malley PM, Kloska DD, Bachman JG. Predicting risk-taking with and without substance use: the effects of parental monitoring, school bonding, and sports participation. Prev Sci. 2012;13:605–15.
22. Fallu J-S, Janosz M, Brière FN, Descheneaux A, Vitaro F, Tremblay RE. Preventing disruptive boys from becoming heavy substance users during adolescence: a longitudinal study of familial and peer-related protective factors. Addict Behav. 2010;35:1074–82.
23. Hill KG, Hawkins JD, Bailey JA, Catalano RF, Abbott RD, Shapiro VB. Person–environment interaction in the prediction of alcohol abuse and alcohol dependence in adulthood. Drug Alcohol Depend. 2010;110:62–9.
24. Hoeve M, Dubas JS, Eichelsheim VI, van der Laan PH, Smeenk W, Gerris JRM. The relationship between parenting and delinquency: a meta-analysis. J Abnorm Child Psychol. 2009;37:749–75.
25. Brook JS, Whiteman M, Balka EB, Cohen P. Parent drug use, parent personality, and parenting. J Genet Psychol. Routledge. 1995;156:137–51.
26. Fals-Stewart W, Kelley ML, Fincham FD, Golden J, Logsdon T. Emotional and behavioral problems of children living with drug-abusing fathers: comparisons with children living with alcohol-abusing and non-substance-abusing fathers. J Family Psychol. US: American Psychological Association. 2004;18:319–30.
27. Scherrer JF, Xian H, Pan H, Pergadia ML, Madden PAF, Grant JD, et al. Parent, sibling and peer influences on smoking initiation, regular smoking and nicotine dependence. Results from a genetically informative design. Addict Behav. 2012;37:240–7.
28. Lee JY, Kim W, Brook JS, Finch SJ, Brook DW. Adolescent risk and protective factors predicting triple trajectories of substance use from adolescence into adulthood. J Child Fam Stud. 2020;29:403–12.
29. Cleveland MJ, Feinberg ME, Bontempo DE, Greenberg MT. The role of risk and protective factors in substance use across adolescence. J Adolesc Health. 2008;43:157–64.
30. Ryan SM, Jorm AF, Lubman DI. Parenting factors associated with reduced adolescent alcohol use: a systematic review of longitudinal studies. Aust N Z J Psychiatry. SAGE Publications Ltd. 2010;44:774–83.
31. Allen M, Donohue WA, Griffin A, Ryan D, Turner MMM. Comparing the influence of parents and peers on the choice to use drugs: a meta-analytic summary of the literature. Crim Justice Behav. SAGE Publications Inc. 2003;30:163–86.
32. Kosty DB, Farmer RF, Seeley JR, Gau JM, Duncan SC, Lewinsohn PM. Parental transmission of risk for cannabis use disorders to offspring. Addiction. 2015;110:1110–7.

33. Hicks BM, Krueger RF, Iacono WG, McGue M, Patrick CJ. Family transmission and heritability of externalizing disorders: a twin-family study. Arch Gen Psychiatry. American Medical Association. 2004;61:922–8.
34. Iacono WG, Carlson SR, Taylor J, Elkins IJ, Mcgue M. Behavioral disinhibition and the development of substance-use disorders: findings from the Minnesota Twin Family Study. Dev Psychopathol. 1999;11:869–900.
35. Krueger RF, Hicks BM, Patrick CJ, Carlson SR, Iacono WG, McGue M. Etiologic connections among substance dependence, antisocial behavior, and personality: modeling the externalizing spectrum. Washington, DC: American Psychological Association; 2009. p. 88.
36. Morgan AB, Lilienfeld SO. A meta-analytic review of the relation between antisocial behavior and neuropsychological measures of executive function. Clin Psychol Rev. 2000;20:113–36.
37. Young SE, Friedman NP, Miyake A, Willcutt EG, Corley RP, Haberstick BC, et al. Behavioral disinhibition: liability for externalizing spectrum disorders and its genetic and environmental relation to response inhibition across adolescence. J Abnormal Psychol. US: American Psychological Association. 2009;118:117–30.
38. Porreca A, Biringen Z, Parolin M, Saunders H, Ballarotto G, Simonelli A. Emotional availability, neuropsychological functioning, and psychopathology: the context of parental substance use disorder [Internet]. BioMed Res Int. Hindawi; 2018 [cited 2020 Sep 2]. p. e5359037. Available from: https://www.hindawi.com/journals/bmri/2018/5359037/.
39. Acheson A, Vincent AS, Cohoon AJ, Lovallo WR. Defining the phenotype of young adults with family histories of alcohol and other substance use disorders: studies from the family health patterns project. Addict Behav. 2018;77:247–54.
40. Agrawal A, Lynskey MT, Madden PAF, Bucholz KK, Heath AC. A latent class analysis of illicit drug abuse/dependence: results from the National Epidemiological Survey on Alcohol and Related Conditions. Addiction. 2007;102:94–104.
41. Conway KP, Compton W, Stinson FS, Grant BF. Lifetime comorbidity of DSM-IV mood and anxiety disorders and specific drug use disorders: results from the National Epidemiologic Survey on Alcohol and Related Conditions. J Clin Psychiatry. 2006;67:247–58.
42. Goldstein RB, Weissman MM, Adams PB, Horwath E, Lish JD, Charney D, et al. Psychiatric disorders in relatives of probands with panic disorder and/or major depression. Arch Gen Psychiatry. American Medical Association. 1994;51:383–94.
43. Lev-Ran S, Roerecke M, Le Foll B, George TP, McKenzie K, Rehm J. The association between cannabis use and depression: a systematic review and meta-analysis of longitudinal studies. Psychol Med. 2014;44:797–810.
44. McCutcheon VV, Scherrer JF, Grant JD, Xian H, Haber JR, Jacob T, et al. Parent, sibling and peer associations with subtypes of psychiatric and substance use disorder comorbidity in offspring. Drug Alcohol Depend. 2013;128:20–9.
45. Rothenberg AW, Lansford JE, Chang L, Deater-Deckard K, Di Giunta L, Dodge KA, et al. Examining the internalizing pathway to substance use frequency in 10 cultural groups. Addict Behav. 2020;102:106214.
46. Buu A, DiPiazza C, Wang J, Puttler LI, Fitzgerald HE, Zucker RA. Parent, family, and neighborhood effects on the development of child substance use and other psychopathology from preschool to the start of adulthood. J Stud Alcohol Drugs. Alcohol Research Documentation, Inc. 2009;70:489–98.
47. Kerr S, Dalrymple K, Chelminski I, Zimmerman M. Depression and substance use disorders in the offspring of depressed parents as a function of the parent's borderline personality disorder symptomatology. Ann Clin Psychiatry. 2018;30:207–14.
48. Marmorstein NR, Iacono WG, McGue M. Associations between substance use disorders and major depression in parents and late adolescent–emerging adult offspring: an adoption study. Addiction. 2012;107:1965–73.
49. Cloninger CR, Bohman M, Sigvardsson S. Inheritance of alcohol abuse: cross-fostering analysis of adopted men. Arch Gen Psychiatry. American Medical Association. 1981;38:861–8.
50. Cloninger CR. Neurogenetic adaptive mechanisms in alcoholism. Science. American Association for the Advancement of Science. 1987;236:410–6.
51. Vuolo M, Staff J. Parent and child cigarette use: a longitudinal, multigenerational study. Pediatrics. American Academy of Pediatrics. 2013;132:e568–77.
52. Fagan AA, Najman JM. The relative contributions of parental and sibling substance use to adolescent tobacco, alcohol, and other drug use. J Drug Issues. SAGE Publications Inc. 2005;35:869–83.
53. Hartman CA, Lessem JM, Hopfer CJ, Crowley TJ, Stallings MC. The family transmission of adolescent alcohol abuse and dependence. J Stud Alcohol. Alcohol Research Documentation, Inc. 2006;67:657–64.
54. Scholte RHJ, Poelen EAP, Willemsen G, Boomsma DI, Engels RCME. Relative risks of adolescent and young adult alcohol use: the role of drinking fathers, mothers, siblings, and friends. Addict Behav. 2008;33:1–14.
55. Hopfer CJ, Stallings MC, Hewitt JK, Crowley TJ. Family transmission of marijuana use, abuse, and dependence. J Am Acad Child Adolesc Psychiatry. 2003;42:834–41.
56. Mayhew KP, Flay BR, Mott JA. Stages in the development of adolescent smoking. Drug Alcohol Depend. 2000;59:61–81.
57. McGue M, Sharma A, Benson P. Parent and sibling influences on adolescent alcohol use and mis-

use: evidence from a U.S. adoption cohort. J Stud Alcohol. 1996;57:8–18.
58. Samek DR, McGue M, Keyes M, Iacono WG. Sibling facilitation mediates the association between older and younger sibling alcohol use in late adolescence. J Res Adolesc. 2015;25:638–51.
59. Stallings MC, Gizer IR, Young-Wolff KC. Genetic epidemiology and molecular genetics. In: Sher KJ, editor. The oxford handbook of substance use and substance use disorders, vol. 1. Oxford: Oxford University Press; 2016.
60. Bot SM, Engels RCME, Knibbe RA, Meeus WHJ. Friend's drinking behaviour and adolescent alcohol consumption: the moderating role of friendship characteristics. Addict Behav. 2005;30:929–47.
61. Cleveland MJ, Feinberg ME, Jones DE. Predicting alcohol use across adolescence: relative strength of individual, family, peer, and contextual risk and protective factors. Psychol Addict Behav. US: American Psychological Association. 2012;26:703–13.
62. Fowler T, Shelton K, Lifford K, Rice F, McBride A, Nikolov I, et al. Genetic and environmental influences on the relationship between peer alcohol use and own alcohol use in adolescents. Addiction. 2007;102:894–903.
63. Harden KP, Hill JE, Turkheimer E, Emery RE. Gene-environment correlation and interaction in peer effects on adolescent alcohol and tobacco use. Behav Genet. 2008;38:339–47.
64. Tang Z, Orwin RG. Marijuana initiation among American youth and its risks as dynamic processes: prospective findings from a National Longitudinal Study. Subst Use Misuse. Taylor & Francis. 2009;44:195–211.
65. Van Ryzin MJ, Fosco GM, Dishion TJ. Family and peer predictors of substance use from early adolescence to early adulthood: an 11-year prospective analysis. Addict Behav. 2012;37:1314–24.
66. Walden B, McGue M, Lacono WG, Burt SA, Elkins I. Identifying shared environmental contributions to early substance use: the respective roles of peers and parents. J Abnormal Psychol. US: American Psychological Association. 2004;113:440–50.
67. Van Den Bree MBM, Whitmer MD, Pickworth WB. Predictors of smoking development in a population-based sample of adolescents: a prospective study. J Adolesc Health. 2004;35:172–81.
68. Cleveland HH, Wiebe R, Rowe DC. Genetic influences on associations with substance using peers – add health. J Genet Psychol. 2005;166:153–69.
69. Burk WJ, van der Vorst H, Kerr M, Stattin H. Alcohol use and friendship dynamics: selection and socialization in early-, middle-, and late-adolescent peer networks. J Stud Alcohol Drugs. Alcohol Research Documentation, Inc. 2012;73:89–98.
70. Kirillova G, Reynolds M, Kirisci L, Mosovsky S, Ridenour T, Tarter R, et al. Familiality of addiction and its developmental mechanisms in girls. Drug Alcohol Depend. 2014;143:213–8.
71. Samek DR, Goodman RJ, Erath SA, McGue M, Iacono WG. Antisocial peer affiliation and externalizing disorders in the transition from adolescence to young adulthood: selection versus socialization effects. Dev Psychol US: American Psychological Association. 2016;52:813–23.
72. Windle M, Windle RC. Sex differences in peer selection and socialization for alcohol use from adolescence to Young adulthood and the influence of marital and parental status. Alcohol Clin Exp Res. 2018;42:2394–402.
73. Leung RK, Toumbourou JW, Hemphill SA. The effect of peer influence and selection processes on adolescent alcohol use: a systematic review of longitudinal studies. Health Psychol Rev. Routledge. 2014;8:426–57.
74. Harris KM, Halpern CT, Whitsel E, Hussey J, Tabor J, Entzel P, et al. The national longitudinal study of adolescent to adult health: research design [internet]. 2009. Available from: https://addhealth.cpc.unc.edu/documentation/study-design/
75. Allen JP, Chango J, Szwedo D, Schad M, Marston E. Predictors of susceptibility to peer influence regarding substance use in adolescence. Child Dev. 2012;83:337–50.
76. Eaves L. The effect of cultural transmission on continuous variation. Heredity. 1976;37:41–57.
77. Eaves LJ, Last KA, Young PA, Martin NG. Model-fitting approaches to the analysis of human behaviour. Heredity. 1978;41:249–320.
78. Cloninger CR, Rice J, Reich T. Multifactorial inheritance with cultural transmission and assortative mating. II. A general model of combined polygenic and cultural inheritance. Am J Hum Genet. 1979;31:176–98.
79. Cloninger CR, Rice J, Reich T. Multifactorial inheritance with cultural transmission and assortative mating. III. Family structure and the analysis of separation experiments. Am J Hum Genet. 1979;31:366–88.
80. Vogler GP. Multivariate path analysis of familial resemblance. Genet Epidemiol. 1985;2:35–53.
81. McGue M, Wette R, Rao DC, MacCluer JW. A Monte Carlo evaluation of three statistical methods used in path analysis. Genet Epidemiol. 1987;4:129–55.
82. Hicks BM, Foster KT, Iacono WG, McGue M. Genetic and environmental influences on the familial transmission of externalizing disorders in adoptive and twin offspring. JAMA Psychiatry. American Medical Association. 2013;70:1076–83.
83. Keller MC, Medland SE, Duncan LE, Hatemi PK, Neale MC, Maes HHM, et al. Modeling extended twin family data I: description of the Cascade model. Twin Res Human Genet. Cambridge University Press. 2009;12:8–18.
84. Maes HH, Neale MC, Martin NG, Heath AC, Eaves LJ. Religious attendance and frequency of alcohol use: same genes or same environments: a bivari-

ate extended twin kinship model. Twin Res Human Genet. Cambridge University Press. 1999;2:169–79.
85. Kendler KS, Ohlsson H, Sundquist J, Sundquist K. Triparental families: a new genetic-epidemiological design applied to drug abuse, alcohol use disorders, and criminal behavior in a Swedish National Sample. AJP. American Psychiatric Publishing. 2015;172:553–60.
86. Reynolds CA, Barlow T, Pedersen NL. Alcohol, tobacco and caffeine use: spouse similarity processes. Behav Genet. 2006;36:201.
87. Eaves L. The use of twins in the analysis of assortative mating. Heredity. Nature Publishing Group. 1979;43:399–409.
88. Eaves LJ, Heath AC, Martin NG. A note on the generalized effects of assortative mating. Behav Genet. 1984;14:371–6.
89. Vanyukov MM, Neale MC, Moss HB, Tarter RE. Mating assortment and the liability to substance abuse. Drug Alcohol Depend. 1996;42:1–10.
90. Agrawal A, Heath AC, Grant JD, Pergadia ML, Statham DJ, Bucholz KK, et al. Assortative mating for cigarette smoking and for alcohol consumption in female Australian Twins and their Spouses. Behav Genet. 2006;36:553–66.
91. Kendler KS, Lönn SL, Salvatore J, Sundquist J, Sundquist K. The origin of spousal resemblance for alcohol use disorder. JAMA Psychiatry. American Medical Association. 2018;75:280–6.
92. Stallings MC, Cherny SS, Young SE, Miles DR, Hewitt JK, Fulker DW. The familial aggregation of depressive symptoms, antisocial behavior, and alcohol abuse. Am J Med Genet. 1997;74:183–91.
93. Saunders GRB, McGue M, Iacono WG, Elkins IJ. Parent–offspring resemblance for drinking behaviors in a longitudinal twin sample. J Stud Alcohol Drugs. Alcohol Research Documentation, Inc. 2016;78:49–58.
94. Falconer DS, Mackay TFC. Introduction to quantitative genetics. 4th ed. Harlow, England: Prentice Hall; 1996.
95. Glantz MD, Leshner AI. Drug abuse and developmental psychopathology. Dev Psychopathol. 2000;12:795–814.
96. Regier DA, Farmer ME, Rae DS, Locke BZ, Keith SJ, Judd LL, et al. Comorbidity of mental disorders with alcohol and other drug abuse: results from the epidemiologic catchment area (ECA) study. JAMA. American Medical Association. 1990;264:2511–8.
97. Compton WM, Thomas YF, Stinson FS, Grant BF. Prevalence, correlates, disability, and comorbidity of DSM-IV drug abuse and dependence in the United States: results from the National Epidemiologic Survey on Alcohol and Related Conditions. Arch Gen Psychiatry. American Medical Association. 2007;64:566–76.
98. Degenhardt L, Hall W, Lynskey M. Alcohol, cannabis and tobacco use among Australians: a comparison of their associations with other drug use and use disorders, affective and anxiety disorders, and psychosis. Addiction. 2001;96:1603–14.
99. Johnston L, O'Malley PM, Bachman JG. Monitoring the future: national results on adolescent drug use : overview of key findings, 2000. National Institute on Drug Abuse, U.S. Department of Health and Human Services, Public Health Service, National Institutes of Health; 2001.
100. McGue M, Hicks BM. Behavioral genetics of adolescent substance use and abuse. In: Zucker RA, Brown SA, editors. The oxford handbook of adolescent substance abuse. Oxford: Oxford University Press; 2019.
101. Young SE, Rhee SH, Stallings MC, Corley RP, Hewitt JK. Genetic and environmental vulnerabilities underlying adolescent substance use and problem use: general or specific? Behav Genet. 2006;36:603–15.
102. Obot IS, Wagner FA, Anthony JC. Early onset and recent drug use among children of parents with alcohol problems: data from a national epidemiologic survey. Drug Alcohol Depend. 2001;65:1–8.
103. Bierut LJ, Dinwiddie SH, Begleiter H, Crowe RR, Hesselbrock V, Nurnberger JI, et al. Familial transmission of substance dependence: alcohol, marijuana, cocaine, and habitual smoking: a report from the collaborative study on the genetics of alcoholism. Arch Gen Psychiatry. American Medical Association. 1998;55:982–8.
104. Volk HE, Scherrer JF, Bucholz KK, Todorov A, Heath AC, Jacob T, et al. Evidence for specificity of transmission of alcohol and nicotine dependence in an offspring of twins design. Drug Alcohol Depend. 2007;87:225–32.
105. Capaldi DM, Stoolmiller M. Co-occurrence of conduct problems and depressive symptoms in early adolescent boys: III. Prediction to young-adult adjustment. Dev Psychopathol. Cambridge University Press. 1999;11:59–84.
106. Disney ER, Elkins IJ, McGue M, Iacono WG. Effects of ADHD, conduct disorder, and gender on substance use and abuse in adolescence. AJP. American Psychiatric Publishing. 1999;156:1515–21.
107. Jessor R, Jessor SL. Problem behavior and psychosocial development: a longitudinal study. New York: Academic Press; 1977.
108. Heath AC, Bucholz KK, Madden PAF, Dinwiddie SH, Slutske WS, Bierut LJ, et al. Genetic and environmental contributions to alcohol dependence risk in a national twin sample: consistency of findings in women and men. Psychol Med. 1997;27:1381–96.
109. Jessor R, Donovan JE, Costa FM. Beyond adolescence: problem behaviour and young adult development. Cambridge University Press: New York; 1994.
110. Hawkins JD, Catalano RF, Miller JY. Risk and protective factors for alcohol and other drug problems in adolescence and early adulthood: implications for substance abuse prevention. Psychol

Bull. US: American Psychological Association. 1992;112:64–105.
111. Young SE, Mikulich SK, Goodwin MB, Hardy J, Martin CL, Zoccolillo MS, et al. Treated delinquent boys' substance use: onset, pattern, relationship to conduct and mood disorders. Drug Alcohol Depend. Elsevier. 1995;37:149–62.
112. McGue M, Iacono WG. The association of early adolescent problem behavior with adult psychopathology. AJP. American Psychiatric Publishing. 2005;162:1118–24.
113. Patterson GR, Reid JB, Dishion TJ. A social learning approach: antisocial boys. Eugene, OR: Castalia Publishing; 1992.
114. Simons RL, Wu C-I, Conger RD, Lorenz FO. Two routes to delinquency: differences between early and late starters in the impact of parenting and deviant peers. Criminology. John Wiley & Sons, Ltd. 1994;32:247–76.
115. Tremblay RE, Pihl RO, Vitaro F, Dobkin PL. Predicting early onset of male antisocial behavior from preschool behavior. Arch Gen Psychiatry. American Medical Association. 1994;51:732–9.
116. Lynskey MT, Fergusson DM, Horwood LJ. The effect of parental alcohol problems on rates of adolescent psychiatric disorders. Addiction. 1994;89:1277–86.
117. Kendler KS, Davis CG, Kessler RC. The familial aggregation of common psychiatric and substance use disorders in the National Comorbidity Survey: a family history study. Br J Psychiatry. London, United Kingdom: Cambridge University Press;. 1997;170:541–8.
118. Markon KE, Krueger RF, Watson D. Delineating the structure of normal and abnormal personality: an integrative hierarchical approach. J Pers Soc Psychol. 2005;88:139–57.
119. Franco S, Olfson M, Wall MM, Wang S, Hoertel N, Blanco C. Shared and specific associations of substance use disorders on adverse outcomes: a national prospective study. Drug Alcohol Depend. 2019;201:212–9.
120. Hesselbrock V, Meyer R, Hesselbrock M. Psychopathology and addictive disorders: The specific case of antisocial personality disorder. Addictive states. New York: Raven Press; 1992. p. 179–91.
121. Korhonen T, van Leeuwen AP, Reijneveld SA, Ormel J, Verhulst FC, Huizink AC. Externalizing behavior problems and cigarette smoking as predictors of cannabis use: the TRAILS study. J Am Acad Child Adolesc Psychiatry. 2010;49:61–9.
122. Sher KJ, Trull TJ. Personality and disinhibitory psychopathology: alcoholism and antisocial personality disorder. J Abnormal Psychol US: American Psychological Association. 1994;103:92–102.
123. Tarter RE, Kirisci L, Mezzich A, Cornelius JR, Pajer K, Vanyukov M, et al. Neurobehavioral disinhibition in childhood predicts early age at onset of substance use disorder. AJP. American Psychiatric Publishing. 2003;160:1078–85.
124. Tarter RE, Kirisci L, Habeych M, Reynolds M, Vanyukov M. Neurobehavior disinhibition in childhood predisposes boys to substance use disorder by young adulthood: direct and mediated etiologic pathways. Drug Alcohol Depend. 2004;73:121–32.
125. Vanyukov MM, Tarter RE, Kirisci L, Kirillova GP, Maher BS, Clark DB. Liability to substance use disorders: 1. Common mechanisms and manifestations. Neurosci Biobehav Rev. 2003;27:507–15.
126. Young SE, Stallings MC, Corley RP, Krauter KS, Hewitt JK. Genetic and environmental influences on behavioral disinhibition. Am J Med Genet. 2000;96:684–95.
127. Zuckerman M. P-impulsive sensation seeking and its behavioral, psychophysiological and biochemical correlates. NPS Karger Publishers. 1993;28:30–6.
128. Gorenstein EE, Newman JP. Disinhibitory psychopathology: a new perspective and a model for research. Psychol Rev US: American Psychological Association. 1980;87:301–15.
129. Bauer LO, Hesselbrock VM. P300 decrements in teenagers with conduct problems: implications for substance abuse risk and brain development. Biol Psychiatry. 1999;46:263–72.
130. Iacono WG, Carlson SR, Malone SM, McGue M. P3 event-related potential amplitude and the risk for Disinhibitory disorders in adolescent boys. Arch Gen Psychiatry. American Medical Association. 2002;59:750–7.
131. Iacono WG, Malone SM, McGue M. Substance use disorders, externalizing psychopathology, and P300 event-related potential amplitude. Int J Psychophysiol. 2003;48:147–78.
132. Iacono WG, Malone SM, McGue M. Behavioral disinhibition and the development of early-onset addiction: common and specific influences. Annu Rev Clin Psychol. 2008;4:325–48.
133. Begleiter H, Porjesz B, Bihari B, Kissin B. Event-related brain potentials in boys at risk for alcoholism. Science. American Association for the Advancement of Science. 1984;225:1493–6.
134. Polich J, Pollock VE, Bloom FE. Meta-analysis of P300 amplitude from males at risk for alcoholism. Psychol Bull US: American Psychological Association. 1994;115:55–73.
135. Brandeis D, Banaschewski T, Baving L, Georgiewa P, Blanz B, Schmidt MH, et al. Multicenter P300 brain mapping of impaired attention to cues in hyperkinetic children. J Am Acad Child Adolesc Psychiatry. 2002;41:990–8.
136. Klorman R. Cognitive event-related potentials in attention deficit disorder. J Learn Disabil. SAGE Publications Inc. 1991;24:130–40.
137. Chen ACH, Porjesz B, Rangaswamy M, Kamarajan C, Tang Y, Jones KA, et al. Reduced frontal lobe activity in subjects with high impulsivity and alcoholism. Alcohol Clin Exp Res. 2007;31:156–65.

138. Begleiter H, Porjesz B. Genetics of human brain oscillations. Int J Psychophysiol. 2006;60:162–71.
139. Bornovalova MA, Hicks BM, Iacono WG, McGue M. Familial transmission and heritability of childhood disruptive disorders. AJP. American Psychiatric Publishing. 2010;167:1066–74.
140. Farmer RF, Kosty DB, Seeley JR, Gau JM, Klein DN. Family aggregation of substance use disorders: substance specific, nonspecific, and intrafamilial sources of risk. J Stud Alcohol Drugs. Alcohol Research Documentation, Inc. 2019;80:462–71.
141. Long EC, Lönn SL, Sundquist J, Sundquist K, Kendler KS. The role of parent and offspring sex on risk for externalizing psychopathology in offspring with parental alcohol use disorder: a national Swedish study. Soc Psychiatry Psychiatr Epidemiol. 2018;53:1381–9.
142. Vrieze SI, Hicks BM, Iacono WG, McGue M. Decline in genetic influence on the co-occurrence of alcohol, marijuana, and nicotine dependence symptoms from age 14 to 29. AJP. American Psychiatric Publishing. 2012;169:1073–81.
143. Epstein M, Hill KG, Roe SS, Bailey JA, Iacono WG, McGue M, et al. Time-varying effects of families and peers on adolescent marijuana use: person-environment interactions across development. Dev Psychopathol. 2017;29:887–900.
144. Kendler KS, Schmitt E, Aggen SH, Prescott CA. Genetic and environmental influences on alcohol, caffeine, cannabis, and nicotine use from early adolescence to middle adulthood. Arch Gen Psychiatry. American Medical Association. 2008;65:674–82.
145. DeFries JC, Plomin R, Vandenberg SG, Kuse AR. Parent-offspring resemblance for cognitive abilities in the Colorado adoption project: biological, adoptive, and control parents and one-year-old children. Intelligence. 1981;5:245–77.
146. Plomin R, DeFries JC. The colorado adoption project. Child [Wiley, Society for Research in Child Development]. 1983;54:276–89.
147. Plomin R, DeFries JC, Knopik VS, Neiderhiser, JM. Behavioral genetics (6th Edition). Worth Publishers: New York, NY; 2013.
148. Stoolmiller M. Implications of the restricted range of family environments for estimates of heritability and nonshared environment in behavior–genetic adoption studies. Psychol Bull. US: American Psychological Association. 1999;125:392–409.
149. McGue M, Keyes M, Sharma A, Elkins I, Legrand L, Johnson W, et al. The environments of adopted and non-adopted youth: evidence on range restriction from the sibling interaction and behavior study (SIBS). Behav Genet. 2007;37:449–62.
150. Cadoret RJ, O'Gorman TW, Troughton E, Heywood E. Alcoholism and antisocial personality: interrelationships, genetic and environmental factors. Arch Gen Psychiatry. American Medical Association. 1985;42:161–7.
151. Cadoret RJ, Troughton E, O'Gorman TW. Genetic and environmental factors in alcohol abuse and antisocial personality. J Stud Alcohol. Alcohol Research Documentation, Inc. 1987;48:1–8.
152. Goodwin DW, Schulsinger F, Hermansen L, Guze SB, Winokur G. Alcohol problems in adoptees raised apart from alcoholic biological parents. Arch Gen Psychiatry. American Medical Association. 1973;28:238–43.
153. Yates WR, Cadoret RJ, Troughton E, Stewart MA. An adoption study of DSM-IIIR alcohol and drug dependence severity. Drug Alcohol Depend. 1996;41:9–15.
154. Huibregtse BM, Corley RP, Wadsworth SJ, Vandever JM, DeFries JC, Stallings MC. A longitudinal adoption study of substance use behavior in adolescence. Twin Res Human Genetics. Cambridge University Press. 2016;19:330–40.
155. Kendler KS, Ohlsson H, Sundquist J, Sundquist K. Transmission of alcohol use disorder across three generations: a Swedish National Study. Psychol Med. Cambridge University Press. 2018;48:33–42.
156. Cadoret RJ, Yates WR, Ed T, Woodworth G, Stewart MA. Adoption study demonstrating two genetic pathways to drug abuse. Arch Gen Psychiatry. American Medical Association. 1995;52:42–52.
157. Langbehn DR, Cadoret RJ, Caspers K, Troughton EP, Yucuis R. Genetic and environmental risk factors for the onset of drug use and problems in adoptees. Drug Alcohol Depend. 2003;69:151–67.
158. Keyes M, Legrand LN, Iacono WG, McGue M. Parental smoking and adolescent problem behavior: an adoption study of general and specific effects. AJP. American Psychiatric Publishing. 2008;165:1338–44.
159. King SM, Keyes M, Malone SM, Elkins I, Legrand LN, Iacono WG, et al. Parental alcohol dependence and the transmission of adolescent behavioral disinhibition: a study of adoptive and non-adoptive families. Addiction. 2009;104:578–86.
160. Kendler KS, Ohlsson H, Edwards AC, Lichtenstein P, Sundquist K, Sundquist J. A novel sibling-based design to quantify genetic and shared environmental effects: application to drug abuse, alcohol use disorder and criminal behavior. Psychol Med. 2016;46:1639–50.
161. Delker E, Brown Q, Hasin DS. Alcohol consumption in demographic subpopulations. Alcohol Res. 2016;38:7–15.
162. Hasin DS, Shmulewitz D, Sarvet AL. Time trends in US cannabis use and cannabis use disorders overall and by sociodemographic subgroups: a narrative review and new findings. Am J Drug Alcohol Abuse. Taylor & Francis. 2019;45:623–43.
163. Merrick MT, Ford DC, Ports KA, Guinn AS. Prevalence of adverse childhood experiences from the 2011-2014 behavioral risk factor surveillance system in 23 states. JAMA. Pediatr American Medical Association. 2018;172:1038–44.

164. Vasilenko SA, Evans-Polce RJ, Lanza ST. Age trends in rates of substance use disorders across ages 18–90: differences by gender and race/ethnicity. Drug Alcohol Depend. 2017;180:260–4.
165. Witbrodt J, Mulia N, Zemore SE, Kerr WC. Racial/ethnic disparities in alcohol-related problems: differences by gender and level of heavy drinking. Alcohol Clin Exp Res. 2014;38:1662–70.
166. Saunders GRB, McGue M, Malone SM. Sibling comparison designs: addressing confounding bias with inclusion of measured confounders. Twin Res Human Genetics. Cambridge University Press. 2019;22:290–6.
167. Liu M, Jiang Y, Wedow R, Li Y, Brazel DM, Chen F, et al. Association studies of up to 1.2 million individuals yield new insights into the genetic etiology of tobacco and alcohol use. Nature genetics. Nat Publ Group. 2019;51:237–44.
168. Dudbridge F. Power and predictive accuracy of polygenic risk scores. PLOS Genetics. Public Library of Science. 2013;9:e1003348.
169. Kong A, Thorleifsson G, Frigge ML, Vilhjalmsson BJ, Young AI, Thorgeirsson TE, et al. The nature of nurture: effects of parental genotypes. Science. American Association for the Advancement of Science. 2018;359:424–8.

Part III

Genomic Studies in Substance Use

Gene Mapping and Human Disease

6

Joseph D. Terwilliger

Introduction

We have known for a century that many psychiatric disorders are correlated in families and that there are likely to be genetic factors underlying these correlations. We also know that gene mapping has been a powerful tool to help us understand the biology of a plethora of simple diseases, both psychiatric and otherwise. The literature these days is full of articles about genetic studies of psychiatric disorders showing tens or hundreds of genetic variants associated with any given disease. As of 2019, more than 1000 single-nucleotide polymorphisms (SNPs) have been significantly associated with psychiatry-related traits [1].

Despite more than a hundred loci having been correlated with schizophrenia after analyzing tens of thousands of patients, they are estimated to explain no more than about 3% of the disease risk [2]. If we increase the sample size to hundreds of thousands or even millions of schizophrenia patients, the number of loci correlated with the disease would probably rise to the thousands or even tens of thousands, with the as-yet-undiscovered loci each having smaller effect size than any of the known loci (if one needs bigger samples to find them, it would be precisely because their effect sizes are individually smaller).

More importantly, these variants correlated with schizophrenia are genetic markers from a genome-wide association (GWA) array, which measures a genome-scanning set of common variants seen in healthy people. These variants most likely are not themselves phenotypically related to schizophrenia but are in linkage disequilibrium with other variants that may do something. In fact, around each of these hundred or so correlated loci, there are usually many correlated SNPs showing statistical association with the disease. Linkage disequilibrium extends over very wide genomic regions, often including multiple genes. What this means is that while we have identified SNPs that are correlated with genetic variants which are influencing schizophrenia risk, we do not know the functional variants, or even what genes the functional variants are in. That means we do not really know the biology underlying these associations, though we can guess at what they might be [2].

A lot of work has been done over the last 3 decades on the genetics of psychiatric disorders, and more than a thousand associations with SNPs have been found, but we have learned very little about the genetics of these disorders, and even less about their underlying biology, as we do not

J. D. Terwilliger (✉)
Columbia University – Department of Psychiatry, Gertrude H. Sergievsky Center, Department of Genetics and Development, New York, NY, USA

New York State Psychiatric Institute – Division of Medical Genetics, New York, NY, USA
e-mail: jdt3@cumc.columbia.edu

M. M. Vanyukov (ed.), *Genetics of Substance Use*, https://doi.org/10.1007/978-3-030-95350-8_6

even know what genes the functional variants are in, which are at the root of these SNP-trait associations.

This may seem obscure to a nongeneticist. Therefore, the purpose of this chapter will be to review the basic principles underlying gene mapping, and why it works when it works, with focus on the successes of this approach in elucidating the biology of diseases for which individual genetic variants contribute a large amount to the risk of disease. While psychiatric traits and addiction do not typically have such strong genetic factors underlying them, the fundamental principles and logic are not different. The difference is that the predictive value of phenotype on genotype in a sample is greatly reduced when we are studying more complex traits. As in any epidemiological study, when the phenotype does not predict the exposure, there is very little power in these approaches. Similarly, when the risk factors do not have much predictive power on the disease, there is very little value in identifying them.

This chapter will cover the fundamental theory underlying gene mapping strategies, including why and how they work; examples where the theory worked for simple monogenic disorders; examples of what happens as the etiology becomes slightly more complex, involving multiple potential causes of the same disorder; a discussion of what evolutionary thinking predicts about the relationship between genetic risk factors and disease; what happens when a disease is influenced by both genetics and environmental exposures; and what we have seen in studies of more complex traits, like schizophrenia and other psychiatric traits, and how that makes sense given our understanding of gene mapping and evolutionary biology. The emphasis on simpler traits in this chapter is motivated by didactic reasons. In order to understand why genetic approaches have underperformed in complex traits, one needs to understand why they did work in the cases where gene mapping revolutionized our understanding of a variety of disorders from Huntington's disease to lactose intolerance.

Background

In a short 150 years, we have progressed from Mendel's initial conceptualization of genes as some unit of inheritance that could be passed from parents to children to being able to sequence entire genomes at a low cost in an amazingly short period of time.

It is anecdotally obvious to everyone that family members resemble each other and that this similarity is attributable in a large part to the genetic variation shared by relatives. Anecdotally, we all recognize that tall parents tend to have tall children, fat parents tend to have fat children, Korean parents have Korean children, and so on. We all understand that there is a genetic component to virtually every trait imaginable but also that genetics do not determine everything about who we are, or what diseases we will eventually suffer from. While the children of fat parents may be at increased risk of obesity, through proper diet and exercise, there is no guarantee they will themselves be fat as adults.

The search for understanding of the ways genetic variation can influence human phenotypic variation has been a primary focus of biomedical research for the past 3 decades. From the beginning, we have had enormous success in identifying single genetic variants that were sufficient to outright cause a number of rare human diseases. Today our understanding of the molecular basis of single-gene disorders includes some 275,716 phenotypically active molecular variants catalogued in the Human Gene Mutation Database as of December 2019 [3], and this number is growing at a rate of more than 2000 per month today.

Now that we can whole-genome sequence individuals at low cost in a very short amount of time, it has become a fairly trivial process to identify new causal variants for the many rare monogenic diseases, which remain to be characterized. To be certain, there are many such diseases remaining for which the etiology is as yet unknown, as evidenced by the large number of orphan diseases seen in every children's hospital in the world. As the cost of whole-genome sequencing decreases, and as the sequencing error rates decrease, it seems inevitable that one day it will be a routine part of prenatal screening, so that genotypes of all known causal molecular variants can be identified from birth.

This is a major accomplishment of modern genetic science and will be a part of routine health care in the coming decades, and it can have a real effect on health. At least some people will be able to predict from birth, to some extent, whether they will be able to digest lactose, metabolize phenylalanine, etc., so that they can adopt appropriate lifestyle modifications.

However, human geneticists have been more motivated in the past quarter century by trying to understand the genetic component of risk for the much more common and complex multifactorial diseases of greatest public health impact in the Western world. Such traits (like diabetes, cardiovascular disease, obesity, schizophrenia, cancer, and so forth) underlie the bulk of morbidity and mortality in the Western world and are often "lifestyle-mediated." What this means is that we assume that genes are involved, but their effects are individually small and contingent on other genetic factors as well as environment and lifestyle factors. The process of identifying such genetic variants has been far less successful to date, having been described aptly as "a relentless catalogue of failed aspirations" in the classic book "The Rise and Fall of Modern Medicine." [4] Yes, as mentioned above, we have found a thousand such variants influencing psychiatric diseases, but altogether they explain only a tiny fraction of the heritable component of variance of those traits – the difference between variants and variance being of paramount importance for medical genetics [5].

The literature is filled with genome-wide association studies of every complex trait imaginable, with page-long author lists hailing from the entire membership of the United Nations and beyond, each reporting to find tens or hundreds of new "loci" associated with each and every trait. As the sample size increases, so does the number of loci associated with every trait, with ever-decreasing individual effects. As predicted 2 decades ago, scientists are finding needles in a needlestack [6], with more and more loci being found, which contribute less and less to the trait, essentially signifying nothing, as statistical significance has almost nothing to do with biological importance, and these effects vary among samples and between populations.

In 1916, Castle wrote that "It seems...very doubtful whether [insanity] is inherited as a Mendelian unit character, but that [it] is inherited is obvious for it occurs much oftener in families than in the general population, where it is between 1 and 2 percent." [7] A century later, after studying tens of thousands of affected individuals across the world, over 100 loci are reported to contribute to the risk of schizophrenia, but these loci combined explain less than 5% of the ***genetic*** component of the risk [8] of schizophrenia. More importantly, each of these 100 loci represents statistical association between schizophrenia and a set of linked single-nucleotide polymorphisms, spanning a small genomic region, which are unlikely to be the active functional variants. For all the GWA studies, which have been done to date, there are precious few molecularly characterized variants (or even which specific gene harbors such variants), which are known to be causal because of the enormous confounding of exposures due to linkage disequilibrium [5].

The reason people began the search for genes 30 years ago was the hope that they would uncover new biological insights into the nature of the disease. Today we have little biological knowledge resulting from all these studies, as we have neither identified most of the relevant functional variants nor do we even know which gene in a region harbors the relevant functional variation.

One of my favorite titles for a "serious" paper published in a respectable journal (Nature) is "Genetic variants in novel pathways influence blood pressure and cardiovascular disease risk" [9]. What would one expect to find in such a paper? Presumably one expects them to have identified specific genetic variants, which are found in specific genes which are in novel (previously unknown) pathways of genes, which are shown to influence blood pressure and cardiovascular disease risk, right? A reasonable assumption given the grandiose title, the authors claim to have identified 28 loci influencing blood pressure but then immediately add that "Most of the 28 blood pressure loci harbour multiple genes, and although substantial research is required to identify the specific genes and variants responsible for these associations, several loci contain highly plausible biological candidates." So, in other words, they have not identified any genetic variants, or even genes which themselves influence blood pressure or cardiovascular disease risk, and not only that, but the genes which are in the associated regions contain "highly plausible biological candidates," which means they are not even in novel pathways. And this paper has a list of contributing authors and affiliations, which takes three pages in a very small font size, for an article that only had three pages of large font size for the actual science. This is typical of the state of GWAS research in complex diseases today.

So what is the explanation for the apparent discrepancy between the empirical data and the hype promised by the promoters of the human genome project 25 years ago? Why have the results, especially in psychiatric traits, been so underwhelming compared to expectations, especially when we have the ability to sequence an individual's entire genome in a trivial amount of time and cost? To understand this problem, let us review the way gene mapping works and why it was so successful in the case of rare monogenic disorders, as a means to understand why it has not generally lived up to the hype for common chronic diseases.

Principles of Gene Mapping

Conceptually gene mapping studies are very straightforward and simple. One collects a set of individuals or families from a population and measures some phenotype(s) on each individual. The hope is that the phenotypes of these individuals will predict some underlying risk genotypes. One then searches across the entire genome, hoping to identify the locus or loci whose genotype frequencies differ according to phenotype. Two factors are essential for successful mapping: (1) The phenotypes in a sample of individuals must be correlated with the underlying risk genotypes. (2) Those functional risk genotypes must be correlated with marker genotypes which have been measured experimentally. For monogenic rare diseases, this was straightforward, as individuals (especially within a single large family) who shared some rare disease phenotype usually shared the same cause of the disease. This was often a single variant of a single gene, which could be identified easily by mapping strategies. For traits that are more common, and/or are affected by multiple segregating variants of multiple loci, things quickly become much less straightforward.

In any epidemiological study, one samples individuals from a population with the hope that the phenotypes are predictive of some underlying risk factor. In the case of a dichotomous trait, like a disease, an important risk factor would be detectable because it would have a different distribution in affected and unaffected individuals. For genetic diseases, there would be different genotype distributions at some causal locus between those affected and unaffected individuals. Because genetic variants are inherited on linear chromosomes, there are correlations in the segregation patterns of alleles at nearby loci caused by this "linkage." Linkage has been a useful tool for reducing the dimensionality of the genome, making it possible to identify disease-predisposing loci without the need to query every potentially variable nucleotide across the entire genome. Even when we have data from whole-genome sequencing, it is not advisable to analyze every single variant independently, because of the curse of dimensionality (too much multiple testing)!

Figure 6.1 schematically outlines the two correlations, which both must be strong for a mapping study to be successful. $\mathbf{G_M}$ represents the vector of observed marker locus genotypes for all individuals, $\mathbf{G_D}$ represents the vector of unobserved disease locus genotypes for all individuals, and **Ph** represents the vector of phenotypes of all individuals in a study. Phenotypes must predict genotypes of some risk locus – that is to

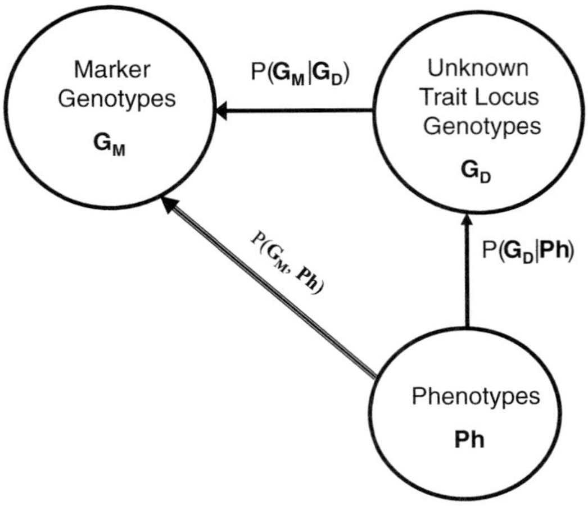

Fig. 6.1 Detectance and power: In a genetic study, one ascertains individuals from the population based on their phenotype (Ph) and hopes to identify correlations with some marker locus genotypes (G_M); i.e., $P(G_M|Ph)$ varies with phenotype. Marker loci themselves, however, are typically assumed not to be directly influencing the phenotype themselves. Individuals who share some disease phenotype are, however, likely to share genotypes at loci that do directly affect disease risk (G_D). The conditional probability $P(G_D|Ph)$ is referred to as the *detectance*. Random genetic marker loci, while phenotypically silent, can be found ubiquitously across the genome, such that some subset of these markers will be located close to any putative risk-influencing locus. In the figure, $P(G_M|G_D)$ is a measure of the statistical correlation between marker and disease genotypes, due to linkage and/or linkage disequilibrium. The convolution of detectance and linkage/linkage disequilibrium determines the strength of the correlation between observed marker locus genotypes and phenotypes. In other words, to detect linkage or association between marker loci and disease phenotypes, it is necessary to have a phenotype (Ph) which predicts the genotypes of the actual predisposing loci (G_D), *and* it is necessary to have strong correlations between G_D and the genotypes of the marker loci which have been genotyped in the study (G_M)

say that $P(\mathbf{G_D}|\mathbf{Ph})$ (the "detectance") must vary with phenotype, and there must be linkage – that is to say that $P(\mathbf{G_M}|\mathbf{G_D})$ must also represent a strong correlation. What one always tests when comparing phenotypes in a sample with genotypes of some marker locus or SNP is the null hypothesis that $P(\mathbf{G_M},\mathbf{Ph}) = P(\mathbf{G_M})P(\mathbf{Ph}) = \sum_{G_D} P(G_M|G_D)P(G_D|Ph)P(Ph)$, which is true whenever either $P(\mathbf{G_M}|\mathbf{G_D}) = P(\mathbf{G_M})$ independent of $\mathbf{G_D}$, or $P(\mathbf{G_D}|\mathbf{Ph}) = P(\mathbf{G_D})$ independent of **Ph**. Phenotypes and marker genotypes can only be correlated if there is both a real predictive value of phenotype on the underlying risk genotype and a strong correlation between the genotypes of the marker under study and genotypes at the risk locus.

Note that here we speak of the predictive value of the phenotype on the genotype, which is quite different from what physicians and epidemiologists are primarily interested in, which would be the predictive value of genotype on phenotype, $P(\mathbf{Ph} \mid \mathbf{G_D})$, which in a population would be the risk or penetrance. It is possible for some risk factor to have a very high probability of causing a disease and yet to have the disease be a very poor predictor of that risk factor. Consider the case of the well-known *BRCA1* locus as a risk factor for breast cancer. *BRCA1* has more than 1600 known variants, each of which significantly increases the risk of cancer, such that roughly 60% of individuals carrying one of those 1600 variants will develop breast cancer by age 70 [10]. So the risk (or "predictance") is very high. However, if we look at all women with breast cancer, less than 10% carry any *BRCA1* mutation, and very few of those share the same identical molecular genotype (as a result of there being 1600 known causal risk alleles!). As a result of this very weak detectance, genome-wide association studies of breast cancer are not typically capable of detecting association with *BRCA1* (unless one is looking at a small population isolate), as each of those 1600 known variants occurs on a different independent haplotype background, so no correlation with nearby SNPs would be expected in the population.

Humans have 22 pairs of autosomes and one pair of sex chromosomes – each such chromosome can be conceptualized as one linear DNA molecule, which they received from one of their parents. In turn, each individual transmits one copy of each of these chromosomes to each of their children. However, during the process of gamete formation, meiosis, genetic material can be reciprocally exchanged between the two copies of each chromosome an individual carries. In this process, the two homologous copies of each

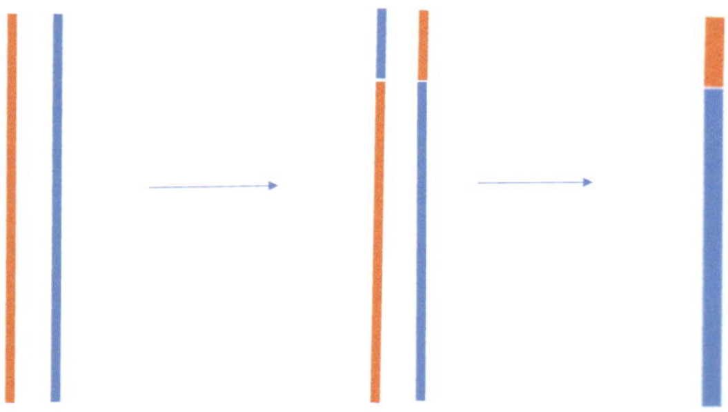

Fig. 6.2 Meiotic recombination: Schematic of meiotic recombination – genetic material is reciprocally exchanged between homologous chromosomes at random locations across the genome in each meiosis, and such recombination gradually, over many generations, breaks down the correlations among genotypes of syntenic loci

chromosome line up next to each other and exchange material as shown in Fig. 6.2. One such recombination event occurs on average once every 100,000,000 base pairs in each meiosis, and one copy of each recombinant chromosome is distributed to each gamete. Because a chromosome is an extremely long linear string, and recombination is a very sparse process, genetic variants at loci close together on the same chromosome will tend to be coinherited in meiosis, a phenomenon known as linkage. For loci that are extremely close together, recombination is so rare that variants at these loci can be coinherited over hundreds or even thousands of generations without recombination, leading to correlation between alleles of linked loci in the population, the phenomenon known as linkage disequilibrium.

Physical linkage is thus the essence of all gene mapping. The number and locations of crossover events are assumed to be largely random and independent in each meiosis. However, some regions are more prone to recombination than others. For this reason, there is an imperfect correlation between physical distance and the frequency of such crossover events. For this reason, we work with genetic maps – in which "genetic distance" is measured in terms of the expected numbers of crossovers between two loci per meiosis, where a span of DNA on which the expected number of recombination events per meiosis is 1 is defined as 1 Morgan, and recombination-based genetic maps are calibrated in that metric. Genetic and physical distance are imperfectly correlated as, for example, there seem to be more recombination events near telomeres, and less near centromeres, and there are many hotspots and cold spots for recombination along the physical length of each chromosome, and there are also differences in the recombination rates between the sexes and even with age.

The correlation among neighboring loci due to linkage is very straightforward to quantify and analyze when one has pedigree data. Remember, however, that linkage is a relationship between genotypes of neighboring loci, not a relationship between genotypes and phenotypes. For simplicity, let us consider the case of a rare dominant disease, for which every individual who has the disease also carries the same causal genetic variant and that this variant is sufficiently rare that the probability of anyone being homozygous for this variant is negligible. In this case, we would have a deterministic detectance relationship in that we can infer that all affected individuals would be heterozygous for this disease-causing variant and that all those unaffected would be homozygous for the normal allele at this locus. Under these assumptions, it is simple to quantify the correlations between the causal locus and neighboring marker loci in families due to linkage.

Consider the family shown in Fig. 6.3, in which all of the affected individuals can be inferred to carry the same risk allele, inherited identical-by-descent (IBD) from their affected father. Because recombination is a sparse process, this means that a very large segment of that same paternal chromosome around the disease locus would also have been received by the three affected children. Recall that recombination occurs only on the order of once every hundred million or so base pairs. In this example, there was one recombination event along this chromosome in the meiosis leading to the first child and another independent recombination event in the meiosis leading to the second affected child, such that all three affected individuals share a very long segment of this chromosome IBD from their father, as indicated by the red arrows in the fig-

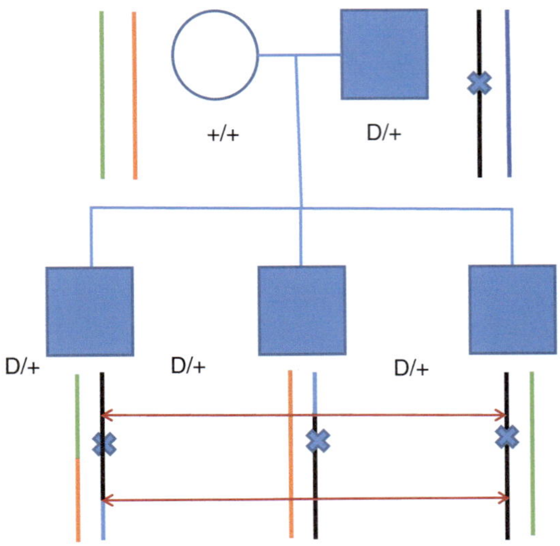

Fig. 6.3 Detectance and Linkage in Rare Dominant Disease: A rare dominant disease pedigree is shown. In this example, because the disease is assumed to be rare, each affected individual is inferred to carry one disease allele and one normal allele (i.e., genotype D/+ at the disease locus). The three affected sons in this pedigree are inferred to have received their disease allele from their father on the same (black) chromosome. In this case, the first and second sons received recombinant chromosomes from their father, while the third son received this entire chromosome with no recombination. The portion of the chromosome where all three sons received the same paternal chromosome is delineated by red arrows. Based on this information, the genomic location of the disease allele can be restricted to this region

ure. The length of the shared segment, which would be inherited IBD by all individuals connected by M meiotic events, is distributed according to an Erlang distribution, E[2,M], with mean length of 2/M Morgans. In the family with three meioses connecting the affected individuals together, the expected length of this shared segment would be 2/3 = 0.67 Morgans.

If each of the affected sons in this pedigree themselves had three affected sons each, then under the detectance model, we assumed all nine of those individuals would have received the same disease-predisposing allele from their grandfather, with nine additional opportunities for meiotic recombination to whittle down the shared region as shown in Fig. 6.4 with the shared segment now having expected length 2/12 = 0.17 Morgans. If several generations later we sampled descendants of these same individuals who were also affected with the disease, it would be parsimonious to assume that they had received the same disease-causing allele IBD from their shared affected ancestor, with many intervening meioses, during which recombination would have further whittled down the shared segment around this causal allele (Fig. 6.5),

Another important principle in genetics is that most copies of the same molecular variant in any given population are typically assumed to be clonal in origin, having descended from one common historical mutation event as in Fig. 6.6. Of course, recurrent mutation does occur, but it is rare, and it is even more unusual for multiple recurrent instances of the same molecular variant to rise to appreciable frequency in the population, as most new mutations quickly go extinct within a small number of generations. For this reason, when we sample two individuals from a population who have the same molecular variant at a given locus, we typically assume that they received that allele identical-by-descent from a common ancestor somewhere in human history.

Generally, the rarer the variant is, the shorter the time to the nearest common ancestor, and accordingly, the smaller the number of meioses in which recombination could have occurred to break down correlations due to linkage with neighboring loci. Especially in the star-shaped genealogies that characterize most modern human populations (characterized by recent rapid population growth after the advent of agriculture), the vast majority of variants in human populations are rare, and most rare variation is of recent origin and is geographically restricted – effectively individuals sharing rare variants at a given locus are likely to have received those variants from a very recent common ancestor, and accordingly very long haplotypes will tend to be shared around said variant.

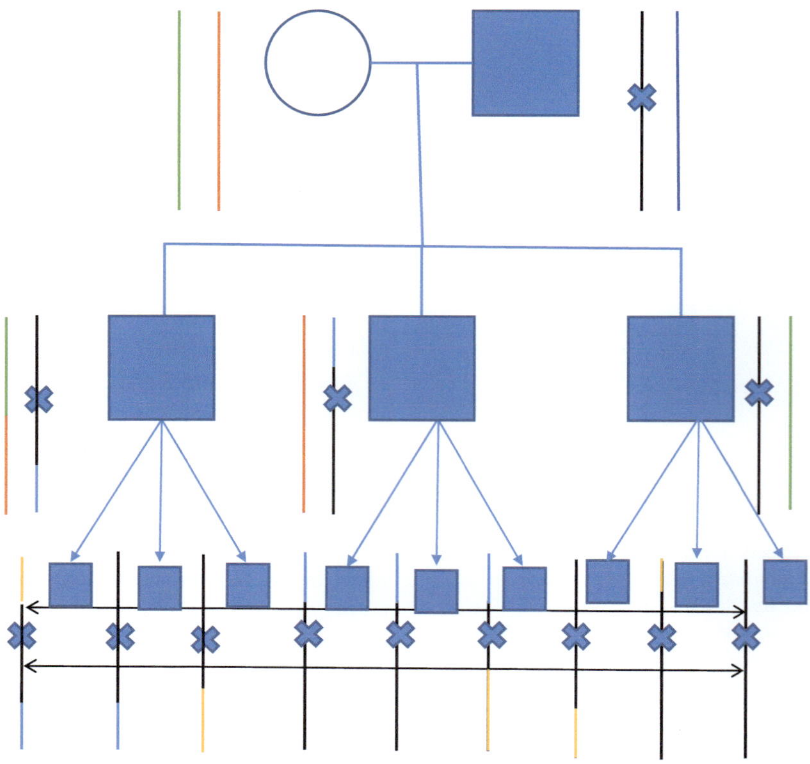

Fig. 6.4 Linkage analysis in large pedigrees: Starting from the pedigree in Fig. 6.3, if each of these three affected sons had three additional affected sons, we would have an additional nine meioses in which recombination could have occurred to further reduce the region of the genome shared by all affected individuals in this family. Based on the observed recombinations, the region is now reduced to the part of the chromosome between the arrows in this figure. As we add more meioses, the shared segment around any clonally inherited disease allele will gradually decrease in size due to this recombination process.

Practical Examples and Successes of Gene Mapping by Linkage in Families

It has long been known that many diseases appear to segregate in families, with inheritance patterns suggesting they were clearly dominant or recessive. In the case of a dominant disease, a single risk allele could be sufficient to cause the disease, while in the case of recessive diseases, both copies of the same gene would need to be disrupted for an individual to become ill. In the case of a dominant trait, one would see affected individuals across multiple generations of a family, with parent and child often both affected with the same disease. For recessive diseases, on the other hand, it would be necessary for each of an individual's parents to carry one risk allele, but since one risk allele is insufficient to cause the disease, those carrier parents would not, themselves, be affected, but siblings of affected individuals would have a 25% chance to be affected, because they would have a 50% chance to receive the disrupted allele from each of their two parents. This leads to clustering of disease among siblings in nuclear families but not correlations between parents and children. Since these diseases are typically quite rare, it is unusual for two unrelated parents to both carry risk alleles in the same gene.

When parents are related, however, it is not unusual for them to have received the same risk allele identical by descent from their nearest common ancestor. Thus, recessive disorders are frequently seen in offspring of consanguineous

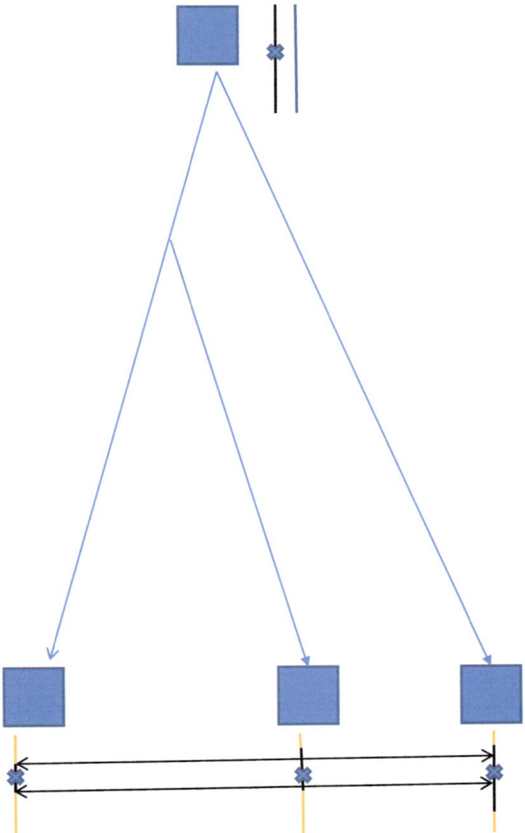

Fig. 6.5 Association analysis = linkage analysis: If we imagine that the process shown in Figs. 6.3 and 6.4 continues over many generations, the segment of the genome shared by this set of affected individuals decreases even further – assuming these affected individuals have inherited their disease-predisposing alleles clonally, from a common ancestor, as shown. When we sample seemingly unrelated individuals for an association analysis, we are hoping that they have received clonal disease-predisposing alleles from a common ancestor, and that they are thus representing the bottom generation of a gigantic pedigree (of unknown size and structure) deep in the history of the population. The deeper the connection, the smaller the shared chromosomal segment will be around the disease locus in which marker loci would be coinherited with the disease allele

matings, and this is one likely reason why inbreeding is frowned upon by a wide variety of cultures. Having said that, in many cultures – especially in the Middle East – cousin marriages are very common for cultural reasons, among which is the tradition of patrilineal inheritance of property, if one has only daughters, but they marry male cousins, the property stays within the family across generations. For this reason, many studies of rare recessive disorders have been conducted in populations with high rates of consanguinity, and others have been successfully performed in small founder populations, for analogous reasons.

One population with both of these characteristics was identified living along the shores of Lake Maracaibo in Northwestern Venezuela [11]. A very high incidence of Huntington's disease, a dominantly inherited neurological disorder of late onset, was found in this population, and affected individuals were linked into one large pedigree of roughly 3000 individuals, with all affected individuals connected to a common founder individual in the early 1800s [12]. By 2004, that pedigree contained over 18,000 individuals, more than 15,000 of which were alive at that time [13]. In 1983, this family, along with another American family, was analyzed jointly, and a marker on chromosome 4 was shown to segregate perfectly with the putative Huntington's disease risk allele in both pedigrees, with no recombination observed [12], and the genetic defect itself was subsequently identified a decade later in 1993 [14]. Interestingly, despite this being one of the first molecularly characterized dominant genetic causes identified for a severe human disease, the function of the gene in which this mutation was identified remains unclear, despite decades of research.

The Finnish population has likewise been a subject of intensive study over the years because it was noticed by Perheentupa and others [14] that a number of rare diseases occurred in Finland that were not seen in neighboring countries. These diseases appeared to be rare genetic diseases that were hypothesized to have increased in frequency in Finland due to the small founder population size and subsequent genetic isolation from neighboring countries. Interestingly, it has also been noticed that many of the most common genetic diseases in Europe, like cystic fibrosis and phenylketonuria, are extremely rare in Finland, so while there is not a higher overall incidence of genetic diseases in Finland, the diseases that occur are different, owing to population bottlenecks and genetic isolation for

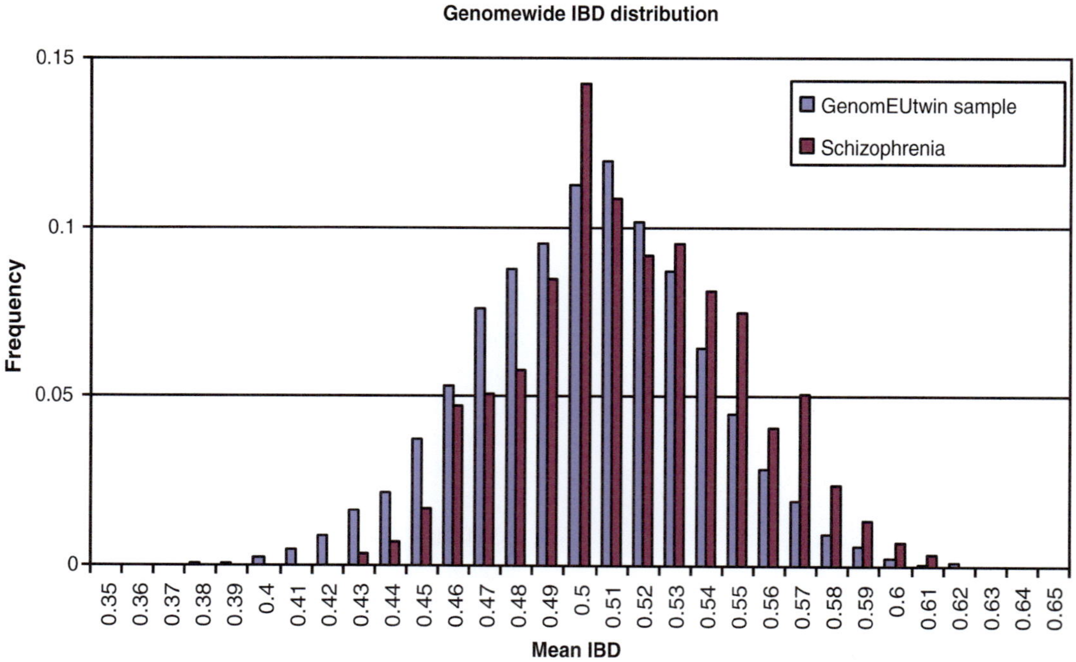

Fig. 6.6 Affected sibpairs share more of their genomes IBD than random sibpairs: Siblings share, on average, 50% of their genetic material identical by descent (IBD) from their parents. However, chromosomal segregation and recombination in meiosis are random processes, such that the actual proportion of their genomes shared IBD by any pair of siblings will not be exactly 50%, but will be a random variable with mean 50%. For a large set of dizygotic twins from Finland [66–68], we estimated the amount of autosomal DNA shared by each pair of siblings based on a microsatellite genome scan, with a histogram of these proportions graphed using the blue bars in the figure (nicely centered around 50% IBD, but with significant variation between 40% and 60%). When we performed the same analysis for sibpairs from Finland in which both sibs had a diagnosis of schizophrenia [52, 59–65], the histogram shown in red was observed. The mean is slightly larger than 50%, and most notably there was a large excess of sibpairs sharing more than 55% of the genome IBD, and a paucity of sibpairs sharing less than 45% of their genome IBD. That is to say that sibpairs who share the disease phenotype tend to share more of their genomes IBD than randomly selected sibpairs, even though no individual single-locus effects were found, as would be expected for a polygenic trait

centuries [15]. Over the years, the genetic variants underlying 35 diseases of the so-called Finnish disease heritage have been identified [16, 17].

Linkage analysis is based on the concept that individuals within a family sharing some rare genetic trait are likely to share the same genetic cause of that trait, identical by descent within the family. However, especially for recessive disorders that typically involve loss of function of a given gene, there is often significant allelic heterogeneity – meaning if there are many different ways a random mutation event could destroy the function of a gene, many different such mutations will have occurred by chance in human history, and as such there will be many different alleles causing the same disorder in different families. This is the general rule, we now realize, on a global scale. For example, cystic fibrosis, one of the most common recessive diseases in Europe, has more than 2000 known causal variants in the same CFTR gene [18], and more than 950 variants have been found in the phenylalanine hydroxylase gene that can cause phenylketonuria [19].

Because of the unique population structure of Finland, however, it was quickly realized that the vast majority of individuals (70%–100%) with diseases of the Finnish disease heritage carried the same molecular variants identical by descent from a recent common ancestor [20–22]. In other words, most individuals with those diseases were the bottom generation of a large pedigree connecting them to common ancestors, much like was the case for the Huntington's disease gene story in Venezuela. To this end, the detectance was almost deterministic, predicting not only that individuals within families shared the same molecular variants but also that individuals within the same population were very likely to have the same molecular variant (which, in the case of Finland, was one very large pedigree going back to many generations), and because of this, individuals sharing some unusual recessive disease in Finland were also very likely to be homozygous for the same molecular variant despite being a culture that generally avoids consanguinity to the extent possible.

Much as described in the theoretical discussion above, individuals sharing diseases from the Finnish disease heritage very often shared the same molecular variants as well, identical by descent within the recent history of the Finnish population, and the extent of this sharing was such that we were able to detect linkage disequilibrium (i.e., to detect linkage within the population between markers and the disease-predisposing allele) over regions ranging from 2.5 to 13 centiMorgans, which is a very large genomic region of millions of base pairs in length, allowing us to very quickly identify the genomic region where the causative genes were located [21].

The difficulty remained that basically everything in those regions of millions of base pairs was shared by all the affected individuals, so it was a complex and laborious task to identify which of these millions of nucleotides was actually causative for each such disease. However, there was a theory that recessive disorders are largely caused by loss-of-function variants, such that neither maternal- nor paternal-derived copies of the gene were functional. All of the genes in each shared haplotype were sequenced to look for molecular variants that likely disrupted one of the genes in the region. Since we know that humans carry loss of function or "knockout" variants in a wide variety of genes without serious complications [23, 24], identifying one potential knockout mutation was considered insufficient to establish that we had found the disease gene. It was typically required that one demonstrate that the same disease could arise from independent mutations disrupting the same gene.

To that end, it was necessary to identify very rare cases of the same genetic disorders from unrelated populations. International collaborations were established to search for independent mutations causing the same phenotype. As an example, the gene underlying one disease of the Finnish Disease Heritage, polycystic lipomembranous osteodysplasia with sclerosing leukoencephalopathy (PLO-SL), was mapped to a small region on chromosome 19 by linkage disequilibrium analysis in the late 1990s [25, 26]. All affected individuals shared a 153 kb haplotype, which carried one large deletion. Another individual from Japan who had the same disease was sequenced and was found to be homozygous for a single-base deletion in exon 3 of the same gene, which appeared to be a loss of function mutation as well [27]. In subsequent years, more loss-of-function mutations in this same gene have repeatedly been shown to cause this rare disease, and a second gene was also later identified that can cause the same disease, also in a recessive mode of inheritance. Interestingly, this second gene, located on chromosome 6, encodes a different subunit of the same receptor signaling complex [28]. Likewise, for this second causal gene, multiple mutations in different populations were identified as part of the required proof that they had identified the actual functional variants causing the disorder.

Heterogeneity and Gene Mapping

Over time it became clear that allelic heterogeneity (different molecular variants in the same gene causing the same disease) and locus heterogeneity (different molecular variants in independent genes causing the same disease) were typical findings. Most recessive disorders carry hundreds or even thousands of disruptive causal variants. When one looks at diseases of the eye, the ear, and the brain, organs known to express an enormous number of genes, there are often numerous independent causes of clinically indistinguishable diseases. For example, nonsyndromic deafness can be caused by molecular variants in more than 400 independent genes [29], nonsyndromic retinitis pigmentosa can be caused by variants in more than 60 known genes [30], and more than 570 genes have been implicated in autosomal recessive intellectual disability [31]. Most of these have been identified by focusing on single families, often from Middle Eastern countries where there are a large number of consanguineous matings. However, it is clear that with so much allelic and locus heterogeneity, if one did not look within individual families, it would have been very difficult to identify any of these loci by traditional mapping approaches in outbred populations.

For disorders like nonsyndromic deafness, the population-level detectance is simply not sufficient for a genome-wide association study of randomly ascertained patients with nonsyndromic deafness in the USA to yield any meaningful results, even though, conditional on having a risk genotype for any of these disorders, the penetrance (or chance to be affected with the disease) is often close to 100%. This is because any given person with nonsyndromic deafness could have it because of risk genotypes in any of 400+ genes, each of which has numerous unique disease-predisposing variants in the population. This is a useful illustration of the difference between detectance and risk, as discussed above for breast cancer. For breast cancer, of course, the genetic risk factor with the greatest difference in detectance between cases and controls is sex, as the vast majority of breast cancer patients are women, even though the risk itself is low – the vast majority of women do not get breast cancer.

When studying rare Mendelian diseases for which there is significant heterogeneity, within a single family, the affected individuals typically share the same risk alleles of the same locus identical by descent within the pedigree. Because of this property, it was possible to perform linkage analysis allowing for a mixture of family types – with some proportion of families carrying risk variants of one gene of interest, and the rest of the families carrying risk alleles at some other locus somewhere else in the genome. As long as each family had a reasonably large number of affected individuals, researchers were still able to map the genes by allowing for this locus heterogeneity as a parameter in the linkage analysis [32–35]. Successful analyses using this model were performed for numerous etiologically heterogeneous Mendelian disorders (e.g., [33, 36–38]).

The success in mapping the genes underpinning such heterogeneous diseases led people to believe it was simply a matter of increasing the sample size to identify the genes underpinning diseases that were more complex, being caused by interactions among variants of several genes acting jointly rather than independently causing the disease outright. Many traits were known to be correlated among relatives yet were clearly not caused outright by genetic variants of single loci. In other words, the search began for loci underlying diseases, which aggregated in families, but did not clearly segregate as dominant or recessive single-gene disorders do.

Some studies of such complex traits were carried out in large families from small populations, when they were available (e.g., [39–43], but for many such diseases, large families were difficult to find, leading researchers to begin focusing their efforts on large collections of very small families – like affected sibpairs [44–55].

Family Studies of Complex Psychiatric and Neurological Traits

Psychiatrists have long been interested in genetics, largely because the biology underlying diseases like schizophrenia has been extremely difficult to get a handle on. It has long been suspected that the disease results from a complex interaction between numerous genetic and environmental factors, the vast majority of which are poorly characterized. For this reason, many psychiatric researchers turned to gene mapping with a hope of getting some clues. Many of the initial group of psychiatric geneticists fully expected to spend a few years looking for genes, to uncover some secrets of the underlying biology, so that they could then go back to clinical research with new insights about the neurobiology of the disease.

This euphoria was driven by the clear successes of gene mapping in disorders which had individual loci contributing to risk in a large way. Monogenic disorders were even easier to map in the Finnish population, because most people sharing the same disorder also shared the same genetic cause, identical-by-descent from a common ancestor. In the northeastern part of Finland, there is a geographically isolated region (Kuusamo) where the incidence of schizophrenia is roughly three times higher than the nationwide average. They also have dramatically higher familial clustering in this region, and all families with two or more affected children could even be traced to common ancestors in the 1600s [56]. If there was ever going to be a chance to map schizophrenia genes by linkage, this would seem to be an ideal natural experiment to address the question.

In Finland, there exist registry data of all hospital discharge diagnoses, all prescription drugs dispensed, and all disability pension recipients. Using these data, back in the late 1990s, 29,124 schizophrenia patients born between 1940 and 1969 were identified, and they were linked together in families using the national population register (which records all family relationships in Finland going back a few centuries). Each of these individuals were then contacted and recruited in a systematic nationwide manner for study. A total of 360 families with at least one schizophrenic were identified from the northeastern Finnish isolate of Kuusamo, including 69 nuclear families with at least two affected siblings. These nuclear families were then connected to common ancestors within the previous 350 years. Using this information, a genome scan was performed to search for linkage and/or linkage disequilibrium – looking for regions that showed excessive haplotype similarity among individuals with schizophrenia as compared with unaffected individuals from the same isolate. Unfortunately, no individual locus in the genome showed significant correlation with schizophrenia [57].

However, it was noticed that the distribution of p-values for all loci in the analysis seemed to be nonuniform (in modern genomics terminology, the "Q-Q plot" showed an excess of small but nonsignificant p-values). To check if this was significantly different from what would be expected by chance, a randomization test was performed. That is to say, the phenotypes of each individual were randomized, and the genome-wide association analysis was repeated. This process was repeated several thousand times to see what the expected number of significant p-values would be if there were no relationship between any genes in the genome and schizophrenia. For every p-value cutoff from 0.05 down to 0.001, there were roughly twice as many positive findings in our dataset than what was seen when we randomized the case and control status, consistent with the idea that there were hundreds of loci affected schizophrenia, scattered all across the genome [57]. This is completely consistent with Fisher's decades old models of polygenic inheritance, in which he proposed that complex quantitative traits that aggregated in families could be explained by a combination of a very large number of genes, each with very small individual effect on the trait [58].

Linkage analysis was also performed in affected sibpairs (both having schizophrenia) from all across Finland, and no evidence of linkage was found to any genomic region in a genome scan [52, 59–65]. On average, pairs of siblings share 50% of their genome, identical by descent, from their parents. Using the same linkage data, the proportion of the entire genome shared IBD by each pair of affected siblings was estimated, as shown in the red bars in the histogram in Fig. 6.6. As a control, the same genome-wide marker set was analyzed in an independent dataset of randomly ascertained Finnish dizygotic twins from the GenomEUtwin project [66–68] (the blue bars in the histogram in Fig. 6.6). For the GenomEUtwin dataset, as expected, there was an average genome-wide sharing of 50%, and the distribution was symmetric around 0.5. The schizophrenic sibpairs, on the other hand, had an average sharing larger than 50%, with a distribution that is skewed upward, with most sibpairs sharing more than 50% of their genomes IBD. More convincingly, there was a huge excess of sibpairs sharing more than 55% of the genome IBD, compared with those sharing less than 45%.

Just as the genome-wide association study suggested, the linkage evidence was most consistent with a polygenic model, in which there were as many as hundreds of loci spread all over the genome, which predisposed an individual to schizophrenia, even in this extreme population isolate. A decade later, large international consortium genome-wide association studies for schizophrenia were conducted with thousands of samples and came to the same conclusion that they "…provide molecular genetic evidence for a substantial polygenic component to the risk of schizophrenia involving thousands of common alleles of very small effect." [69] This idea of looking at the distribution of genome-wide p-values and empirical IBD sharing along the genome has subsequently become a popular approach in complex disease genetics, as it has been generalized in the concepts of "Q-Q plots" and "polygenic risk scores," which are ubiquitous in GWA papers today.

Over the years, for complex multifactorial traits, family studies were able to isolate several loci of large effect, like the relationship between apolipoprotein E and Alzheimer's disease [70, 71] or that between HLA or the insulin gene regions and type I diabetes [55]. Similarly, for many complex disorders, there are subsets of cases that cluster in families more than others, behaving in a quasi-Mendelian manner, for which traditional linkage analysis was especially effective – e.g., maturity-onset diabetes of the young [37], early-onset Alzheimer's disease [72, 73], familial breast cancer [38], and many more. Still, these major risk factors explained only a small fraction of the risk in the general population. Geneticists were seduced by the possibility that with a large enough sample size and the technology to cheaply and rapidly sequence whole genomes, we would be able to explain a much larger proportion of these diseases of public health importance, and so the quest continued. Again, the primary objective was to uncover unknown aspects of the underlying biology of these diseases by finding causal genes, which changed our view of these disorders on a molecular level.

It is important to remember that in most areas of medicine, identifying the causes of disease is not strongly related to treatments or cures. Infectious disease is the big exception, and our advances in understanding the cause of communicable diseases was one of the big successes of modern medicine. Improvements in sanitation, vaccines, and antibiotics dramatically changed the balance of power in our struggle against pathogens, though as the current Covid-19 pandemic clearly illustrates, the war has not been (and probably cannot be) won completely. Pathogens are subject to the same evolutionary forces as every other species, and they are constantly adapting in their own battle for survival [74], and we have to keep ourselves engaged in that fight, lest we end up losing the incredible advantage we have developed in that war over the last century.

For monogenic disorders, we have known the causal variants for decades in some cases, and yet very scant few treatments based on our knowledge of genetics has been developed. Though knowing the genetic cause in some cases can allow people to avoid risky exposures – i.e., phenylketonurics can avoid many symptoms by avoiding dietary phenylalanine, and those with hypolactasia can avoid consuming lactose.

Much of the interest in genetics, however, has been with the idea that cause leads to cure, which is not the case for most chronic disorders. When one has a headache, one takes aspirin, which relieves the headache. When one has cancer, one tries to remove or destroy the cancerous tissue. When one has a broken leg, splints, casts, and the like are used to immobilize the bone and allow it to heal. When one has schizophrenia, they might take lithium to treat the symptoms, and if you have clogged arteries you might get stents inserted to alleviate the problem. These are not related to the cause of those diseases but are the ways we try to cure them.

CDCV and the Case for GWAS

A quarter century ago, Risch and Merikangas first proposed that the future of genetic studies of complex diseases might be focused on unrelated individuals, taking advantage of short-range linkage disequilibrium which exists [75] around very common alleles, owing to their clonal identity at some point prior to the exodus of humans from the African continent [76] (all humans are ultimately related if we go back far enough in evolutionary time). The main rationale was that collecting unrelated individuals would be easier than collecting families or even pairs of affected siblings (a popular study design at that time), at least for common variants (10% to 80% frequency) of what was then considered to be small effect size (genotype relative risks of 1.5 to 4). The crux of the argument for why it would be useful to identify such risk factors was because "despite the small effects of such genes, the magnitude of their attributable risk (the proportion of people affected due to them) may be large because they are quite frequent in the population, making them of public health significance." Eric Lander subsequently agreed that common complex diseases might be caused by common variants with fairly substantial effect sizes, using several well-known examples back in 1996, arguing that "The Apolipoprotein E gene has three major variants (E2, E3, and E4) that explain a large fraction of the risk for Alzheimer's disease, as well as the risk for cardiovascular disease. The MTHFR, Factor V, ACE, and CKR-5 genes each have common variants associated with, respectively, homocysteine levels, risk of thrombosis, heart disease, and resistance to HIV." [77]

This inference was based on the so-called common disease-common variant (CDCV) hypothesis, which stated that "most of the genetic risk for common, complex diseases is due to loci where there is one common variant (or a small number of them)" [78]. Under this model, there would have been common variants shared across populations, predating the exodus of humans from Africa, which would be responsible for most of the genetic portion of the risk of multifactorial diseases, at least in European and Asian populations. In other words, the argument was that common variants of large effect, like ApoE and Alzheimer's disease (OR > 10 for homozygous E4 carriers), likely existed for most other complex traits, but we simply had not looked for them and therefore had not found them yet.

There were a number of counterarguments made at the time, but the bottom line was that human evolution is a complex history, and we surely did not know the truth. Although arguments were made suggesting that allelic and locus heterogeneity was likely to be the rule and not the exception – much as had been the case for simple monogenic disorders, – the usual response was to say that we just do not know, and so we should do the experiment and find out [32]. The reason this mattered is because GWAS would only succeed at elucidating the bulk of the genetic portion of the etiology of common complex disorders if CDCV turned out to be true, which from hindsight we now know does not seem to be the case.

In reality, the main motivation for performing genome-wide association studies for complex traits was the advent of technological advances rather than any genuine belief in CDCV. Humans are very good at engineering, and biochemists developed fantastic technologies for SNP genotyping in the 1990s, and later for exome and even whole-genome sequencing. The problem was that the only samples available for applying those technologies at the time were pre-existing population-based epidemiological studies, on which blood samples had been collected and stored in someone's freezer. This made it very attractive to apply the new technologies to available samples, and scientists quickly realized that the only way this would work in practice would be under the CDCV hypothesis and ideally also would be conducted in small, homogeneous populations, which were as close as possible to being the bottom generation of one very large pedigree, like Finland had been for simple monogenic traits.

Euphoria enveloped the field, and to motivate the allocation of money to this large-scale initiative in the late 1990s and early 2000s, leading scientists made quite remarkable predictions. For instance, in 1999, former NIH director Francis Collins suggested that a hypothetical doctor's visit in 2010 could lead a patient to learn that "his risk of contracting prostate cancer and Alzheimer's diseases are reduced because he carries low-risk variants of the several genes known in 2010 to contribute to these illnesses," and "a prophylactic drug regimen based on knowledge of [his] personal genetic data can be precisely prescribed to reduce his cholesterol and the risk of coronary artery disease to normal levels" [79]. By 2005, he was even more confident, suggesting that by 2010, "predictive genetic tests will be available for as many as a dozen common conditions" and that by 2020, "new gene-based designer drugs will be developed for diabetes, heart disease, Alzheimer's disease, schizophrenia, and many other conditions…" [80].

Perhaps the most accurate prediction from the late 1990s was by John Bell, who suggested that "considering the current rapid acquisition of genetic information relating to common disease and the dramatic technological developments that continue to fuel the field, it would be surprising if most of the major genetic factors involved in human diseases were not defined over the next 5-10 years." [81] All of these predictions were based on different sets of assumptions about what the genotype-phenotype relationships underlying complex multifactorial traits were likely to be. But what does evolutionary theory predict about these phenogenetic relationship?

Evolution and Phenogenetics

Evolution is a fairly simple conceptual idea that was first proposed less than 2 centuries ago by Darwin [82, 83]. The basic concept in evolutionary biology is that all living organisms have descended from a common ancestor, with the process of divergence being driven by random mutation events that occur during reproduction. These mutation events lead to an increase in genetic variation over time, some of which has phenotypic effects. In each generation, some organisms will survive to reproductive age, and others will not. Of those which survive to reproductive age, some will have more offspring than others. This process is largely random but can be influenced by natural selection. Natural selection refers to the idea that individuals with different phenotypes have different relative probabilities and frequencies of reproducing and thus differentially contribute their genetic material to the next generation. Obviously, in order to reproduce, the first requirement is that they survive to reproductive age.

Equally important is the fact that once an individual has reached the age where they have finished reproducing, and raising their young, their phenotypes are no longer directly subjected to natural selection. In ancient times, people did most of their reproducing before age 35, such that if one was predisposed to a disease of later onset, this would never have been filtered out by natural selection, as such individuals would have already passed their genes (or not) to the next generation before becoming ill. In a sense that has a lot to do with why it is all downhill for most of us after our 30s, as we are living on extra time after that from an evolutionary perspective.

Natural selection does not care about what traits society perceives to be "positive" or "negative." It only cares about differential survival to reproductive age and differential reproductive success. Perhaps more importantly, it acts on phenotypic variation, not genotypic variation. The smaller the effect of any given genetic variant on the phenotype, which influences reproductive success, the less its frequency will be influenced by selection.

So what does this mean in practice? It means that diseases that lead to infertility or death in childhood will be strongly selected against, while diseases that do not affect fertility or fecundity (typically mild diseases or diseases of late onset) will not be subjected directly to natural selection. For example, for monogenic recessive disorders, for which individual variant alleles can cause severe childhood diseases with high probability, risk alleles are typically very rare [32], since homozygous individuals do not normally reproduce.

Of course, in human populations, the vast majority of variants are extremely rare, independent of their phenotypic effects. Consider that the meiotic mutation rate per nucleotide per generation is on the order of 10^{-8} [84] and that a haploid genome is on the order of 3 x 10^9 nucleotides in length [85], implying that each newborn individual carries roughly 30 new germline mutations from each parent, somewhere in the genome. The world population is almost 8 x 10^9 individuals, comprising 1.6 x 10^{10} haploid genomes, which translates to 4.8 x 10^{11} de novo singleton mutations, or something on the order of 160 de novo mutations at each nucleotide position in the genome in the currently living population of our species. Basically, every nucleotide in the genome is likely varied, if variation at that site is compatible with life. However, as of March 9, 2020, the ALFA (Allele Frequency Aggregator) website at NCBI lists roughly 447 million sites at which variation has been detected, of which roughly nine million (roughly 3.5%) have minor allele frequencies over 0.01 worldwide [86]. Most sequenced variation in the human genome is thus known to be rare, and most variation has not even been detected yet, as fewer than 100,000 individuals have been analyzed included in that analysis to date. Again, the fact is that most variation is rare, independent of its phenotypic consequences.

Variation that deterministically causes diseases of early onset that negatively impact reproductive fitness will be kept rare by natural selection. However, this does NOT mean that variation that is rare will necessarily have large phenotypic impacts, since the overwhelming majority of variants in our population are extremely rare, and most of them have negligible phenotypic effect at best. If we subtract out the 275,000 or so variants in the Human Gene Mutation Database that are hypothesized to have direct and significant phenotypic consequences, it is likely that most of the remaining 446 million variants described in the ALFA project are selectively neutral or at least "nearly neutral" [87, 88].

For most chronic diseases of public health importance, the effect of the disease state on reproduction are minimal, as they have their largest morbidity and mortality in older post-reproductive populations and thus have not been subjected to significant reproductive selection. It is therefore reasonable to assume that the frequency distribution of genomic variants that influence these traits would be very similar to the overall allele frequency distribution in the genome, where the overwhelming majority will be very rare, and maybe 3.5% of such phenotypically relevant variants would have allele frequencies over 0.01 worldwide. If this were true, then 96.5% of variants that are phenotypically impacting any given trait would be less than 1% frequent, and more than 95% of variants would have frequencies less than 0.001, as in random sequence data across the genome.

To be sure it is not really that simple. It is well known that protein coding regions show systematically less variation than noncoding regions and that the amount of variation in a given gene is related to how essential the gene structure and function is to life. Some essential genes are ubiquitously expressed across tissues, performing housekeeping roles in fundamental cellular processes. Those genes show extremely limited variation, suggesting that protein altering mutational variation may not be compatible with life and may lead to spontaneous abortion. Other genes, when destroyed, can be sufficient to cause a number of monogenic diseases. These diseases, however, are less severe, as they do not prevent birth, and may negatively impact only certain tissues (as in the aforementioned cases of nonsyndromic deafness or intellectual disability). Those generally show somewhat more natural variation than essential housekeeping genes, while other less critical genes can be mutated without serious phenotypic consequences and thus show the highest levels of variation. This is all consistent with the previous discussion of how selection works. This generally means, however, that coding sequences will have an even larger proportion of rare variation than noncoding sequences, because of these selective effects.

Furthermore, we know that severe alterations in protein structure can (and often do) cause monogenic diseases outright, as can regulatory variants that prevent a gene from being transcribed, for example. But more subtle changes in protein structure or regulation often have smaller phenotypic effects. These more subtle variants are likely to be the main players in most normal variation and in common chronic diseases, and as outlined above, most of the variants that affect such traits must be rare, though more common ones may explain more of the variance. Of course, we cannot forget that somatic changes in DNA sequence during development, as well as epigenetic modifications, can modify the already small effects that inherited variation does have.

GWAS Results

It is obvious that the technological innovations of the past quarter century have been extremely valuable, and we have learned a lot about human variation and the genetics of human disease. With today's technological capability, the process of identifying the variants that cause rare recessive diseases can be reduced from a decade to weeks, and we can quickly sequence an individual's entire genome and screen for all the known variants that can have known functional effect on human phenotypes – and there are almost 300,000 of those as stated above. This is real progress and is a testament to the ability of human beings to solve engineering problems, analogous to when our scientists worked together to find a way to split the atom or to put a man on the moon. In the future, when clinical quality sequencing becomes affordable and widely available, we will absolutely be sequencing people at birth, because then we will be able to screen everyone for all of the known functional variants for which there are real phenotypic consequences, some of which could be avoided through early lifestyle interventions. But will it be useful for prediction or treatment of complex traits? The jury is very much still out on that, but surely a few thousand SNPs have already been correlated weakly with various chronic diseases. But it is important to remember that knowing about correlations between SNPs and disease does not imply that we know the functional variants or even the genes which are directly involved, which would be a necessary step before meaningful biological interventions would be possible.

At the beginning of the euphoria for such association studies, the "poster child" example used to justify the proposal was the aforementioned relationship between variation at the ApoE gene and the risk of Alzheimer's disease. In one of the first large-scale association studies of Alzheimer's disease, back in 2007, the only significant conclusion was summarized by the title, "A high-density whole-genome association study reveals that APOE is the major susceptibility gene for sporadic late-onset Alzheimer's disease" [89]. In this study, a p-value of less than 10^{-34} was found with one single SNP located 14 kb away from the known functional variant in APOE, and no other variant in the entire genome reached statistical significance with the second most significant SNP giving a p-value 27 orders of magnitude less significant than the ApoE-linked SNP. Rather than making the logical conclusion that there are not further common variants contributing significantly to sporadic late-onset Alzheimer's disease in an important way, the authors instead argued that this lack of positive findings meant that more funding was needed to do even bigger studies to find the rest of the genes. This phenomenon has been likened to a form of Western Zen (in which no means yes) [5], the failure of a study to find something does not imply that the hypothesis motivating the study was inaccurate but rather that even bigger studies should be done, since important things would be found if they had more patients and markers. Modern "big data" science lacks stopping rules, especially when projects become "too big to fail."

A decade later, researchers from 292 different research institutes around the world combined forces and did a meta-analysis of 94,437 individuals with 9.45 million "common" variants [90] and claimed to have found genome-wide significant evidence for 25 loci, which combine to explain less than 1/3 of the genetic component of variance in AD risk. Note that APOE by itself explains roughly 25% of the genetic variance, while all other significant loci combined explain just over 5% [91], meaning that most of this variance would be due to loci that are either too rare or have too small of an individual effect size to be identified even with this enormous study sample. In other words, very little additional understanding of the genetics of Alzheimer's disease came from a decade's worth of work collecting and genotyping tens of thousands of additional samples. As future studies become bigger, additional loci will surely be found, but they will contribute an ever-decreasing amount to the variance (if the effect size were not smaller than the one's we have already identified, you would not need an even larger sample to detect them). It should be noted that other than ApoE, very little is known about the specific molecular variants or even which genes they are in, just as in the blood pressure analysis described in the introductory section of this chapter.

Obesity is another major object of genome-wide association studies. One study which examined 249,796 individuals was able to identify 18 new loci associated with body mass index, in addition to 14 previously known loci [92]. According to the authors, "…the variants identified by this large study explain only 1.45% of the variance in BMI." But because the study is so large, one of the identified SNPs, rs29941, gave a significant p-value of 3×10^{-9} yet explained an estimated "0.00%" of the variance. This is a great example to illustrate the gulf of difference between statistical significance and "importance." With large enough samples, you can detect vanishingly small effects. Of the 18 newly discovered loci in that genome-wide association study, the largest effect of all of them was estimated to explain only 0.06% of the variance in BMI.

The story is similar for most complex traits – more and more SNPs are identified with larger and larger samples, explaining less and less of the variance of the traits they are associated with. And yet scientists lament the "missing heritability," meaning that even with enormous studies, most of the genetic variance remains unexplained by all the GWAS and linkage studies combined. This is not really surprising. Evolution creates heterogeneity. Most genetic variants are rare, and we can clearly see that identifiable common variants contribute very little to the genetic variance of most complex traits. The difference between "variants" and "variance" is as critical as the difference between "significance" and "importance." With many different contributing genes, genetic "causation" itself may be a misleading concept, as it tends to imply genes *for* the trait.

Despite the paucity of important findings, the technocrats behind the HapMap project who pushed for a shift from family studies to GWAS a quarter century ago strangely claimed that the controversy about the CDCV hypothesis was "... ultimately resolved by the remarkable success of the genetic association studies enabled by the HapMap project." [93] They went on to list a massive table of "successful" studies, including loci for such traits as bipolar disorder, Parkinson's disease, and schizophrenia, and even ApoE and Alzheimer's disease was included, even though it had been found by family studies decades earlier.

Despite these claims of success, Parkinson's disease researchers later that year claimed that "Taken together, studies appear to provide substantial evidence that none of the SNPs originally featured as PD loci [sic: from GWAS studies] are convincingly replicated and that all may be false positives...it is worth examining the implications for GWAS in general." [94] Today, 24 loci have been confirmed, but the heritability explained by all the known loci is only 0.033 [95]. The case of schizophrenia today has already been discussed in the Introduction of this chapter, with 100 loci now known, which together explain less than 5% of the genetic component of the risk. And the list goes on and on of the traits for which very little has been found, with researchers interpreting this to mean they need more money for bigger studies with more markers.

One major point that is often forgotten is that Risch and Merikangas [75] compared the number of singleton affected individuals needed to achieve 80% power to identify a genotyped functional variant by association analysis both under simple random sampling and when sampling a pair of affected siblings. In all models that they have considered, the required sample size was dramatically smaller if one sampled affected sib-pairs rather than unrelated affected individuals – with the caveat that the rarer the variant, the greater the advantage of sampling affected relatives.

Why would this be the case, that sampling families with two affected children would ***always*** give higher power than sampling random affected individuals? Remember that complex traits are assumed to be multifactorial – that is to say, they are influenced by a large number of both genetic and nongenetic factors. If you sample a nuclear family with two affected individuals, it increases the probability that they are affected because of shared risk factors, and genes are shared by siblings according to regular quantifiable mathematical rules. Environments can be shared as well – for example, if mom cooks a lot of bacon, it is likely that both are eating bacon, but there are no rules to quantify this correlation in exposures.

Every nucleotide in the genome is varied somewhere in the human population if it is compatible with life, as discussed above. Many of those variants do have phenotypic effects. Given that allelic and locus heterogeneity are very common for monogenic disorders, it is inevitable that there will be an enormous number of variants in most loci influencing complex traits as well. Within any single family, however, etiological complexity will necessarily be reduced, simplifying the problem substantially. Studying smaller, more homogeneous populations should likewise be more powerful than studies of cosmopolitan heterogeneous ones – more signal and less noise (cf. [96, 97]). Whether these sampling strategies simplify the genetic architecture sufficiently to make gene identification possible is another story, as in the Finnish schizophrenia study illustrated above.

There is no mathematical basis (even when there is allelic homogeneity and CDCV holds) for suggesting that sampling unrelated individuals is either more powerful or more efficient than sampling families – the only claim was that it is simpler to do, making it possible to collect a sufficiently large sample to compensate for the lower power of the ascertainment scheme. This is the same rationale used to justify the shift from studying large extended pedigrees to affected sib-pairs in the early 1990s – the idea that you could make up for the reduction in power (owing to increased etiological heterogeneity) by increasing the sample size. Of course, if it is really that difficult to find families with more than one affected individual, it is fair to question why one expects the trait to have a genetic basis in the first place. In the past, one first had to demonstrate that a trait was heritable before getting funded to look for genes, and heritability can only be demonstrated by showing that families with multiple affected individuals exist at greater frequency than would be expected by chance.

Gene-Environment Interactions

As described above, natural selection is a very weak filter that acts on phenotype, not on genotype. The process of mutation generates lots of variation over time, most of which is not filtered by selection, as it has little direct phenotypic effect. Nevertheless, mutation is the source of all genetic variations, and that variation can become important when environments change. Individual genetic variants can then become beneficial or harmful, but their existence allows a species to adapt, as some individuals will survive and reproduce more efficiently when the environment changes. Substance abuse, the topic of this book, is all about differential responses to an exogenous environmental factor. And there are some reasons why such traits could be simpler than we might expect. To illustrate the idea, let us examine closely the story of lactase persistence.

Mammals typically breastfeed their young, and lactose is the predominant sugar in milk. The enzyme lactase is used to break the disaccharide lactose into the simple sugars glucose and galactose. If a child were to receive dysfunctional copies of the lactase gene from both of its parents, it would be unable to digest lactose, which can lead to diarrhea, dehydration, weight loss, and ultimately death. For this reason, while there are many loss-of-function variants in the lactase gene (because there are many ways to randomly knock out any given gene), each of them is extremely rare due to strong negative selection against homozygotes in the past, before the advent of lactose-free substitutes for breast milk [98].

Adult-type hypolactasia is a different story, in which individuals who were able to digest milk just fine when they were infants cannot digest it as adults. This trait also appears to be recessively inherited and segregates in families but is obviously not due to loss-of-function mutations in the lactase gene, as those are well-known to cause congenital lactase deficiency, and these individuals were able to digest lactose when breastfeeding as children [99]. The initial expectation was that some gene would be knocked out in the copies inherited from each parent, and therefore allelic heterogeneity might be expected. For reasons discussed above, Finland seemed to be an ideal population to look for the gene. Furthermore, even adults in Finland often drink glasses of milk with their meals, such that exposure to lactose is ubiquitous.

Surprisingly, it was found that all individuals who were lactase nonpersistent carried the identical C/C genotype at a single SNP located 13,910 bp before the start of the lactase gene, in an intron of a different gene, while all individuals who expressed lactase as adults had a C/T genotype at this position [100]. The same result was found in samples from several other Eurasian populations showing that all individuals with lactase persistence had the C/T genotype at this one specific site. This is the exact opposite of the case for most recessive disease traits. Why? Well, it turns out that the T allele is the new mutation rather than the "disease-related" C allele. Most sub-Saharan Africans are C/C, as are most East Asians. When also including other primate species in the analysis, C was clearly the ancestral allele. In this case, a novel mutation within our species created the "beneficial" T allele, which conferred a new function that was not normally needed – it prevented lactase from being turned off after weaning.

In early humans, like most other mammals, once weaning is complete, milk was not normally consumed, and therefore, the lactase enzyme was no longer needed. Obviously not producing unneeded enzymes would be advantageous for an organism, to conserve resources. Mutation is the engine that powers evolution, and over time, variation has arisen in mammalian genomes to allow the enzyme to stop being produced after weaning. Dairy culture was a human innovation that began in earnest only a few thousand years ago. The idea of drinking milk produced by another species is a uniquely human innovation. Chimpanzees do not drink horse milk, and dogs do not drink bear milk. In populations that developed dairy culture and obtained a significant portion of their daily caloric intake from milk, there likely was a selective advantage to being able to digest lactose throughout life. Over a scant few thousand years, one variant particularly increased substantially in frequency, coevolving with dairy culture in the Middle East and Central Asia, and that variant moved with them into Europe, together with dairy culture itself. Positive selection allowed this single molecular variant to increase enormously over time as dairy culture spread into Europe [101].

Random mutations that cause loss of function are typically numerous in any given gene, as there are many ways mutations can knock out a gene causing loss of function. Mutations are random and lots of loss-of-function mutations therefore exist, as seen for congenital lactose intolerance [98]. However, the number of ways a random mutation can add a new function are far fewer. There are very few sites in the human genome where specific random mutations would have prevented the lactase gene from being turned off after weaning, while there are very many sites where random mutation would knock the gene out from infancy. In Europe, there is just this one single variant, which causes the vast majority of lactase persistence. However, dairy culture has arisen elsewhere at different times in human history, and further analysis has shown that there are indeed additional variants in the same genomic region that can also prevent lactase from being turned off after weaning, which are found in other parts of the world [102, 103].

Adult-type hypolactasia is just one simple example of a trait for which natural selection acted on existing genetic variation in the presence of a novel environmental exposure. Many other traits of interest involve similar genetic responses to new environmental exposures. Consider alcohol metabolism, for example. The aldehyde dehydrogenase 2 enzyme normally works to catalyze the conversion of acetaldehyde to acetic acid in the process of alcohol metabolism. There is a common variant allele of this gene in East Asia, which carries a loss-of-function mutation. Individuals carrying this defective allele fail to properly metabolize acetaldehyde leading to a series of adverse phenotypic consequences that can make alcohol consumption an unpleasant experience. In East Asians, there is a strong correlation between genotype of this locus and alcohol dependence [104]. Another example would be in pharmacogenetics, which is the study of genetic influences on variation in response to exposure to a novel pharmaceutical intervention, a topic deserving of an entire chapter of its own, but which could also be of significant relevance to people studying substance abuse.

As I write this book chapter, we have just begun quarantine-like conditions in the entire world because of the addition of a new exogenous exposure – that of Covid-19. Many investigators have already begun to search for genetic variants in the human genome, which may influence which individuals have good or bad outcomes from infection with this novel coronavirus. In Western society, we have become preoccupied with genetic studies of lifestyle-driven chronic diseases of late onset, to the detriment of infectious disease research [74], but the technologies we have developed may provide useful insights into the differential outcome of infection. Much like lactase persistence, it is very possible that individuals with different genotypes may respond differently to this new exposure, and so it is rational to search for them.

The main topic of this book is another example of this – that of substance abuse and addiction. The exposure to such a wide variety of readily available addictive substances is relatively new in evolutionary history. Just as animal milk production and dairy culture increased because of demand, so did large-scale production and distribution of alcohol and various other addictive drugs. Exposure to these substances can produce different responses in different individuals, and some individuals develop addiction, while others appear to be quite resistant. It is not unlikely that genetic variation exists in the population, which influences these individual variations in response. Alcohol dependence is a good example, as outlined above. But while alcohol has been abused throughout the world for millennia, other abused substances have been introduced into our population much more recently or have been geographically localized in the past and only recently have expanded to be available worldwide to people of all genetic backgrounds. It is quite possible that existing genetic variation responds in a variety of ways to such compounds.

I have no expertise in the biology of substance abuse, but like everyone else, I have seen friends respond very differently to their battles with addiction. In his bestselling book, Aiming High [105], Darren Prince described the very different paths he and basketball player Dennis Rodman had in their respective battles with substance abuse and addiction. Darren suffered from a long-term battle with opiate addiction, while Dennis has had his own well-documented struggles with alcohol. These two men both had access to resources and had the support of friends and family in their struggles with addiction, but while Darren was extremely successful in overcoming his addiction (despite his daily struggles, he never relapsed), Dennis has had a much more difficult struggle. Similarly, we all know life-long smokers who were able to wake up one day, and quit cold turkey, while others can struggle for years without breaking their addiction. There must be interesting biological factors that influence these different responses, just as there must be variation in who becomes addicted in the first place – obviously not everyone who has a couple beers now and then becomes an alcoholic. Having said that, there is no reason to believe that it has to be etiologically simple.

Lactase nonpersistence was an easy trait to study in Finland, because milk consumption is virtually ubiquitous, so there was no variation in exposure. Traits like substance abuse are far more complicated as not everyone is exposed. And much like lactose intolerance, the environmental exposure is required to express the phenotype of interest. For example, I have never tried smoking tobacco or any other recreational drug besides alcohol, so it is impossible to know how I would respond to those, while the one time I was prescribed opiates for a bad cough, I strongly disliked the physiological effects (other than successfully suppressing the cough). Pharmacogenetics is even more difficult as still fewer people are exposed to any given pharmaceutical. One can, of course, look at the set of all people with exposure and look at differences in responses. This can certainly be done in population studies, though family studies are unfortunately difficult as not all individuals in a family would have the same experience with substance use, in contrast to lactase nonpersistence, as milk consumption was effectively ubiquitous in Finland.

As an alternative approach to studying only those individuals who have been exposed, one might want to think about what other traits might be worth studying in relatives of people suffering from substance abuse and addictive behavior. Every first-degree relative of an affected individual shares half his genetic material. The molecular variants, which might predispose to substance abuse, do not "cause" substance abuse, but rather they typically change the structure or regulation of a protein. That variation, in concert with other genetic and environmental factors, eventually leads to the bad outcome. But half of all first-degree relatives will share any given molecular variant allele with the affected individual. The question is what the effect is in individuals who do not have the other requisite risk factors. I would hypothesize that every person reading this chapter is far more expert than I am when it comes to substance abuse and addiction, so in the interests of not illustrating the depths of my ignorance, let me illustrate how one might choose alternative phenotypes for study, contrasting the typical clinician's disease-oriented thinking with a geneticist's biologically focused thinking.

The trait I will use to illustrate this concept is one that I suffer from and that has a necessary and novel exogenous exposure – being a professional tuba player. If one is not presented with a tuba in elementary school, there is no chance they will end up with the trait. Furthermore, like substance abuse, it is difficult to find families with multiple affected individuals because it is very unusual for relatives to share the exposure.

A clinician's approach to this "disorder" might be to do a detailed study on a set of probands who are professional tuba players in order to find diagnostically meaningful subsets of the disease. For example, in studies of hypertension, it can be important to separate salt-sensitive from non-salt-sensitive hypertensives in a study to reduce heterogeneity, or with lung cancer, the etiology might be expected to be quite different in smokers and nonsmokers. In the case of tuba playing, one might choose to contrast individuals who have a better high range with those who have a better low range, or you might contrast individuals who have better intonation vs those who do not, etc. The former might have relationships to mouth size and lung function, while the latter might be more influenced by hearing, such that one could focus on more biological phenotypes in this way. The problem with subdividing your set of exposed individuals, however, is that it reduces the potential sample size rather than increasing it. When dealing with a rare complex trait, which requires an exogenous exposure that is far from ubiquitous, this may be a suboptimal design for a research study.

On the other hand, a geneticist who is not clinically oriented might be more interested in thinking about what biological traits might put one at risk for becoming a professional tuba player, and given that the relatives of the affected person share half his genes, one could study those background traits rather than outcome variables. Figure 6.7 shows an example of different factors that are related to success at playing the tuba. For example, tooth and jaw structure have a big influence, as does lung capacity, or ability to hear subtle variations in pitch, or finger dexterity, etc. Each of those trait categories could then be investigated by looking for measurable phenotypes which could be related to performance. For example, to study lung function, one might measure vital capacity, or exhalation rate, or air flow pressure or ability to regulate the said pressure; for hearing, one might test how sensitive an individual is to detect subtle differences in pitch; for tooth structure, one might measure the size of

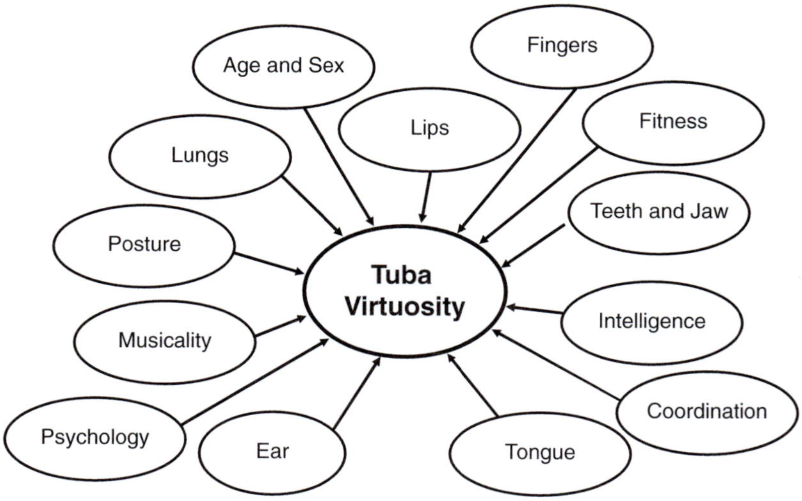

Fig. 6.7 Endophenotypes for a complex trait requiring a rare environmental trigger: When studying a complex phenotype that requires a rare environmental exposure, it can be difficult to identify multiplex families, even when there is a strong genetic component of the trait. Another way to identify potential "genetically correlated" traits of interest would be to examine first degree relatives of affected individuals (who share roughly half their genes), and see how they differ phenotypically from random individuals selected from the population for related traits. In this example, the "rare disease" is being a tuba virtuoso, which requires the rare environmental risk factor of having been given a tuba to play. There are many reasons to suspect there is a genetic component of variation in this trait, as many other heritable traits are correlated with success at playing the tuba. Several such organ systems and/or traits are shown in this figure, each of which could be studied in relatives of the "affected" proband as a means of studying the genetic component of tuba virtuosity. Substance abuse is an analogous problem, in which exposure to the substance is required. Close phenotypic examination of first-degree unaffected relatives of patients in comparison with a random sample of controls might provide a way to use genetic thinking to expand the phenotypic search-space.

the teeth or shape of the mouth in various dimensions; and so on. In other words, the approach would be to identify genetically-mediated biological covariates which could themselves be studied in a sample of individuals who had not been exposed to the environmental "insult".

One would then first demonstrate that the trait of interest is, in fact, differently distributed between professional tuba players and a cohort of random individuals from a population. This does not prove that the trait is a risk factor for success at playing the tuba, however, as it can be difficult to separate cause from effect. Obviously, training affects lung function and hearing and posture and many other potentially related measurements. However, if the trait is causally related to the outcome, and predated the initial exogenous exposure (in this case to a tuba), and was genetically influenced, relatives of tuba players would also be expected to have a different phenotypic distribution from relatives of the random cohort, given that they share 50% of their genetic material. If one identifies such traits, then one can do a family study looking for the genetic (and environmental) factors, which affect variation in the trait. The end result is a way to increase the informative sample size, as information can now be gleaned from studying these alternative phenotypes in individuals lacking the requisite environmental exposure.

The geneticist's approach to complex traits thus focuses on thinking about what potential susceptibility genes might do biologically in the absence of the required exposures. How do biological relatives of an affected person differ from random individuals in a population? I might suggest that healthy first-degree relatives of affected persons are an understudied population, which might provide key insights into the genetics of such difficult to study poorly understood complex traits such as substance abuse, autism, schizophrenia, among others.

Conclusions

As whole-genome sequencing becomes cheaper and faster every year, an ever-increasing fraction of the population of the developed world has access to their own individual genome sequence. On paper, this seems like something that would be of value in predicting one's predisposition to a variety of phenotypes, and understanding the nature of human variation and its response to environmental exposures.

Many traits are caused outright by deleterious variants of a single gene, and our ability to screen whole genomes at low cost will eventually prove very useful in screening everyone for all of these known conditions. Now that the cost of whole-genome sequencing is trivial compared to the other medical costs associated with childbirth, it seems likely that in the coming decades, this will be routinely done on all newborns to screen for each of the hundreds of thousands of known deleterious variants.

Despite the enormous successes we have had in identifying the pathological variants for these monogenic disorders, orphan rare diseases of unknown etiology are still enormously common, with hundreds of such diseases seen in every major hospital in the world, with an obvious bias towards understudied ethnic populations. However, we know that our genetic methods work very effectively for identifying the causes of simple monogenic conditions. Every children's hospital in the country sees a surprisingly large number of patients with orphan diseases of unknown etiology, many of which turn out to be inborn genetic defects. Individuals coming from underserved minority populations are more likely to present with unknown orphan diseases precisely because they are understudied. The causes and classifications of these diseases will also become trivial as we begin whole-genome sequencing in clinical settings.

In the Western world, however, there is a disproportionate emphasis on applying the new technological advances to common multifactorial traits, because of their enormous public health impact. Today, for example, there is a huge investment in a project called "All Of Us," which aims to collect genetic and medical history data from a million Americans [106]. The sampling is being conducted using the classical and mathematically well-characterized ascertainment scheme of advertisement in the New York City Subway system and other such haphazard approaches, hoping to end up with a quasi-random self-selected sample of the country.

There are significant reasons to doubt the effectiveness of such a big data strategy when applied to a rather haphazardly collected sample with reliance on externally measured electronic medical records for phenotype data, especially given the weak genotype-phenotype relationships seen to date in well-characterized case-control samples. Perhaps a wiser approach would be to select patients from children's hospitals around the country who have some orphan disease and then collect DNA and medical records from their parents as well. In this way, you would have a reasonable chance of getting some medically significant results about genetic contribution to these orphan diseases, while also getting a sample of unrelated individuals from the general population – the healthy parents of the sick child. And this sample would also be biased in the desired way towards underserved populations in the US, for obvious reasons.

Identification of such pathological variants of very high impact is now a routine engineering exercise, however, and because this works so effectively, it is clear that population-level screening for these simple disorders will be the most important long-term impact of the human genome project. This is a very valuable tool, but we need to be careful to remember that great tools for solving one type of problem are not always valuable for others.

For common complex chronic diseases of the greatest public health impact, there is scant reason to believe that all the genotyping in the world will make them meaningfully predictable, treatable, or understandable. While we have related a few thousand SNPs with various chronic diseases, in most of those cases, we have not identified the functional molecular variants nor even what genes they are found in. This means that we have not learned much about their underlying biology compared to the hype and the promises.

There are very few examples of specific functional variants being identified, which directly affect any of these common complex human traits of interest, even though thousands of SNP associations have been found with very small effect sizes. These days, it is routine to have studies with tens or even hundreds of thousands of subjects in genome-wide association studies, sampled from consortia of investigators from all over the world – often with lists of authors that are as long as the entire paper itself. Much of this is motivated by attempts to fulfill promises made 25 years ago, about predicting disease risks of complex diseases from birth and developing prophylactic drug regimens tailored to each individual's personal genotype information. Such personalized medicine was the justification for the enormous investment of private and public funds in this endeavor, but to date, the results have been far less than promised. Basically, we keep trying to square this circle, by taking the square peg that is a complex disease and trying to force it into the round hole of CDCV, primarily because there is a lot of money in round holes, not because we have a good scientific reason.

References

1. Horwitz T, et al. A decade in psychiatric GWAS research. Mol Psychiatry. 2019;24(3):378–89.
2. Schizophrenia Working Group of the Psychiatric Genomics, C. Biological insights from 108 schizophrenia-associated genetic loci. Nature. 2014;511(7510):421–7.
3. Stenson PD, et al. The human gene mutation database: towards a comprehensive repository of inherited mutation data for medical research, genetic diagnosis and next-generation sequencing studies. Hum Genet. 2017;136(6):665–77.
4. Le Fanu J. The rise and fall of modern medicine. New York: Carroll and Grf Publishers; 1999.
5. Terwilliger JD, Weiss KM. Confounding, ascertainment bias, and the blind quest for a genetic 'fountain of youth'. Ann Med. 2003;35(7):532–44.
6. Weiss KM, Terwilliger JD. How many diseases does it take to map a gene with SNPs? Nat Genet. 2000;26(2):151–7.
7. Castle WE. Genetics and eugenics. Cambridge, MA: Harvard University Press; 1916.
8. Corvin A, Sullivan PF. What next in schizophrenia genetics for the psychiatric genomics consortium? Schizophr Bull. 2016;42(3):538–41.
9. International Consortium for Blood Pressure Genome-Wide Association, S, et al. Genetic variants in novel pathways influence blood pressure and cardiovascular disease risk. Nature. 2011;478(7367):103–9.
10. Tuncel G, Ergoren MC. Functional coding and non-coding variants in human BRCA1 gene and their use in genetic screening. Med Oncol. 2019;36(8):71.
11. Negrette A. Corea de Huntington: Estudio de Una Sola Familia a Traves de Varias Generaciones. Maracaibo, Venezuela: University of Zulia; 1955.
12. Gusella JF, et al. A polymorphic DNA marker genetically linked to Huntington's disease. Nature. 1983;306(5940):234–8.
13. Wexler NS, et al. Venezuelan kindreds reveal that genetic and environmental factors modulate Huntington's disease age of onset. Proc Natl Acad Sci U S A. 2004;101(10):3498–503.
14. A novel gene containing a trinucleotide repeat that is expanded and unstable on Huntington's disease chromosomes. The Huntington's Disease Collaborative Research Group. Cell. 1993;72(6):971–83.
15. Kaariainen H, et al. Genetics in an isolated population like Finland: a different basis for genomic medicine? J Community Genet. 2017;8(4):319–26.
16. Polvi A, et al. The Finnish disease heritage database (FinDis) update-a database for the genes mutated in the Finnish disease heritage brought to the next-generation sequencing era. Hum Mutat. 2013;34(11):1458–66.
17. Kestila M, Ikonen E, Lehesjoki AE. Finnish disease heritage. Duodecim. 2010;126(19):2311–20.
18. De Boeck K. Cystic fibrosis in the year 2020: a disease with a new face. Acta Paediatr. 2020;
19. Blau N. Genetics of phenylketonuria: then and now. Hum Mutat. 2016;37(6):508–15.
20. Varilo T. The age of the mutations in the finnish disease heritage: a genealogical and linkage disequi-

librium study. In: Department of Medical Genetics. Helsinki: University of Helsinki; 1999. p. 99.
21. Peltonen L, Jalanko A, Varilo T. Molecular genetics of the Finnish disease heritage. Hum Mol Genet. 1999;8(10):1913–23.
22. Varilo T, et al. The age of human mutation: genealogical and linkage disequilibrium analysis of the CLN5 mutation in the Finnish population. Am J Hum Genet. 1996;58(3):506–12.
23. Bartha I, et al. Human gene essentiality. Nat Rev Genet. 2018;19(1):51–62.
24. Chen WH, et al. OGEE v2: an update of the online gene essentiality database with special focus on differentially essential genes in human cancer cell lines. Nucleic Acids Res. 2017;45(D1):D940–4.
25. Pekkarinen P, et al. Fine-scale mapping of a novel dementia gene, PLOSL, by linkage disequilibrium. Genomics. 1998;54(2):307–15.
26. Pekkarinen P, et al. Assignment of the locus for PLO-SL, a frontal-lobe dementia with bone cysts, to 19q13. Am J Hum Genet. 1998;62(2):362–72.
27. Paloneva J, et al. Loss-of-function mutations in TYROBP (DAP12) result in a presenile dementia with bone cysts. Nat Genet. 2000;25(3):357–61.
28. Paloneva J, et al. Mutations in two genes encoding different subunits of a receptor signaling complex result in an identical disease phenotype. Am J Hum Genet. 2002;71(3):656–62.
29. Yan D, et al. The genetic basis of nonsyndromic hearing loss in Indian and Pakistani populations. Genet Test Mol Biomarkers. 2015;19(9):512–27.
30. Fahim A. Retinitis pigmentosa: recent advances and future directions in diagnosis and management. Curr Opin Pediatr. 2018;30(6):725–33.
31. Hu H, et al. Genetics of intellectual disability in consanguineous families. Mol Psychiatry. 2019;24(7):1027–39.
32. Terwilliger JD, Weiss KM. Linkage disequilibrium mapping of complex disease: fantasy or reality? Curr Opin Biotechnol. 1998;9(6):578–94.
33. Musarella MA, et al. Multipoint linkage analysis and heterogeneity testing in 20 X-linked retinitis pigmentosa families. Genomics. 1990;8(2):286–96.
34. Ott J. Linkage probability and its approximate confidence interval under possible heterogeneity. Genet Epidemiol Suppl. 1986;1:251–7.
35. Ott J. Linkage analysis and family classification under heterogeneity. Ann Hum Genet. 1983;47(4):311–20.
36. Pajukanta P, et al. Linkage of familial combined hyperlipidaemia to chromosome 1q21-q23. Nat Genet. 1998;18(4):369–73.
37. Vaxillaire M, et al. A gene for maturity-onset diabetes of the young (Mody) maps to chromosome 12q. Nat Genet. 1995;9(4):418–23.
38. Hall JM, et al. Linkage of early-onset familial breast cancer to chromosome 17q21. Science. 1990;250(4988):1684–9.
39. Pajukanta P, et al. Genomewide scan for familial combined hyperlipidemia genes in Finnish families, suggesting multiple susceptibility loci influencing triglyceride, cholesterol, and apolipoprotein B levels. Am J Hum Genet. 1999;64(5):1453–63.
40. Ginns EI, et al. A genome-wide search for chromosomal loci linked to bipolar affective disorder in the old order Amish. Nat Genet. 1996;12(4):431–5.
41. Hovatta I, et al. A genome-wide search for schizophrenia genes in an internal isolate of Finland suggesting multiple susceptibility loci. Am J Med Genet. 1998;81(6):453–4.
42. Kuokkanen S, et al. Genomewide scan of multiple sclerosis in Finnish multiplex families. Am J Hum Genet. 1997;61(6):1379–87.
43. Tienari PJ, et al. 2-locus linkage analysis in multiple-sclerosis (Ms). Genomics. 1994;19(2):320–5.
44. Penrose LS. The detection of autosomal linkage in data which consists of pairs of brothers and sisters of unspecified parentage. Ann Eugenics. 1935;6:133–8.
45. Perola M, et al. Genome-wide scan of predisposing loci for increased diastolic blood pressure in Finnish siblings. J Hypertens. 2000;18(11):1579–85.
46. Liu JJ, et al. A follow-up linkage study supports evidence for a bipolar affective disorder locus on chromosome 21q22. Am J Med Genet. 2001;105(2):189–94.
47. Williams NM, et al. A systematic genomewide linkage study in 353 sib pairs with schizophrenia. Am J Hum Genet. 2003;73(6):1355–67.
48. International Psoriasis Genetics, C. The International Psoriasis Genetics Study: assessing linkage to 14 candidate susceptibility loci in a cohort of 942 affected sib pairs. Am J Hum Genet. 2003;73(2):430–7.
49. Larsen F, et al. Linkage analysis of a candidate region in Scandinavian sib pairs with multiple sclerosis reveals linkage to chromosome 17q. Genes Immun. 2000;1(7):456–9.
50. A complete genome screen in sib pairs affected by Gilles de la Tourette syndrome. The Tourette Syndrome Association International Consortium for Genetics. Am J Hum Genet. 1999. 65(5): p. 1428–36.
51. Ghosh S, et al. Type 2 diabetes: evidence for linkage on chromosome 20 in 716 Finnish affected sib pairs. Proc Natl Acad Sci U S A. 1999;96(5):2198–203.
52. Ekelund J, et al. A genome scan for schizophrenia loci in affected sib-pairs collected in Finland. Am J Med Genet. 1997;74(6):559.
53. Bray MS, Boerwinkle E, Hanis CL. OB gene not linked to human obesity in Mexican American affected sib pairs from Starr County, Texas. Hum Genet. 1996;98(5):590–5.
54. Tiret L, et al. Evidence, from combined segregation and linkage analysis, that a variant of the angiotensin I-converting enzyme (ACE) gene controls plasma ACE levels. Am J Hum Genet. 1992;51(1):197–205.
55. Davies JL, et al. A genome-wide search for human type 1 diabetes susceptibility genes. Nature. 1994;371(6493):130–6.
56. Hovatta I, et al. Schizophrenia in the genetic isolate of Finland. Am J Med Genet. 1997;74(4):353–60.
57. Hovatta I, et al. A genomewide screen for schizophrenia genes in an isolated Finnish subpopulation,

suggesting multiple susceptibility loci. Am J Hum Genet. 1999;65(4):1114–24.
58. Fisher RA. The correlation between relatives on the supposition of mendelian inheritance. Trans R Soc Edinb. 1918;53:399–433.
59. Paunio T, et al. Genome-wide scan of an extended Finnish schizophrenia study sample. Am J Med Genet. 2000;96(4):O1.
60. Paunio T, et al. Genome-wide scan in a nationwide study sample of schizophrenia families in Finland reveals susceptibility loci on chromosomes 2q and 5q. Hum Mol Genet. 2001;10(26):3037–48.
61. Paunio T, et al. Genome-wide scans provide evidence for schizophrenia loci on 1q, 2q and 5q in a nationwide study sample from Finland. Am J Hum Genet. 2001;69(4):120.
62. Ekelund J, et al. Genome-wide scan for schizophrenia in the Finnish population: evidence for a locus on chromosome 7q22. Hum Mol Genet. 2000;9(7):1049–57.
63. Peltonen L, et al. Search for schizophrenia genes in Finnish families reveal a locus on Chromosome 1q. Am J Hum Genet. 2000;67(4):181.
64. Ekelund J, et al. Genome-wide scan for schizophrenia in the Finnish population: evidence for a locus on chromosome 7q22. Am J Hum Genet. 1999;65(4):1378.
65. Hovatta I, et al. Linkage analysis of putative schizophrenia gene candidate regions on chromosomes 3p, 5q, 6p, 8p, 20p and 22q in a population-based sampled Finnish family set. Mol Psychiatry. 1998;3(5):452–7.
66. Silander K, et al. Analysis of genetic variation in the GenomEUtwin project. Twin Res. 2003;6(5):391–8.
67. Litton JE, et al. Data modeling and data communication in GenomEUtwin. Twin Res. 2003;6(5):383–90.
68. Peltonen, L. And GenomEutwin GenomEUtwin: a strategy to identify genetic influences on health and disease. Twin Res, 2003. 6(5): p. 354–360.
69. International Schizophrenia, C, et al. Common polygenic variation contributes to risk of schizophrenia and bipolar disorder. Nature. 2009;460(7256):748–52.
70. Strittmatter WJ, et al. Apolipoprotein E: high-avidity binding to beta-amyloid and increased frequency of type 4 allele in late-onset familial Alzheimer disease. Proc Natl Acad Sci U S A. 1993;90(5):1977–81.
71. Pericak-Vance MA, et al. Linkage studies in familial Alzheimer disease: evidence for chromosome 19 linkage. Am J Hum Genet. 1991;48(6):1034–50.
72. Rogaev EI, et al. Familial Alzheimer's disease in kindreds with missense mutations in a gene on chromosome 1 related to the Alzheimer's disease type 3 gene. Nature. 1995;376(6543):775–8.
73. Sherrington R, et al. Cloning of a gene bearing missense mutations in early-onset familial Alzheimer's disease. Nature. 1995;375(6534):754–60.
74. Terwilliger JD. Mother Nature and globalization to blame for Covid-19 crisis. In Asia Times. 2020 Hong Kong.
75. Risch N, Merikangas K. The future of genetic studies of complex human diseases. Science. 1996;273(5281):1516–7.
76. Reich DE, Lander ES. On the allelic spectrum of human disease. Trends Genet. 2001;17(9):502–10.
77. Lander ES. The new genomics: global views of biology. Science. 1996;274(5287):536–9.
78. Pritchard JK, Cox NJ. The allelic architecture of human disease genes: common disease-common variant...or not? Hum Mol Genet. 2002;11(20):2417–23.
79. Collins FS. Shattuck lecture–medical and societal consequences of the human genome project. N Engl J Med. 1999;341(1):28–37.
80. Collins FS. Personalized medicine: a new approach to staying well. In Boston globe. 2005.
81. Bell J. The new genetics in clinical practice. BMJ. 1998;316(7131):618–20.
82. Darwin C. On the origin of species by meand of natural selection, or the preservation of favoured races in the struggle for life. London: John Murray; 1859.
83. Darwin C. The descent of man and selection in relation to sex, vol. 2. London: J. Murray; 1871. In Boston Globe, 2005. http://archive.boston.com/news/globe/editorial_opinion/oped/articles/2005/07/17/personalized_medicine/.
84. Campbell CD, Eichler EE. Properties and rates of germline mutations in humans. Trends Genet. 2013;29(10):575–84.
85. Piovesan A, et al. On the length, weight and GC content of the human genome. BMC Res Notes. 2019;12(1):106.
86. Phan L, et al. "ALFA: Allele Frequency Aggregator." [2020 March 9, 2020]. Available from: www.ncbi.nlm.nih.gov/snp/docs/gsr/alfa/.
87. Ohta T. Slightly deleterious mutant substitutions in evolution. Nature. 1973;246(5428):96–8.
88. Kimura M. The neutral theory of molecular evolution. Sci Am. 1979;241(5):98–100, 102, 108 passim.
89. Coon KD, et al. A high-density whole-genome association study reveals that APOE is the major susceptibility gene for sporadic late-onset Alzheimer's disease. J Clin Psychiatry. 2007;68(4):613–8.
90. Kunkle BW, et al. Genetic meta-analysis of diagnosed Alzheimer's disease identifies new risk loci and implicates Abeta, tau, immunity and lipid processing. Nat Genet. 2019;51(3):414–30.
91. Ridge PG, et al. Assessment of the genetic variance of late-onset Alzheimer's disease. Neurobiol Aging. 2016;41:200 e13–20.
92. Speliotes EK, et al. Association analyses of 249,796 individuals reveal 18 new loci associated with body mass index. Nat Genet. 2010;42(11):937–48.
93. Manolio TA, Brooks LD, Collins FS. A HapMap harvest of insights into the genetics of common disease. J Clin Invest. 2008;118(5):1590–605.
94. Myers RH. Considerations for genomewide association studies in Parkinson disease. Am J Hum Genet. 2006;78(6):1081–2.

95. Chang D, et al. A meta-analysis of genome-wide association studies identifies 17 new Parkinson's disease risk loci. Nat Genet. 2017;49(10):1511–6.
96. Terwilliger JD, Goring HH. Update to Terwilliger and Goring's "Gene mapping in the 20th and 21st centuries" (2000): gene mapping when rare variants are common and common variants are rare. Hum Biol. 2009;81(5–6):729–33.
97. Terwilliger JD, Goring HH. Gene mapping in the 20th and 21st centuries: statistical methods, data analysis, and experimental design. Hum Biol, 2009. 2000;81(5–6):663–728.
98. Diekmann L, Pfeiffer K, Naim HY. Congenital lactose intolerance is triggered by severe mutations on both alleles of the lactase gene. BMC Gastroenterol. 2015;15:36.
99. Sahi T. Genetics and epidemiology of adult-type hypolactasia. Scand J Gastroenterol Suppl. 1994;202:7–20.
100. Enattah NS, et al. Identification of a variant associated with adult-type hypolactasia. Nat Genet. 2002;30(2):233–7.
101. Enattah NS, et al. Evidence of still-ongoing convergence evolution of the lactase persistence T-13910 alleles in humans. Am J Hum Genet. 2007;81(3):615–25.
102. Enattah NS, et al. Independent introduction of two lactase-persistence alleles into human populations reflects different history of adaptation to milk culture. Am J Hum Genet. 2008;82(1):57–72.
103. Segurel L, Bon C. On the evolution of lactase persistence in humans. Annu Rev Genomics Hum Genet. 2017;18:297–319.
104. Luczak SE, Glatt SJ, Wall TL. Meta-analyses of ALDH2 and ADH1B with alcohol dependence in Asians. Psychol Bull. 2006;132(4):607–21.
105. Prince D. Aiming high. Los Angeles: Light Hustler; 2018.
106. National Institutes of Health (NIH) – All of us. [cited 2020 4/20/2020]; Available from: http://allofus.nih.gov/.

Linkage and Association Studies of Substance Use Disorders

7

Brion Maher

Introduction

As discussed elsewhere in this volume, twin, family, and adoption studies provided evidence of significant genetic influences on substance use and substance use disorders (SUD), with heritability estimates generally ranging from 0.4 to 0.6 (Chap. 4) and modest sibling recurrence risks (Chap. 5). This is greater than the heritability found for most other common psychiatric disorders, including anxiety disorders [1] or depression [2]. Consistent with the field of human disease genetics since the start of the molecular era, studies examining the genetics of substance use have focused on identifying mutations or genetic variants that are "linked" or "associated" with a particular disease or disorder. The overall goal is to identify genes linked or associated with these outcomes to identify novel pathways or biological mechanisms that will translate to clinical practice.

The field of SUD genetics has transitioned through study designs, driven largely by the technologies, approaches, and expectations of each time period [3]. The gene-mapping approach common in each era was heavily influenced by assumptions about the genetic architecture (i.e., the number of genes responsible for variation in disease risk) of a given disease and the available technology for measuring genetic variation. The 1990s, researchers largely applied linkage analysis in large pedigrees and later candidate gene approaches. Since ~2005, the field has moved toward performing genome-wide association scans.

This chapter has two parts. First, it discusses several important topics that have not been detailed elsewhere in this volume and are somewhat unique to substance use genetics or are important to understanding the content of this chapter. These issues include the following: the measures and methods used in genetic studies of substance use disorder, the definition of "cases" and "controls" in studies of SUDs, and the commonly studied SUD candidate gene systems. Second, it reviews the important genetic linkage and association findings in the field of substance use genetics for the most frequently studied substances (alcohol, nicotine, cannabis, opioids, and cocaine) and for general (common) liability (the continuous trait underlying risk for addiction across substance classes) [4, 5] over the past three decades, primarily highlighting those with evidence, as of this writing, for replication. Furthermore, it discusses the possible future of these areas of research for substance use and other behavioral traits.

B. Maher (✉)
Department of Mental Health, Johns Hopkins Bloomberg School of Public Health, Baltimore, MD, USA
e-mail: brion@jhu.edu

M. M. Vanyukov (ed.), *Genetics of Substance Use*, https://doi.org/10.1007/978-3-030-95350-8_7

Part I: Issues in Molecular Genetic Studies of Addiction

Methods and Measurement

Genetic Variation

Linkage and association analyses rely on genetic polymorphism, or interindividual variation in the genomic sequence, to represent specific regions or sites in the genome and formally (statistically) test for a relationship between that region and a disease or trait. There are several types of genetic polymorphisms, or markers, scattered throughout the genome, and their use in the field has increased or decreased, depending on both the interest in a type of polymorphism and the availability of technology to assess that type. After blood groups (starting with the polymorphism of the ABO gene, readily genotyped based on the ABO system blood type phenotype), the first widely used markers were restriction fragment length polymorphisms (RFLPs), which were identified by variable length DNA fragments caused by differential digestion by restriction enzymes, visualized as the characteristic "DNA fingerprint" on Southern blots via gel electrophoresis [6]. In retrospect, RFLPs were frequently the result of single nucleotide substitutions, which disrupted the DNA sequence recognized by the restriction enzyme, leading to different length fragments when recognized and cut by the enzyme. Variable number of tandem repeats (VNTR) and short tandem repeats (STR) were subsequently discovered [7, 8]. These are repeat polymorphisms, where a segment of DNA is repeated multiple times, in tandem, along a chromosome. The length of that repeated DNA segment is the distinguishing feature between VNTRs (10+ nucleotides) and STRs (<10 nucleotides).

Prior to 2005, the vast majority of genetic studies of substance use disorders relied on RFLPs, VNTRs, or STRs in linkage analysis. The assumption was that there would be genetic variants that would exhibit a large or "major gene" effect by nearly perfectly co-segregating in a Mendelian fashion (e.g., dominant, recessive) with addiction. More recently, single nucleotide polymorphisms (SNPs) have become the most widely utilized genetic markers. SNPs are substitutions of one nucleotide for another. SNPs usually consist of two alleles in the population (i.e., biallelic) and occur at tens of millions of sites throughout the genome.

Massive investment in discovery of variation in 2002 in the human genome through an international consortium (HapMap Project) led to the discovery of millions of single nucleotide polymorphisms (SNPs) [9]. This work was not without its detractors, who argued that many of the assumptions regarding the value of the project for mapping genetic associations with disease were unrealistic or optimistic [10]. Nevertheless, after genome-wide array technology became affordable to most researchers, several hallmark genome-wide association studies were published [11, 12]. Investment in diverse reference population samples and development of novel methods provide the ability to impute the entire genome's known common SNP across studies which used different genotyping arrays [9, 13, 14].

Gene-Mapping Approaches

Linkage analysis is a statistical approach in which, using samples of family members with and without disease or disorder, an investigator formally tests for linkage between risk for that disease and polymorphisms (variations at chromosomal loci) in known locations throughout the genome. "Linkage" refers to the violation of Mendel's law of independent assortment, under which we expect the alleles (variants) at two different genes to sort independently into separate gametes. Linkage is the result of those two genes residing close together on the same chromosome. In the case of linkage analysis in human pedigrees, the two "genes" being tested are the risk for disease and a genetic polymorphism. Thus, if we know the genomic location of the polymorphism (e.g., a specific base-pair position on chromosome 4), then we have an estimate of the location of a gene linked to risk for the disorder.

Linkage Disequilibrium

Geneticists assume the substitution mutations that create SNPs have occurred once in population history at a particular location in the genome. These single mutation events are important to understanding the concept of linkage disequilibrium (LD), or the correlation between polymorphisms in close proximity along a chromosome. When a new mutation occurs, that allele is perfectly correlated with the haplotype, or set of neighboring nucleotides, on which it occurred. Over generations, recombination will reshuffle those haplotypes and diminish the strength of LD, but SNPs tens, hundreds, or even millions of base pairs apart will remain correlated, "associated," or "in linkage disequilibrium" for many generations and across human populations.

Association Testing

The phenomenon of linkage disequilibrium allows for LD or *association mapping*, which generally involves testing for differences in the frequency of one allele of a SNP versus the other, in case versus control populations, or for a correlation between an allele or genotype and a quantitative trait in population-based samples. Family-based association methods test for association as an excess (over the expected 50%) transmission of a particular allele from parents to an offspring with the disorder (affected). A significant case-control difference in frequency of an allele, excess transmission of the allele to cases, or correlation between the presence of an allele and a quantitative trait is taken as evidence that the SNP tested is itself, or is in linkage disequilibrium with, a variant that is at least partly causal of the disease or outcome.

Genome-Wide Association Scans (GWAS)

Since 2005, the field of human genetics has moved largely into GWAS as a method for testing the association of specific SNPs with disease. GWAS rely on millions of SNPs measured using microarray or sequencing technology to test associations with disease at sites spanning the entire genome. The rationale for moving genetics into the genome-wide association study era was built largely on the common-disease/common-variant (CDCV) hypothesis, while the previous focus on linkage analysis was predicated on the assumption that variants with relatively large effects would contribute to disease risk variation in large pedigrees with multiple affected individuals. The CDCV hypothesis [15] posited that complex disease liability varies due to multiple genetic variants that are of modest effect (odds ratios of ~1.5–2.0) but relatively frequent (allele frequency > 5%) in the population. This view of complex traits grew from the failure of linkage approaches to detect rare and highly penetrant (frequently manifest phenotypically) variants in families with multiple affected individuals. These common variants, if they exist, would be generally detectable in association frameworks.

Indeed, many of the early GWAS successes for nonpsychiatric disorders have implicated common variants of modest effect (odds ratios <1.2). In most cases, these variants account for less than 50% of the cases of disease. However, the early round of GWAS results for psychiatric traits, including substance use, included modest sample sizes and did not yield the promising, novel signals [16, 17] seen in biologically relevant genes in many other diseases [11, 18]. For example, the Wellcome Trust Case-Control Consortium [12] performed the first large-scale GWAS study of multiple complex diseases, which revealed statistically significant association at multiple SNPs for five of the seven diseases studied. The lone psychiatric phenotype, bipolar disorder, was among those for which no robust signals were observed. Of course, this failure did not provide exhaustive evidence that CDCV is not true among psychiatric disorders but did adjust expectations for the individual effect sizes pertaining to complex diseases like addiction.

An important caveat of genome-wide studies is the need to correct for multiple statistical tests, as millions of statistical tests are performed and false-positive findings will result without adjustment of the usual p-values levels for statistical significance. In general, p-values smaller than .05 are considered "statistically significant." Applying methods such as Bonferroni correction, genome-wide studies are usually deemed significant only at p-values smaller than $\sim 5 \times 10^{-8}$. This, coupled with the reality of small effect sizes for addiction-related traits, has led to large GWAS meta-analysis consortium studies, the common current approach, with sample sizes now exceeding one million subjects. Consequently, large case-control genome-wide association studies have dominated the 2010s, across all of human disease genetics.

Work by the Psychiatric Genomics Consortium (PGC) has generated genome-wide significant results in many independent regions using a very large, combined sample for schizophrenia [19, 20]. However, the effect sizes are very small (<1.1, less than 10% increase in the risk). This raises two questions: (1) "Does meaningful (i.e., impacting protein quantity or quality) variation in the gene exist?" and (2) "Does the GWAS framework provide adequate detection power for important and meaningful variants?" These questions have been debated, and the consensus in the field has been to pursue larger samples in the interest of detecting variants of very small effect on a given disease or trait. More recently, polygenic approaches, which create composite of SNP effects across many variants or chromosomal regions, have given rise to concepts such as "molecular heritability", or the amount of variation in a trait attributable to measured genetic variation, and have allowed examination of genetic correlation, using results at measured genotypes, between trait GWAS.

Polygenic Approaches

Genome-wide association studies showed the relatively small individual effect sizes of the most strongly statistically associated variants. That was not unexpected. R.A. Fisher is widely regarded as the father of several disciplines, including modern statistical inference in medicine. His contributions to genetics are equally important. In Fisher's seminal work, he proved that familial resemblance could be due to many factors inherited in a Mendelian fashion [21]. Fisher's intent was to resolve a key dispute between biometricians, who believed that discrete genes could not explain quantitative variation in traits, and the Mendelians. His work led to many core statistical techniques still in use today and to the widespread acceptance that the high heritability observed for many human traits was likely due to the effects of many genes. However, many barriers, such as sample size, the availability of markers across the genome, and computing power necessary to perform genome-wide analyses, limited the molecular analysis of genetic variance. Single gene or variant approaches, where one genetic marker or region is individually tested for its relationship with a phenotype of interest, was the dominant paradigm from linkage analysis through candidate genes and even early GWAS. While the GWAS approach has now identified thousands of variants contributing to liability variance for hundreds of diseases, statistically detectable at stringent significance thresholds, these variants individually explain only a trivial amount of trait variance.

Polygenic scoring is a method which relies on genome-wide SNP data and attempts to capture the polygenic trait architecture described by Fisher by indexing "associated" variation across the genome. It has been shown that while the expected rank of any one risk-increasing SNP, given the usual effect sizes of common disease SNPs, would not likely be among the top findings in a typical GWAS, there is an expectation that the SNPs in the upper tail of the distribution of test statistics will be enriched with the tens or hundreds of true risk SNPs accounting for the heritability of a trait [22]. Consequently, investigators now frequently use polygenic risk scores to index the genetic risk for a disease or outcome. Polygenic scores are constructed using the results, *below* some p-value threshold, of large existing discovery GWAS of a trait to calculate test statistic-weighted sum scores of risk alleles in a test dataset. The resulting scores are interchangeably referred to as "polygenic scores" (PGS), "genetic risk scores" (GRS), or "polygenic risk scores" (PRS). These terms describe a measure comprising a large number of SNPs pooled together to represent a measured set of variants underlying genetic variation in a particular SUD-related trait and will typically refer to the coefficient of variation representing the variance accounted for in a trait by a particular polygenic score.

Molecular Heritability Approaches

In addition to approaches which create polygenic sum scores, multiple additional approaches have been developed to examine multi- or polygenic contributions to disease, including genome-wide complex trait analysis (GCTA) [23]. GCTA allows the estimation of SNP-heritability, or the phenotypic variance accounted for by genome-wide measured SNPs. Bivariate GCTA analysis can also estimate the SNP covariance of two phenotypes. This is a more powerful approach than that using sum scores [24] and has been applied to estimate both the SNP heritability of individual disorders and their SNP covariances [23].

Observed genetic correlations between groups of traits may be reflective of the fact that the neurobiological systems underlying etiologic pathways through drug use to addiction, that involve drug-related reinforcement, the psychological characteristics reflecting behavior regulation, and natural reinforcement and motivation may overlap. However, differences in behavior dysregulation and nonnormative behavior associated with licit and illicit drug abuse may explain the respective genetic groupings.

Pathway or Systems Approaches

Pathway analysis is an approach where polymorphisms in multiple genes are simultaneously tested for evidence of association. This approach can be used for a large biological process comprising hundreds of genes or even within a single gene (i.e., gene-based). Common pathway approaches, including gene set enrichment analysis (GSEA) [25], Disease Association Protein-Protein Link Evaluator (DAPPLE) [26], and Association LIst Go AnnoTatOR (ALIGATOR) [27], test whether statistical signals preferentially cluster in specific molecular pathways. These methods are able to identify pathways whose component genes and/or proteins might be etiologically relevant even in the absence of associations with genome-wide significance. This could shed light on the biological process underlying drug use and/or related phenotypes.

Case-Control Definition

Human disease geneticists (a shorthand for researchers involved in studies of genetic mechanisms of variation in liabilities to disorders) pay varying degrees of attention to known *environmental* factors influencing trait variation. This is an important consideration, since many human behavioral traits have a heritability of ~50% (i.e., the residual trait variation is due largely to environmental influences) [28]. This is especially germane to substance-use-related traits, where many environmental factors, including parental supervision, peer deviance, and drug availability during adolescence, are strongly associated with initiation of drug use [29]. More critically, drug use itself can be considered an environmental exposure. This may seem like a subtle point, but this is central to understanding the findings of some studies.

In twin and family studies, the role of the environment is usually either estimated or accounted for in the design. However, in case-control studies, the importance of appropriate control selection to allow for accurate inference is recognized [30–32], and it is generally held that cases and controls should be drawn from the same "base," but in genetics the "efficiency principle" is usually applied [31]. That is, given a fixed time and budget, control selection should seek to maximize power. However, it is important to recognize how control definition shapes the questions individual studies can answer. The discussion here is limited to factors specific to substance use genetics, where exposure to a substance is a key and necessary event in the development of a substance use disorder. Studies in substance use genetics will generally use one of three definitions of controls: unscreened, screened for absence of problematic use, or screened for exposure. Unscreened controls, drawn randomly from the population, are the least frequently used and are generally used when convenient as a means for increasing sample size. Controls screened for the absence of lifetime problematic use are frequently used. More recently, studies have relied on "exposed controls," or those who have used the substance being studied some arbitrarily defined number of times [33]. Each approach has its individual strengths and weaknesses. Moreover, as should be apparent from the discussions of common and specific liability elsewhere in this volume, there is a high likelihood that different genes will be involved in different stages of the addiction process from initiation, through regular use, and ultimately addiction. The use of different control types can answer questions about the genetic contributions at different points in the addiction process.

Unscreened controls are readily available in large numbers. However, given the high frequency of SUD in the population, many cases will inadvertently be included in the unscreened control sample and lead to a reduction in power (i.e., risk alleles will be more common in unscreened control datasets than in screened SUD-control sets). The greater the prevalence of a particular substance's use in the population, the greater this reduction in power to detect differences in the frequency of a particular variant between cases and unscreened controls. For example, a random sample of adults in the USA will include >10% of individuals who meet lifetime criteria for an alcohol use disorder. If unscreened, this large number of cryptic cases will have a substantial impact on power.

Controls who are free of use disorders are also frequent in the population, depending on the definition of problematic use given by the investigators. Since these subjects lack problematic use (usually for all substances), they will fall low in the distribution of general liability, that continuous trait reflective of an individual's risk for developing any SUD. That is, they are general liability controls. This can complicate interpretation of a study where cases are selected for a particular drug use disorder but controls are selected for absence of any use disorder, as many of the cases will also exhibit disordered use of other substances.

Controls screened for positive exposure to a substance are usually required to have used that specific substance some minimum number of times without developing problematic use or dependence. Examples of this include "100 lifetime cigarettes without developing nicotine dependence," or "10 opioid exposures without developing an OUD" [34]. Exposed controls are likely to fall below average on the liability distribution specific to that drug but above average on the general liability distribution and are best characterized as "specific liability controls." Consequently, these controls will be useful for studies of the specific drug to which they were exposed, yet did not develop a use disorder, as they are less likely to harbor risk variants for that specific substance but will be less useful as general liability controls if their exposure to one drug indicates broader drug use.

It is important to note that, as discussed at length in Chap. 1 of this volume, most of genetic and other etiological research has been focused on the risk aspect of liability, i.e., factors, including genetic variants, that elevate risk. Symmetric to risk, however, resistance factors, i.e., those that lower the probability of the undesired behavior or disorder, may be more amenable to practical implementation, particularly when they are malleable. Search for resistance factors requires different sampling approaches than the case-control settings common for risk-related research. These factors potentially include the so-called protective genetic variants. Because of focus on risk, they are detected mostly serendipitously, as observed at lower frequencies in affected individuals than in controls. Interestingly, many protective variants have been discovered in studies using exposed controls. Users who do not develop a disorder, thus displaying resistance to it, are more likely to harbor variants protective from disorder than those who do not use the drugs at all, thus displaying resistance to drug-taking as such.

In summary, genetic association studies of substance use disorders, which screen controls for any problematic use of any substance, will generally yield results on the genetic contributions to variation in both the common and, less so, the specific liability to that drug. Studies screening for exposed controls will yield the genetic contributions specific to that drug class [35, 36].

Candidate Genes/Systems

Candidate Genes

As the field progressed near the turn of the millennium, drafts of the Human Genome Project were published, complete with known locations of most genes [37]. Eventually many polymorphisms "at," "in," or "near" the coding region (the portion of the gene that will eventually be transcribed to mRNA and translated to protein, usually the exons) or promoter region (immediately upstream from the gene where transcription factors bind) of genes were discovered, filling the knowledge base of the field.

For decades, evidence has mounted that many neurobiological systems contribute *functionally* to the drug reward and behavior regulation associated with SUD risk. Based on this evidence, Koob and Volkow [38] proposed a theoretical model of drug use disorders that comprises three repeating states/stages: compulsion to use, acute intoxication, and withdrawal. Each stage is underlain by specific behavioral dimensions (impulsivity or loss of executive function, incentive salience or motivation for reward, and negative affect, respectively), and each behavior is underlain by a specific neural substrate (prefrontal cortex, basal ganglia, and amygdala, respectively). In turn, substantial changes in expression or activity of specific neurotransmitter systems are associated with specific stages of use or exhibit substantial differences in expression or activity across drug use stages. For example, serotonin and dopamine transmission mechanisms are significantly dysregulated during each stage [38], while GABA is increased in acute intoxication, norepinephrine is increased in withdrawal, and glutamate is increased during craving/anticipation.

Given decades of prior research on the neurobiological and biochemical bases of addiction, a logical next step was simply to select known genetic variants near "candidate" genes in the biological systems perturbed by drugs of abuse as candidates for association testing in families or in case-control comparisons. Information of this kind could allow investigators to focus on variation in relevant candidate genes in a hypothesis-driven fashion. Candidate gene studies have examined genes in biological pathways believed to be related to the phenotype in question. In SUDs, these candidates have historically been derived from existing biochemical or neurobiological work highlighting the pathways involved in drug metabolisms or the brain pathways impacted by the drug. Targeted investigation of the major neurobiological systems known to be involved mechanistically in the addiction process provides the advantages of hypothesis-driven research while mitigating some of the limitations of the original candidate gene approach that usually targets only known variation. In the GWAS era, we could assay all known functional variation across an entire system of interest and perform gene-based, haplotype-based, or set-based tests to examine the role of a gene or system in a particular disease. Until recently, candidate gene studies involving one or few, frequently unrelated, genes have been the mainstay of association research. Importantly, the GWAS approach does not render the candidate system approach obsolete. In fact, GWAS results are frequently viewed through a candidate lens, with findings emerging from candidate genes known to be expressed in the brain more frequently accepted as "true" or meaningful. The expected result of a GWAS study is to reduce the entire genome to a few candidate genes. In the current post-GWAS era, candidate gene selection is more frequently driven by the mounting evidence generated via atheoretic examination of the genome. This information may ultimately enable the elucidation of developmentally informed causal chains connecting neurobiology, behavior, and psychopathology, including SUD.

As described in other chapters of this book, SUDs share a significant portion of genetic variation influencing liability across drug classes. A host of candidate biological systems may underlie this commonality. The dopaminergic, serotonergic, glutamatergic, and GABAergic systems have each garnered interest as candidate *nonspecific* contributors to SUD risk variation. Several have survived replication attempts, as genes within those systems continue to yield evidence for common and specific contributions to substance abuse liability.

Dopamine System

No gene system has garnered more interest in the substance abuse literature than the dopamine system. The dopamine system is a major component in the mechanisms of substance abuse risk variation and has consequently been the primary target of SUD candidate gene searches [39]. The function of dopamine is mediated by the two groups of dopamine receptors (the D_1-like and D_2-like families of receptors), which work in concert to produce a specific biochemical or behavioral effect [40]. In addition to the receptors, *DRD1–DRD5*, the "dopamine system" of genes includes the dopamine transporter (*SLC6A3*) and the genes for the two primary enzymes responsible for dopamine catabolism in the brain, catechol-O-methyltransferase (*COMT*) and monoamine oxidase (*MAOA*). Virtually all drugs of abuse stimulate dopaminergic neurons, and their rewarding effects are associated with dopamine release [41–44]. Consequently, dopamine system genes were among the most studied candidate gene set for substance use disorders and a host of behavioral correlates, such as attention deficit hyperactivity disorder (ADHD), impulsivity, and novelty seeking. Early work tended to focus on using tandem repeat polymorphisms in the genes, transitioning to SNPs as discovery and technology permitted. The putative functionality of those variants is of continued recent interest [45].

Early work on *DRD2* [46] suggested that the gene is nonspecifically associated with various liabilities to addictive, compulsive, and impulsive disorders [47]. Moreover, intravenous amphetamine administration was used to demonstrate the central role of the dopamine D2 receptor levels in drug reinforcement [48]. As presented later in this chapter, variants in *DRD2* have been associated, and the findings replicated, in very large GWAS, with a variety of substance-use-related outcomes.

The dopamine transporter (*SLC6A3*) provides an attractive candidate gene for SUD liability given that it is the target of methylphenidate, a psychostimulant that is the treatment of choice for ADHD [49], a known risk factor for SUD. An early case-control study reported an association between ADHD and a VNTR in *SLC6A3* [50], results which were later confirmed by others [51–54].

DRD4 is among the frequently studied SUD candidate genes. Ebstein et al. [55] reported a population-based association between the long allele (7-repeat) of a VNTR in exon 3 of the *DRD4* and questionnaire-measured novelty seeking, a trait associated with SUD risk. Following the reported association between novelty seeking and *DRD4*, LaHoste et al. [56] reported a similar association of *DRD4* and ADHD in children and noted that the seven-repeat allele has brain functional implications in a blunted response to dopamine. This result was replicated using both population- and family-based association methods for both ADHD and SUD [57–63]. Meta-analyses supported the role of *DRD4* in ADHD [54, 64], novelty seeking [65], and alcoholism [66]. Recent work demonstrated that the exon 3 VNTR is not in linkage disequilibrium with the surrounding SNPs, highlighting the limits of SNPs in tagging some functional variation and explaining the discordant results in *DRD4* between the candidate gene work, which largely focused on this polymorphism, and the ADHD GWAS literature [64].

Other genes in the dopamine system have been less frequently studied in SUDs, but reports of associations exist for polymorphisms in *COMT* [67], *MAOA* [45], *DRD3* [68] and *DRD5* [54, 69, 70], and SUD and related traits [45, 68]. At the start of the millennium, the dopamine system was the most promising candidate gene system for explaining the common liability to substance use disorders. To date, only *DRD2* has generated consistent results for association with SUD and related traits [45, 71–74].

Serotonergic System

Serotonin (5-HT) is a brain active neurotransmitter throughout the life span and is known to play an essential role in hedonic tone, motivation, learning, and memory. The substantial impact of drugs of abuse on 5-HT activity and 5-HT receptor function is also known largely from research not only in model organisms [75] but also in humans [76, 77]. Consequently, genes in the serotonin system have been central targets of candidate gene studies.

GABAergic System

Gamma-aminobutyric acid (GABA) is the primary inhibitory neurotransmitter in the brain and functions by binding postsynaptically to ion channel-regulating GABA receptors and inhibiting transmission of action potentials. GABA primarily binds to two different types of receptors: $GABA_A$ and $GABA_B$, both of which inhibit action potentials by distinct mechanisms [78]. The $GABA_A$ receptor is comprised of 19 distinct subunits, while the $GABA_B$ receptor is comprised of just two subunits, each coded for by a distinct gene [79, 80]. Each of these genes coding for receptor subunits and genes involved in the presynaptic synthesis and release of GABA can be considered as components of the GABA system.

Glutamatergic System

Glutamate is the primary excitatory neurotransmitter in the nervous system [81]. Glutamate binds postsynaptically to one of four types of neurotransmitter receptors: N-methyl-D-aspartate (NMDA), α-amino-3-hydroxy-5-methyl-4-isoxazolepropionic acid (AMPA), kainate, and metabotropic glutamate receptors (mGluR). Glutamate receptors are widely distributed throughout the nervous system and binding of glutamate promotes activation. The glutamatergic system includes the genes which encode for proteins involved in the metabolism of glutamate and those encoding for the four classes of glutamate receptors, the glutamatergic system comprises nearly 50 genes [82].

Summary of Candidate Genes

While the candidate gene era in psychiatric and behavioral genetics has been considered by many to be a failure [83], several SUD candidate gene associations that were initially discovered during that era now rank among the strongest and most consistent findings for any psychiatric diagnosis (e.g., aldehyde dehydrogenase 2 [*ALDH2*], nicotinic acetylcholine receptor genes, dopamine D2 receptor [*DRD2*], μ1 opioid receptor [*OPRM1*]). Moreover, the possible functional relevance of polymorphisms other than SNPs has seldom been considered [45].

In many ways, the jury is still out on the candidate gene era of human genetics. Several important factors, including the lack of meaningful variation in tested genes, unrealistic expectations about expected effect sizes and sample sizes needed to detect them, and the failure to account for population stratification, surely played a role in the apparent false positives and negatives of the era.

As scientists, we are limited in testing what exists in human populations to observational studies. Much of our knowledge of neurobiology derives from preclinical, animal studies, where genetic engineering is common. A mainstay of these studies has been the knockout model, where a gene's expression is modified and the phenotypic consequences are observed. Nonetheless, a gene for which overwhelming preclinical evidence exists may lack any variation that meaningfully impacts its function in human populations. Failure to detect replicating associations in these genes is frequently seen as an indictment of the candidate approach, whether correctly or not. However, several factors need to be considered when judging the success of the candidate gene approach relative to later approaches. First, large-scale variant discovery efforts, such as HapMap or 1000 Genomes, commenced after the peak of the candidate gene era and discovered millions of previously unknown variants throughout the human genome, including many functional genic variants. Second, the impact of population stratification and differences in allele frequency by population stratum were not yet fully described and subsequent concerns regarding spurious association due to population stratification were addressed with novel methods [84, 85]. Lastly, studies in the candidate gene era were largely underpowered, with samples sizes of a few hundred subjects designed to detect modest to large effects in a range now known to be unrealistic. In spite of these limitations that impacted the candidate gene era, new technologies were developed which allowed for relatively cheap genome-wide SNP genotyping, which drove the field full force into the GWAS era.

Part 2. Current Evidence of Specific Genetic Contributions to Variation in SUD Liability

Alcohol Use and Alcohol Use Disorders (AUD)

Alcohol use and related disorders (i.e., "alcoholism") are common in the population and, consequently, are among the most studied substance use disorders in the genetic literature. There are many linkage and association studies stretching from the advent of the molecular genetics era to the present day.

The metabolic pathways for alcohol metabolism have been well characterized for decades. Alcohol is metabolized by isozymes of alcohol dehydrogenase (ADH) to acetaldehyde which is, in turn, metabolized to acetate by several forms of aldehyde dehydrogenase (AlDH). Genes coding for those enzymes are obvious candidates for contribution to variation in individual response to alcohol. Indeed, variation in genes coding for the ADH and AlDH enzymes has been known for decades to impact alcohol metabolism and risk of alcohol use disorders. Mutations increasing ADH activity or reducing AlDH activity may each lead to a toxic buildup of acetaldehyde and to the characteristic aversive alcohol-flushing response [86]. The most common of the ADH variants, *ADH1B**2, is present in the majority of East-Asian individuals and is protective from alcohol use disorders. A missense SNP at rs1229984 leads to the substitution of the amino acid arginine for histidine at the 48th position in the protein sequence [87]. In the literature, *ADH1B* was previously referred to as *ADH2*. In addition to this variant, another SNP, rs2066702, which leads to the substitution of arginine to cystine at position 370 of *ADH1B*, is associated with a reduced risk for alcohol use disorders in populations of African ancestry [88]. Low activity variants at *ALDH* genes are also associated with a decreased risk for alcohol use disorders [86]. The most common of these variants is rs671, commonly referred to as the *ALDH2**2 variant, that significantly impacts the enzyme structure and reduces activity [88]. Additional genes coding for ADH subunits and AlDHs are the primary drug class specific candidate genes for alcoholism. The alcohol dehydrogenases (*ADH1A*, *ADH1B,* and *ADH1C*) and aldehyde dehydrogenase 2 (*ALDH2*) have been the focus of candidate gene studies of alcohol-use-related phenotypes [88].

In addition to genes involved directly in the metabolism of alcohol in the periphery, several genes active in the brain have been implicated in alcohol use disorders. Primary among these is *GABRA2*, a gene encoding for a subunit of the GABA-A receptor, one of a class of ligand-gated chloride channels which bind the inhibitory neurotransmitter gamma-aminobutyric acid (GABA). GABA has been a target of alcoholism research for decades, primarily because its activity is enhanced by alcohol [89–91]. The initial evidence for the relationship of GABA system genes to AUD in humans was a linkage study, which generated a significant peak on chromosome 4p12, the region harboring the *GABRA2* gene [92].

Linkage Studies of Alcohol Use Disorders and Related Traits

Early linkage studies detected significant linkage in the Collaborative Studies on the Genetics of Alcoholism (COGA). A pedigree study of 987 subjects in 105 pedigrees found significant linkage on chromosome 4 in regions including the *ADH* cluster and *GABRA2*, although there was stronger evidence on chromosomes 1, 2, and 7 [92]. A contemporary linkage analysis performed by Long and colleagues [93] reported significant evidence for linkage on chromosome 4, also near *GABRB1*, and on chromosome 11, near dopamine system genes *DRD4* and *TH*, in a sample of 172 Native American sibling pairs. In a sample of 139 sibling pairs, Wilhelmsen et al. [94] performed a genome-wide linkage study of low-level response to alcohol, a trait that has been linked with an increased risk for later AUD [95] and identified several findings, which were deemed "suggestive" by the authors. In a sample of 243 Mission Indians, Ehlers et al. performed a genome-wide linkage scan and reported linkage peaks for alcohol use severity, on chromosomes 4 and 12, and alcohol withdrawal, on chromosomes

6, 15, and 16 [96]. In the Irish Affected Sib Pair Study of Alcohol Dependence (IASPSAD) sample of 474 Irish pedigrees, Prescott et al. reported a genome-wide significant on chromosome 4 [97]. Subsequently, Gelernter and colleagues reported evidence of significant linkage on chromosome 10 in a sample of African-Americans with alcohol dependence [98]. This study was noteworthy in that it was the lone linkage study of AUD performed in an African-American sample. Findings of significant or suggestive linkage generally implicates a broad chromosomal region, sometimes containing tens or hundreds of genes, in increasing the risk for the trait or disease. Additional approaches, such as genetic association testing using denser sets of genetic markers, are usually needed to pinpoint the specific genes linked or associated with the outcome.

Candidate Gene Studies of AUD

An exhaustive examination of candidate gene studies of AUD and related phenotypes would be a volume in itself. Here, we focus on those genes/variants for which there is compelling evidence for replication or for which large meta-analyses have confirmed significant associations.

In a large candidate gene meta-analysis of the association between rs1229984 in *ADH1B*, Bierut et al. [99] found a significant protective effect (OR = 0.34, $p = 6.6 \times 10^{-10}$) of the minor (lower frequency) allele. Li et al. [100] reported similar results in a separate large meta-analysis. Li et al. [101] reported a protective association of rs698 in ADHIC in a meta-analysis of 53 studies and 13,734 subjects [$p = 1 \times 10^{-8}$]. Similarly, Zaso and colleagues [102] found a significant protective effect [OR = 0.46] of the minor allele at rs698 in *ADH1C* for AUD. Li and colleagues [103] in a meta-analysis, including 17,009 subjects, found a significant protective effect at rs671 in *ALDH2* (OR = 0.22).

There have also been compelling findings from large (sample sizes exceeding 10,000 subjects) meta-analyses of AUD with variants other than the alcohol-metabolizing genes. Daurio [66] found a protective effect of the DRD4 VNTR [7 or more repeats] with AUD severity. Significant associations (OR = 1.24) between rs1800497 in *DRD2* [73] with alcohol dependence in a large meta-analytic sample (*N* = 18,730) and with AUD (OR = 1.23) in a separate large sample (*N* = 16,295) have been reported [73]. Li et al. [104] reported a significant association of rs2229944 in *GABRB2* (OR = 1.33) with AUD, and Cao et al. [105] reported a significant association between rs6313 in *HTR2A* and AUD. Ma [106] reported an association [OR = 1.12] in a large meta-analytic sample [*N* = 5929] between a VNTR in *SLC6A3* and alcohol dependence.

Genome-Wide Association Studies of Alcohol Use Disorder

The first GWAS of AUD, Treutlein and colleagues [17], conducted in a relatively small sample of early-onset (before age 28) male cases (*N* = 487) and controls (*N* = 1358), did not report any significant results after correction for multiple testing. However, replication was attempted among the top 121 SNPs plus 19 additional candidates, with significant findings in the region on chromosome 2, previously reported to be linked to AUD in COGA [92]. The authors also reported additional association with SNPs in *ADH1C*. It should be noted that based on current recommendations for multiple test correction in GWAS, these results would not be considered significant. Moreover, this amplifies the need for larger sample sizes to detect the usual effect sizes seen in GWAS [107]. Subsequent larger-scale GWAS have identified more associations [108–111], and, as sample sizes have increased from hundreds to hundreds of thousands, the statistical significance and replicability of top findings has increased.

In subsequent large meta-analyses (*N* = 26,316 [108]; *N* = 105,000 [109]), a significant relationship was found between alcohol consumption quantity and rs6943555 in the *AUTS2* gene, which has also been implicated in autism spectrum disorders and intellectual disabilities. It is worth noting that this has not been replicated in subsequent large GWAS of alcohol use disorders.

Adkins and colleagues [112] performed a genome-wide association scan for alcohol consumption in 2162 individuals ascertained in population-based studies of development in adolescence and young adulthood. While the sample size is relatively modest when compared to more current studies, a strength of this study is that it captures an important developmental period, when alcohol use typically escalates. The investigators use an alternative to the common Bonferroni approach to correction for multiple testing, called the false discovery rate (FDR). This approach was developed in the context of large-scale genomic testing and relies on the observed distribution of test statistics to estimate statistical significance while controlling for the false discovery rate, or the proportion of tests deemed significant which are false positives. Using this approach, the investigators reported genome-wide significant findings in the GABA transporter 1 (*SLC6A1*) and adrenoceptor alpha 2A (*ADRA2A*) region [112].

In a large (N = 86,627) multiethnic sample, Jorgenson and colleagues [113] performed GWAS on two alcohol consumption traits, drinker vs. nondrinker and, among drinkers, average consumption. The investigators observed ethnic-specific patterns of association between *ALDH2* and *ADH1B* and alcohol consumption.

Walters et al. [110], in what was the initial publication of the Psychiatric Genomics Consortium Substance Use Disorder group, performed GWAS for alcohol dependence, meta-analyzing 28 different studies, with large samples of European (n = 46,568) and African (n = 6280) ancestry. The primary finding of this study was consistency, across both ancestries and in the combined group meta-analysis, in significant associations in the ADH region on chromosome 4, with the most strongly associated SNPs in the meta-analysis across ancestry groups implicating *ADH1B*. Using polygenic approaches, Walters et al. [110] also examined other available GWAS summary statistics on substance-use-related traits and found significant genetic correlations with cannabis and smoking initiation, nicotine dependence, and alcohol consumption quantitative traits, as well as behavioral/psychological traits (neuroticism, delay discounting, risk taking) and psychiatric traits/disorders (depressive symptoms, major depressive disorder [MDD], ADHD, and schizophrenia).

In collaboration with the direct-to-consumer genetics company, Sanchez-Roige [114] performed a GWAS in 20,328 European ancestry subjects using the Alcohol Use Disorder Identification Test (AUDIT). The most significant signal, albeit modest in its effect size, was in the *ADH1C* gene ($p = 4.4 \times 10^{-7}$; ß = −0.05; SNP: rs141973904), located in the chromosome 4 *ADH* gene cluster. Additional suggestive associations were discovered near the gene *KCNJ9* (*GIRK3*), which has been implicated in rodent models of alcohol consumption. Using a polygenic approach employing correlation between GWAS p-values across studies [114], significant positive genetic correlations were found between AUDIT score and high alcohol consumption (r_g = 0.89), alcohol dependence (r_g = 0.68), and lifetime cigarette smoking (r_g = 0.42). There was a particularly interesting negative correlation between total AUDIT score and ADHD (r_g = −0.29). The investigators also used two different approaches to estimate the "chip heritability" of AUDIT score. These approaches were GREML (commonly referred to as GCTA) and LD score regression, which yielded estimated chip heritabilities of 12.05% and 8.8%, respectively, markedly lower than other studies of AUD and of twin studies of alcohol use, indicating that the 23andMe sample (volunteers not ascertained for AUD) may be exhibiting less genetic enrichment for alcohol problems or that AUDIT total score was not adequately measuring alcohol use disorders.

In a subsequent study, Sanchez-Roige and colleagues meta-analyzed the 23andMe sample with an AUDIT GWAS performed in the UK Biobank sample [115]. The investigators combined their previous analysis of the AUDIT in 23andMe (n = 20,328) with UK Biobank (n = 121,604) on the AUDIT total score. An important difference between this and their previous work [114] was that genetic correlation analyses were performed for the AUDIT total score and also on the AUDIT subscales, the 3-item consumption score (AUDIT-C) and the 7-item problematic consequences of alcohol use score (AUDIT-P) separately. AUDIT total score GWAS discovered the strongest signal across 4q23 and 4q24, the region harboring the *ADH* locus, and 4p14, in the *KLB* gene. Gene-based analyses implicated additional genes including *DRD2*, *CRHR1*, and *CADM2*. Genetic correlations (LDSC) were estimated separately for the AUDIT total score, AUDIT-C, and AUDIT-P and found to be significant with alcohol consumption, AD, lifetime smoking, and lifetime cannabis use. There was a noteworthy discordance in the genetic correlation between neuropsychiatric traits and AUDIT scores, with AUDIT-P but not AUDIT total score and AUDIT-C correlated with ADHD and mood disorders. This result suggests that risk for problematic alcohol use is genetically correlated with liabilities to psychiatric illness while consumption alone is not. It is important to note that these were not clinically ascertained samples, where typically heavy alcohol use is associated with psychiatric disease.

The GWAS and Sequencing Consortium of Alcohol and Nicotine use (GSCAN) [116] was a large GWAS of 1.2 million subjects for multiple drinking and smoking phenotypes. The alcohol phenotypes used included drinker vs. nondrinker (total N = 806,607) and drinks/week (total N = 695,160). This study implicated over 500 variants in substance-use-related phenotypes. Among them, "drinks per week" was independently associated with 11 variants across *ADH1B*. Variants across *DRD2* were associated with drinks per week (and also smoking-related phenotypes). Lastly, unique signals were found in the region containing the *CRHR1* gene (corticotropin-releasing hormone receptor 1), which is involved in stress response. Pathway analyses consistently revealed enrichment in association signal in glutamate pathways and in carbohydrate metabolic pathways.

Kranzler and colleagues [117] performed GWAS in a sample of 274,424 subjects ascertained from the Million Veteran Program (MVP) for AUDIT-C and for the dichotomous clinical diagnosis of AUD. Alcohol-related diagnoses were drawn from the Veterans Health Administration electronic health records and represent longitudinal repeated measures drawn from 11 years of care. The sample consisted of 55,584 cases and 218,807 controls and included subjects of European, African, Latino, East Asian, and South Asian ancestries. Meta-analysis across ethnicities yielded genome-wide significant findings in the *ADH* cluster, *DRD2*, and *FTO* with AUD, as well as novel findings in *GCKR* and *SIX3*. Meta-analysis for AUDIT-C across ethnic groups yielded genome-wide significant findings not only in the *ADH* cluster, *GCKR*, and *FTO* but also in *VRK2* (chromosome 2), *KLB*, *DCLK2*, and *ISL1*, on chromosome 4, and *IGF2BP1* (insulin-like growth factor 2 mRNA binding protein 1) and *BAHCC1*, on chromosome 17. Not surprisingly, pathway analysis revealed significant associations in the ethanol oxidation pathway. SNP-based heritability estimates were modest, in the range of 6–11%, depending on the ethnicity and sex of the selected sample. Cell-type group partitioning heritability enrichment analyses implicated the central nervous system (CNS) for AUD and AUDIT-C. A striking finding from the paper was the difference in genetic correlations using LDSC. AUD was positively correlated with psychiatric traits and negatively associated with reproductive (e.g., age at first birth), cognitive (IQ), and educational (years of education) indicators, while AUDIT-C was negatively genetically correlated with obesity-related traits but positively correlated with age at first birth and years of education. The authors concluded that genetic risk for heavy drinking is not sufficient to account for the genetic risk for AUD.

Zhou and colleagues [111] performed the largest GWAS meta-analysis to date, combining the PGC, MVP, and UK Biobank samples (total N = 435,563) in a GWAS of "problematic alcohol use." In addition to replicating the previously published associations, the authors reported 19 novel genome-wide significant findings, 11 of which were located in or near gene regions including *CADM2* (cell adhesion molecule 2) and *SLC39A13* (solute carrier family 39 member 13). A novel finding was a rare variant in *ADH1B*, which causes an amino acid substitution and is in the same codon as a known risk variant (rs2066702).

An important point is that the large samples enable detection of new associations even in genes with prior positive findings, allowing for the discovery of novel functional units of the gene. There was a substantial overlap with the previous GSCAN study and the UKB sample, and most of the "novel" findings had been associated with alcohol use phenotypes in GSCAN. The researchers also performed gene-based analyses, chip-heritability estimates, examined genetic correlations, and performed an approach called Mendelian randomization (MR) to examine causal relationships between other phenotypes and problematic alcohol use. MR uses genetic variation known to be associated with only one trait to examine the causal relationships with other traits [118]. The full sample meta-analyses yielded a molecular (chip) heritability of 0.068, which is far from accounting for twin-based heritability estimates. Gene-based analyses, which jointly examine polymorphisms across a gene, found a significant association in 66 genes, including *ADH4*, *ADH5*, *ADH7*, *ADH1B*, *ADH1C*, *SYNGAP1*, *BDNF*, and *DRD2*. LD score regression was used to examine genetic correlation with summary statistics from 715 phenotypes, which have already been GWAS analyzed in the UKB sample. Among those phenotypes, 138 were significantly genetically correlated with problematic alcohol use. Mendelian randomization showed that risky behavior polygenic risk [119] was positively correlated with problematic alcohol use, which in turn had a bidirectional relationship with educational attainment.

Nicotine Use and Nicotine Dependence

Nicotine is a commonly used substance. Moreover, because of health consequences associated with the most common route of nicotine administration, smoking, nicotine use is commonly assessed in large cohort studies, making it amenable to consortium analysis.

An obvious candidate gene pathway for nicotine dependence is the cholinergic system, the neuronal pathway that primarily utilizes acetylcholine as its neurotransmitter [120]. The primary receptors in the cholinergic system are the muscarinic and nicotinic acetylcholine receptors, so named because of the exogenous compounds, muscarine and nicotine, respectively, which activate them and have been widely used in research. Neuronal nicotinic acetylcholine receptors (nAChRs), which differ from muscle receptors and are encoded by different genes, are expressed in the brain. Nicotine selectively binds to nAChRs. They are composed of five subunits, and a particular neuronal receptor can be composed of one type or some combination of 11 types of subunits, α2–7, α9, α10, and β2–4 (only α7 and α9 can be homopentameric, whereas heteropentamers are formed by two α and three β units) [121]. The unique subunits are each coded for by separate genes. These genes have long been candidates for nicotine addiction and smoking behaviors, since the impact of nicotine in the brain is mediated by its binding to these receptors. Large meta-analyses of candidate gene studies confirmed associations between nicotinic receptor subunit genes *CHRNA3* [122] and *CHRNA5* [122, 123] and smoking quantity and nicotine dependence.

The cytochrome P450 enzymes, a large family of mono-oxigenases encoded by many *CYP* genes, are involved in oxidation of many compounds, primarily functioning as the last oxidase enzyme in the electron transport chain. P450s play a major role in all drug metabolism. Moreover, some P450s interact with, and are up- or downregulated by, some drugs of abuse. Among P450s, CYP2A6 is the major enzyme in nicotine metabolism, and variation in this gene can impact an individual's ability to metabolize nicotine. The gene resides on chromosome 19q, where it is part of a cluster of other cytochrome p450 genes.

Candidate gene studies have been published for a variety of smoking-related behaviors. Polymorphisms impacting activity level of *CYP2A6* were associated with smoking initiation and cigarettes per day in a very large meta-analysis [124]. Outside of the metabolism genes, there is meta-analytic support for the Taq1A polymorphism of the *DRD2* gene, multiple variants in *GALR1* (galanin receptor 1), and rs22236709 in *TTC12* (tetratricopeptide repeat domain 12) [71, 125, 126].

Meta-analyses have been performed for smoking cessation phenotypes, and a handful of significant associations have been reported, including *CYP2A6* [127]. Candidate genes for the serotonin system, the promoter polymorphism of the serotonin transporter (*SLC6A4*/HTTLPR) [127] and the dopamine system, *DRD2,* have been associated with smoking cessation via meta-analysis [74].

Linkage Studies of Nicotine Dependence and Smoking-Related Behaviors

Several genome-wide linkage scans have been performed suggesting loci linked to smoking behavior and ND. Since smoking is a frequently measured trait, an important note is that these studies are diverse in terms of population studied, age, design, ascertainment, and phenotype measured. Results from the linkage era were largely inconsistent and generated "suggestive" (a term used by scientists when a finding did not reach strict statistical significance thresholds) signals on nearly every chromosome. However, there was some converging evidence around a few loci for smoking and smoking-related behaviors.

Straub and colleagues [128] performed a genome-wide linkage analysis in a sample of 343 subjects (308 with nicotine dependence) from 130 families from NZ and a separate sample of 264 subjects (211 with nicotine dependence) from 91 families in the USA. Despite performing follow-up analyses on regions exhibiting suggestive linkage, no regions reached genome-wide significance. However, regions on chromosomes 2 and 10 were the most significant. In a sample of 592 Dutch sibling pairs from 192 families, linkage analysis was performed for smoking initiation and number of cigarettes smoked per week [129]. A significant peak was observed on chromosome 6 for smoking initiation, and converging evidence was found on chromosome 10 for both smoking initiation and number of cigarettes smoked. In a sample of 158 nuclear families, comprising 607 members, a genome-wide linkage analysis was performed for nicotine dependence as measured by the Fagerström Test for Nicotine Dependence (FTND) [130]. The peak evidence for linkage was observed on chromosome 6 for FTND. Additional exploratory analyses were conducted for other measures, including cigarettes per day and smoking cessation, which yielded evidence across multiple chromosomes. Li et al. [131] conducted linkage analysis for nicotine dependence in a sample of 1261 African-American individuals drawn from 402 nuclear families. Significant linkage evidence was generated on chromosome 10q22, with suggestive findings across multiple other chromosomes, notably 9, 11, and 13. In 973 subjects from 105 COGA families, linkage analysis was performed for a quantitative phenotype of cigarettes smoked per day. Strong evidence for linkage was found for chromosome 5q and suggestive evidence for chromosomes 4, 15, and 17. The authors were cautious in their enthusiasm because of the wide distance between the most significant markers on chromosome 5 [132]. Morley and colleagues performed a series of within-sex genome-wide linkage analyses of smoking in a large Australian twin sample [133]. Analyses were performed both with and without subjects who had reported never smoking. The investigators identified suggestive linkage on chromosomes 6p12 and 11p12. Gelernter and colleagues [134] performed genome-wide linkage analysis in a sample of 42 genotyped individuals from 12 families across 416 markers, performing single and multipoint analyses. The investigators reported significant linkage evidence on chromosomes 11p and 9 and noted that the region on chromosome 11 was at or near a region where previous studies had identified linkage to alcohol dependence and illicit drug use. In a sample of 67 multigenerational families and 154 sibling pairs drawn from the COGA sample, Bierut and colleagues [135] performed genome-wide linkage analysis of habitual smoking (one or more packs per day for at least 6 months). The best evidence for linkage was on chromosome 9, and evidence for a comorbid alcohol smoking and alcohol phenotype was on chromosome 2 [135].

Genome-Wide Association Scans of Nicotine Dependence and Smoking Phenotypes

GWAS have significantly contributed to our knowledge of the genetics of smoking behaviors, owing to the ease with which large samples of smokers can be collected and the frequency with which these behaviors are measured in large cohort studies.

At the outset of the GWAS era, Bierut and colleagues [136], using a pooled genotyping approach, followed by targeted genotyping of ~32,000 SNPs in 1050 cases and 879 controls, found evidence for an association of *NRXN1* and smoking. Subsequently, multiple groups, in large samples, reported strong genome-wide significant associations with the region on chromosome 15q25 harboring *CHRNA5*, *CHRNA3*, and *CHRNB4*, three nAchR genes [137–139]. Thorgeirsson et al. [138] performed GWAS of CPD and smoking initiation in a sample of 46,481 subjects, with replication samples totaling over 50,000 subjects. The investigators identified genome-wide significant findings in the 15q25 region, with rs1051730, in the nicotinic acetylcholine receptor alpha 3 subunit (*CHRNA3*) gene, yielding the strongest association. In addition, significant signals were also identified on chromosomes 19q13 (rs4105144) and 8p11 (rs6474412) in regions near nicotine metabolizing genes (*CP2A6* and *CYP2B6*) and nicotinic acetylcholine receptor subunit genes.

Liu and colleagues [137] performed GWAS in a sample of 41,150 subjects collected for genetic studies of 20 diseases as part of the Oxford-GlaxoSmithKline study (Ox-GSK) and reported a genome-wide significant association with smoking quantity on chromosome 15q25, in the nAChR gene region (*CHRNA5*, *CHRNA3*, and *CHRNB4*). Conditioning on this discovery, the investigators also found a significant relationship with a SNP (rs6495308) in *CHRNA3*. The Tobacco and Genetics Consortium (TGEN), in a sample of 74,053 subjects, performed GWAS of smoking initiation and cigarettes per day [139]. In the same report, an expanded meta-analysis with large, existing samples, increasing the sample size to more than 140,000 subjects, identified strong associations in *CHRNA3* ($p \approx 10^{-73}$) and two additional loci for cigarettes per day. For smoking initiation, the researchers identified eight genome-wide significant associations, including in *BDNF* (chromosome 11). *DBH* (chromosome 9) was significantly associated with smoking cessation.

The GWAS and Sequencing Consortium of Alcohol and Nicotine use (GSCAN) [116] was a large GWAS of 1.2 million subjects and was described previously in this chapter. The smoking phenotypes used included nicotine initiation (N = 990,750), nicotine initiation age (N = 260,253), CPD (N = 262,291), and nicotine cessation (N = 477,066). This study implicated hundreds of variants in these phenotypes, including 406 independently associated with smoking phenotypes. Those included each of the brain-expressed neuronic nicotinic receptors, except *CHRNA7*. Gene-based tests implicated *DRD2* and *DBH* in cigarettes per day and cessation, both genes in the dopamine system. Lastly, the finding of the association between *CYP2A6* and cigarettes per day was replicated.

Multiple subsequent large-scale GWAS, with samples ranging from 5000 to 40,000, have consistently implicated nicotinic receptors, including *CHRNA4*, *CHRNB4*, and *CHRNA3*, among their top findings [140–142]. Hancock et al. [143] also reported an association between *DNMT3B* and nicotine dependence in a meta-analysis of 15 cohorts for a total sample size of 38,602.

Genetic Studies of Cannabis Use and Cannabis Use Disorder

Unlike alcohol and nicotine, the genetic studies for other substances tend to be smaller and fewer in number and have produced fewer definitive, replicating findings. Candidate gene systems for cannabis and cannabis use disorder include primarily the genes of the endocannabinoid system. To date, no candidate gene meta-analyses have supported associations with cannabis use or use disorder specifically.

Linkage Studies of Cannabis Use and Cannabis Use Disorders

In the UCSF Family Study, Ehlers et al. [144] reported linkage to chromosomes 3 and 9 for a phenotype of cannabis withdrawal and craving. Hopfer [145] also reported linkage to these chromosomes for cannabis dependence in a sample of adolescents from Colorado. Ehlers [146] reported linkage of a phenotype comprising severe cannabis use disorder and antisociality to chromosomes 16 and 19 in a sample of Native Americans.

Genome-Wide Association Studies of Cannabis Use and Cannabis Use Disorders

In the first GWAS of CUD, Agrawal [147], in a sample of 708 cannabis-dependent cases and 2346 cannabis-exposed controls, reported association on chromosome 17 in *ANKFN1* gene. Sherva and colleagues [148] reported detecting three independent associations in a sample of 14,754 participants, in the *RP11-206 M11.7, SLC35G1,* and *CSMD1* genes. Subsequently, Demontis et al. [149] performed GWAS of CUD in 2387 cases versus ~50,000 controls, with a replication sample of 5501 cases and ~ 300,000 controls and reported genome-wide significant evidence and replication for a signal in *CHRNA2*.

The International Cannabis Consortium conducted GWAS meta-analysis of lifetime cannabis use in a combined meta-analytic sample of 17 cohorts and more than 38,000 subjects. While no individual SNPs reached genome-wide significance, gene-based tests were significant at four genes: *NCAM1*, *CADM2*, *SCOC*, and *KCNT2* [150]. In subsequent work [151] in an expanded sample (N = 184,765), the ICC investigators repeated single SNP association tests, gene-based analyses, and LD score regression to examine genetic correlation with related phenotypes and used Mendelian randomization to test causal relationships between cannabis use and schizophrenia. Significant associations were detected in the *CADM2*, *SDK1*, *ZNF704*, *NCAM1*, *RABEP2*, and *SMG6* genes. SNP-based heritability was estimated at 0.13 by LD score regression, and there was a significant genetic correlation (r_g = 0.83) between lifetime cannabis use and lifetime cigarette smoking. In addition, the researchers showed a causal relationship between schizophrenia polygenic risk influencing lifetime cannabis use.

Johnson et al. [152] reported a large GWAS meta-analysis of CUD in a total sample of 20,916 cases and 363,116 controls. The investigators found a novel genome-wide significant signal on chromosome 7, at rs7783012 [OR = 1.11 (95% confidence interval, 1.07–1.15)] in the *FOXP2* gene, and replicated a signal on chromosome 8 near *CHRNA2* [rs4732724; OR = 0.89 (0·86–0·93)]. The authors also reported significant genetic correlations between CUD and CU but differing patterns of genetic correlations between these two and other phenotypes. Most notably, cannabis use disorder was more genetically correlated with psychiatric disorders, indicating that the variation in liability to develop a use disorder shares genes in common with other psychiatric outcomes.

Opioid Use and Opioid Use Disorders

The genetic contributions to variation in the risk of opioid use disorders is an area of intense interest in the literature because of the substantial consequences of opioid use, most notably fatal overdose. In addition to the genes impacting the common liability to substance use disorders (e.g., *DRD2*, *DRD4*, *SLC6A4*, cytochromes P450), the specific genes coding for the opioid receptors are the common candidate genes for OUDs. It should be noted that opioid receptors participate in the rewarding effects of drugs other than opioids, including alcohol.

In candidate gene studies, Haerian et al. [153] confirmed association via meta-analysis between rs6265 in *BDNF* and heroin dependence in a sample of 2383 subjects. Multiple meta-analyses have confirmed associations between variants in *DRD2* and opioid dependence in meta-analytic samples ($N > 5000$) [72, 154, 155]. Hancock and colleagues [156], in a meta-analysis including 10,575 subjects, confirmed association at multiple SNPs in *ZNF804A* with opioid use disorder.

Linkage Studies of Opioid Use Disorders

Linkage studies on opioid use and opioid use disorders have been relatively limited. Gelernter and colleagues [157] performed cluster analysis on opioid use disorder symptoms measured in 393 nuclear families and linkage analysis using several cluster types as phenotypes. The investigators reported significant linkage on chromosome 17 with the heaviest use cluster phenotype in a combined European and African-American Sample [157]. Lachman and colleagues performed linkage analysis using 305 opioid-dependent sibling pairs and reported significant linkage to chromosome 14q in a region including the gene *NRXN3*, which encodes for the protein neurexin 3 [158]. Glatt et al. in a Han Chinese sample of 397 sibling pairs reported linkage on chromosome 4q31.2 with heroin dependence [159].

GWAS of Opioid Use Disorders

The first GWAS of an OUD was performed in a sample of 104 European ancestry heroin-dependent subjects and 101 matched controls [160]. These authors reported a "suggestive" association with *GABRA3* (gamma-aminobutyric acid, receptor subunit alpha 3) and an additional SNP on chromosome 1 (rs965972), which is not in a gene but survived multiple test correction. Nielsen and colleagues [160] expanded their sample to 200 European-American (EA) cases, with 150 EA controls, and added 125 African-American (AA) cases and 100 AA controls. In the novel analyses, their most significant signal was identical to their previous signal, due to sample overlap. In the small AA subsample, the most significant SNP was in the gene *DUSP27* (cytosolic dual specificity phosphatase 27), but it did not reach the threshold for significance after multiple test correction.

Gelernter and colleagues [161] reported a GWAS on opioid dependence in a sample comprising 3000 EA opioid-dependent cases, 3800 EA controls, 1500 AA dependent cases, and 6400 AA controls. The AA sample yielded more interesting results, and the combined sample yielded positive results in *APB2*, *PARVA*, *KCNC1*, and *KCNG2*. Pathway analyses implicated calcium signaling and synaptic long-term potentiation.

Nelson and colleagues [33] conducted an important study, limiting their control sample to opioid misusing controls who had never progressed to dependence, with the goal of identifying loci important for later stages of the addiction process. This allowed identification of a significant protective variant in *CNIH3*, which needs to be replicated.

Kalsi and colleagues [162] performed GWAS in a sample of 370 Han Chinese subjects with heroin dependence and 134 controls who were screened to absence of mental health problems. No individual SNPs were significant, but gene-based (an approach where all variation in the gene is tested simultaneously) testing revealed a genome-wide significant results in *CCDC42*. This gene was later replicated with modest evidence ($p = 1 \times 10^{-6}$) for association with quantitative alcohol consumption in the past year in a large study. PRS analyses of smoking-related and psychiatric disorders previously analyzed by the PGC did not yield significant results.

Polimanti et al. [163] recently explicitly addressed exposed cases/controls in a sample with a large number of exposed and unexposed controls. The investigators performed analysis in 4503 opioid-dependent controls vs. 4173 opioid-exposed controls, 32,500 unexposed controls (all controls combined and exposed alone). The samples were also diverse. The investigators, using genetic ancestry information, identified 9591 individuals of African ancestry and 31,585 of European ancestry in their sample. Cases were defined as meeting criteria for DSM-IV opioid dependence. Multiple GWAS analyses were performed, including opioid dependence vs. exposed controls, opioid dependence vs. unexposed controls, and exposed controls vs. unexposed controls. Nothing reached genome-wide significance, and specific signals detected by previous GWAS were not replicated. The largest signal was in the comparison among exposed vs. unexposed controls, in the European ancestry subset. A SNP rs9291211 was examined by bioinformatic follow-up and found to be a significant expression quantitative trait locus (eQTL), a SNP shown to impact expression of some behaviorally relevant genes in the brain and associated in the UK Biobank with taking dietary supplements.

Additional analyses were performed at the gene level, resulting in additional findings. Comparing exposed and unexposed controls, the authors reported a significant association between *SDCCAG8* and opioid exposure. This gene has also been previously associated with educational attainment and risk-taking behaviors, possibly contributing to the relationship with propensity to become exposed to opioids. The most important finding was between a relatively rare (allele frequency of 0.039) indel (insertion/deletion polymorphism) on chromosome 18, rs201123820, about 2 kb upstream of *LINC02837* (OD cases vs. unexposed controls). This indel is also associated with musculoskeletal disorders. The authors also created a polygenic risk score from a very large GWAS of risk taking [119] and found the expected significant relationships between risk-taking polygenic risk and opioid exposure, comparing the OD cases to unexposed controls or exposed controls to unexposed controls.

Zhou and colleagues [164] performed a GWAS using the MVP EHR sample combined with the Yale-Penn study, yielding a total sample of 10,544 EA cases; 72,163 EA controls; 5212 AA cases; and 26,876 AA controls. Controls in this sample were opioid-exposed. The primary finding from this study was a genome-wide significant association between OUD and the functional coding variant rs1799971 (Asn40Asp) in *OPRM1*, with replication in two independent samples. The authors also performed a series of secondary analyses. Chip heritability was estimated using LDSC to be 0.113, meaning that approximately 11.3% of the variability in the trait is due to measured SNPs. LDSC was also used to examine genetic correlations with 232 published and 483 previously unpublished traits. There were strong genetic correlations between OUD and ever smoking (r_g = 0.51), alcohol dependence, alcohol use quantity, and an inability to stop smoking. Mendelian randomization was performed to examine causality and showed a positive causal correlation of OUD genetic risk, with never smoked regularly, major depressive disorder, and neuroticism, and a negative causal correlation with educational attainment.

Using electronic health records from a large US healthcare system, Song and colleagues [165] identified 1039 OUD cases and 20,271 controls (10,744 of whom were opioid-exposed) and performed GWAS using the entire control set and then just the opioid-exposed controls (identified as having been prescribed an opioid). The authors found genome-wide significant results in a region on chromosome 4 when using all controls and chromosome 16 when using just exposed controls. Chip heritability was estimated to be 0.06. The investigators found significant correlations of 0.59 and 0.65, respectively, between OUD polygenic risk and alcohol use disorder and nicotine dependence.

Cocaine Use and Cocaine Use Disorders

Linkage Studies of Cocaine Use Disorders

Gelernter et al. [166] performed linkage analysis in a sample of 309 nuclear families, which yielded 528 full and 155 half sib pairs, 55% of whom were AA. Analysis for cocaine dependence produced only suggestive results. The authors then performed subgroup analyses by ethnic group and by phenotypic cluster, which was identified by multiple correspondence analysis, a multivariate approach aimed at identifying the underlying correlation structure of a dataset. They reported a significant result on chromosome 12 in the EA sample for heavy cocaine use and also on chromosome 18 for moderate use of cocaine and opioids.

GWAS of Cocaine Use Disorder

Gelernter et al. [167] performed a GWAS of cocaine use disorder in a sample which overlapped with a previous GWAS of OUD [167]. The discovery sample was 5697 subjects (2482 AA CD cases, 1809 EA DC cases, 800 AA controls, and 485 AA cases). A large, diverse replication sample (N = 4063) drawn from publicly available data was also used. The authors reported a significant result in the gene *FAM53B*, which was discovered in the combined EA + AA analyses. A sample limited effect in *NCOR2* was discovered in the EA sample.

Genetic Studies of the General Liability to Substance Use Disorders

Studies have been performed examining the general liability, or the shared risk across substances, of substance use disorders. These have generally been conducted by combining studies or samples ascertained for different drugs of abuse or by collecting case who have a use disorder for any drug of abuse.

Candidate Gene Association Studies of General Liability

Multiple studies have reported confirmed associations between SNPs in BDNF and substance use disorder. Most recently, and in the largest sample ($N = 9419$), Haerian [153] reported a significant association [OR = 1.36] between rs6265 in *BDNF* and a combined sample of alcohol, nicotine, heroin, methamphetamine, or general substance dependence. Deng et al. [72] reported significant association [OR = 1.55] between rs1800497, also known as the Taq1a RFLP, in *DRD2* and substance dependence in a meta-analysis of 25 studies, with a total $N = 6519$, but the authors concluded that the results were largely driven by samples ascertained for opioid dependence. Li et al. [104] found, when combining studies of heroin, methamphetamine, and alcohol dependence, significant association between variants in GABRA6 (rs3219151, OR = 1.5) and *GABRG2* (rs211013, OR = 1.21; rs211014, OR = 1.39) and substance dependence. Lastly, Schwantes-An and colleagues [168], in a very large GWAS of nearly 17,000 subjects, found a significant relationship between rs1799971 and substance dependence.

Genome-Wide Association Studies of General Liability

The first GWAS of general liability was performed by McGue and colleagues [169] in a sample of 2300 families (7188 individuals) from a longitudinal study at the Minnesota Center for Twin and Family Research (MCTFR). Separate GWAS were performed for multiple substance-use-related behaviors, including a composite index of use frequency and DSM-IV symptoms of 11 different illicit drugs. A SNP rs1868152 on chromosome 3q27.3 in the 3′ region of the *CRYGS* gene yielded a borderline genome-wide significant result. The investigators estimated a chip heritability of 0.37 for illicit drug use using GCTA.

Johnson and colleagues performed GWAS in a sample of cases drawn from the Urban Health Study with controls drawn from publicly available data [170]. A replication sample from publicly available data was also utilized. The sample was diverse and totaled over 10,000 subjects. The investigators reported a significant finding in the *KAT2B* gene that was limited to the African-American sample. Functional follow-up of the SNP (rs9829896) in postmortem dlPFC found that it was associated with expression of *KAT2B* and other substance use relevant genes, *CREBBP* and *OPRM1*.

Wetherill [171] performed GWAS of qualitative and quantitative measures of substance dependence in 2322 subjects drawn from 118 EA COGA families. The qualitative score was constructed based on the endorsement of DSM-IV dependence of alcohol, cannabis, cocaine, or opioids, and the quantitative index was constructed by factor analysis of symptoms across those four substances. The investigators reported a genome-wide significant signal for any dependence at rs2952621 in *LOC151121* and in rs2567261 in *ARHGAP28* for the quantitative index across substances.

Summary and Future Directions

The molecular era of SUD genetics, evolving through linkage analysis to candidate gene association testing and to genome-wide association analysis, has yielded findings that followed somewhat consistent themes. When researchers investigate the genetic contribution to variation in the risk for specific substance use disorders, the largest, replicating effects are discovered in the known metabolic pathways of the drug. In some settings, those findings can also identify protective variants, which, for instance, reduce the drug's ability to induce intoxication or generate an aversive reaction in the drug taker. This is especially true when controls have been exposed to the drug or when quantity of use (e.g., cigarettes per day) phenotypes are used. This has held true for nicotine, alcohol, and opioids. As sample sizes have grown, signals in the general liability pathways have been observed (for example, *DRD2* and other dopamine system genes).

There is, however, an important caveat of discoveries in larger samples. As the sample size grows, the power to detect smaller effect sizes increases. Sample sizes in the millions will yield statistical evidence for SNPs or genes with very small effect sizes, generating concerns about the clinical relevance of such findings. Advocates for continued use of larger GWAS will argue that these findings will provide evidence for new biological pathways, as small signals pile up [172]. An important finding of polygenic approaches is that the genetic architecture for "use" of some common substance, such as alcohol, may differ from "problematic use", with the latter being more strongly correlated with psychiatric diagnosis.

While there have been obvious successes of the GWAS approach, much of the genetic variation underlying many common diseases, including drug addiction, remains unaccounted for by specific polymorphisms. There are multiple complementary avenues the field can use moving forward. Continued use of genome-wide association scans is expected and will contribute some additional knowledge regarding the architecture of SUD genetics. That may highlight some specific "translatable" or "druggable" pathways which could inform the development of future pharmacotherapeutics. In addition, polygenic scores generated from GWAS may allow the use of genome-wide information to evaluate risk. Lastly, advances in the scale of DNA sequencing allow it to proceed at a quick enough pace to make whole exome (the complete exonic, i.e., coding, content of the genome) or whole genome sequencing a reality for relatively large samples. Using these approaches, an investigator can examine case-control frequency differences for moderately rare (1–5% frequency) or very rare (<1%) variants that are not adequately covered by traditional GWAS chips and in genes where common, functional variation is not present. In addition, large multiplex pedigrees previously collected for linkage analysis breathe new life as investigators are now searching for rare sequence variants shared among affected pedigree members. As inexpensive genome sequencing becomes a reality in the foreseeable future, the application of sequencing approaches to interrogate the impact of rare variation on complex human behavior phenotypes will become commonplace.

A consideration which has not been discussed is incorporation of the environment, or other potential risk modifiers, in studies of the genetic contributions to addiction risk. To date, no large-scale GWAS meta-analytic studies have been performed in which known environmental contributors to SUD risk (e.g., childhood adversity) are included as covariates or interactors, in spite of the knowledge that heritability for substance use disorders is largely less than ~50%. The next generation of SUD genetics studies must include measures of the environment to account for non-genetic variation in SUD risks. Importantly, the "environments" associated with SUDs, such as peer delinquency [173, 174] and familial relationship quality [175], are often themselves heritable, requiring thoughtful analytic approaches.

As scientists, we must consider lessons learned from the past few decades of research. Possibly the most important questions are: "did the candidate gene era fail to yield replicable results and why?", "why do human genetic findings frequently not overlap with preclinical animal models?", and "what lessons can be learned from the successes (e.g., nicotinic receptors and alcohol-metabolizing genes) of genetic mapping for SUDs?" These questions are related. Genetic studies are not a direct approach to understanding mechanism. When the approaches work, it is because polymorphisms exist in humans which impact gene function, and the variant alleles are frequent enough to allow us to detect case vs. control differences. Geneticists' ability to study and understand mechanism is limited by the presence of common functional variation in genes in that "mechanism." Why is it that a *DRD2* knockout mouse displays markedly different drug use behavior but there are no "major gene" associations between *DRD2* polymorphisms and an SUD? This is simply due to the lack of equivalent gene-silencing common variation in human populations. In interpreting the results of human genetics studies, it is very important to understand that the absence of evidence of association between variation in a particular gene and a behavior is not evidence for the absence of the neurobiological role played by the protein encoded by that gene. Instead, it is important for us to recognize human genetic studies for what they are – examinations of the impact of genetic variations present in human populations on variation in the trait of interest.

References

1. Hettema JM, Neale MC, Kendler KS. A review and meta-analysis of the genetic epidemiology of anxiety disorders. Am J Psychiatry. 2001;158:1568–78.
2. Sullivan PF, Neale MC, Kendler KS. Genetic epidemiology of major depression: review and meta-analysis. Am J Psychiatry. 2000;157:1552–62.
3. Spence MA, Greenberg DA, Hodge SE, Vieland VJ. The emperor's new methods. Am J Hum Genet. 2003;72:1084–7.
4. Falconer DS. The inheritance of liability to certain diseases, estimated from the incidence among relatives. Ann Hum Genet. 1965;29(1):51–76.
5. Vanyukov MM, Tarter RE, Kirisci L, Kirillova GP, Maher BS, Clark DB. Liability to substance use disorders: 1. Common mechanisms and manifestations. Neurosci Biobehav Rev. 2003;27(6):507–15.
6. Botstein D, White RL, Skolnick M, Davis RW. Construction of a genetic linkage map in man using restriction fragment length polymorphisms. Am J Hum Genet. 1980;32:314–31.
7. Nakamura Y, Leppert M, O'Connell P, Wolff R, Holm T, Culver M, et al. Variable number of tandem repeat (VNTR) markers for human gene mapping. Science. 1987;235:1616–22.
8. Weber JL, May PE. Abundant class of human DNA polymorphisms which can be typed using the polymerase chain reaction. Am J Hum Genet. 1989;44(3):388–96.
9. International HapMap Consortium. The International HapMap Project. Nature. 2003;426:789–96.
10. Terwilliger JD, Hiekkalinna T. An utter refutation of the "fundamental theorem of the HapMap". Eur J Hum Genet. 2006;14(4):426–37.
11. Fisher SA, Abecasis GR, Yashar BM, Zareparsi S, Swaroop A, Iyengar SK, et al. Meta-analysis of genome scans of age-related macular degeneration. Hum Mol Genet. 2005;14(15):2257–64.
12. Burton PR, Clayton DG, Cardon LR, Craddock N, Deloukas P, Duncanson A, et al. Genome-wide association study of 14,000 cases of seven common diseases and 3,000 shared controls. Nature. 2007;447:661–78.
13. 1000 Genomes Project Consortium, Durbin RM, Abecasis GR, Altshuler DL, Auton A, Brooks LD, et al. A map of human genome variation from population-scale sequencing. Nature. 2010;467:1061–73.
14. Taliun D, Harris DN, Kessler MD, Carlson J, Szpiech ZA, Torres R, et al. Sequencing of 53,831 diverse genomes from the NHLBI TOPMed program. Nature. 2021;590(7845):290–9.
15. Reich DE, Lander ES. On the allelic spectrum of human disease. Trends Genet. 2001;17:502–10.
16. Frank J, Cichon S, Treutlein J, Ridinger M, Mattheisen M, Hoffmann P, et al. Genome- wide significant association between alcohol dependence and a variant in the ADH gene cluster. Addict Biol. 2012;17(1):171–80.
17. Treutlein J, Cichon S, Ridinger M, Wodarz N, Soyka M, Zill P, et al. Genome-wide association study of alcohol dependence. Arch Gen Psychiatry. 2009;66(7):773–84.
18. Smyth DJ, Cooper JD, Bailey R, Field S, Burren O, Smink LJ, et al. A genome-wide association study of nonsynonymous SNPs identifies a type 1 diabetes locus in the interferon-induced helicase (IFIH1) region. Nat Genet. 2006;38(6):617–9.
19. Schizophrenia Psychiatric Genome-Wide Association Study (GWAS) Consortium. Genome-wide association study identifies five new schizophrenia loci. Nat Genet. 2011;43(10):969–76.
20. Schizophrenia Working Group of the Psychiatric Genomics Consortium. Biological insights from 108 schizophrenia-associated genetic loci. Nature. 2014;511(7510):421–7.
21. Fisher RA. The correlation between relatives on the supposition of Mendelian inheritance. Transactions – Royal Society of Edinburgh; 1918.
22. Zaykin DV, Zhivotovsky LA. Ranks of genuine associations in whole-genome scans. Genetics. 2005;171:813–23.
23. Yang J, Lee SH, Goddard ME, Visscher PM. GCTA: a tool for genome-wide complex trait analysis. Am J Hum Genet. 2011;88(1):76–82.
24. Purcell SM, Wray NR, Stone JL, Visscher PM, O'Donovan MC, Sullivan PF, et al. Common polygenic variation contributes to risk of schizophrenia and bipolar disorder. Nature. 2009;460:748–52.

25. Subramanian A, Tamayo P, Mootha VK, Mukherjee S, Ebert BL, Gillette MA, et al. Gene set enrichment analysis: a knowledge-based approach for interpreting genome-wide expression profiles. Proc Natl Acad Sci U S A. 2005;102(43):15545–50.
26. Rossin EJ, Lage K, Raychaudhuri S, Xavier RJ, Tatar D, Benita Y, et al. Proteins encoded in genomic regions associated with immune-mediated disease physically interact and suggest underlying biology. PLoS Genet. 2011;7(1):e1001273.
27. Holmans P, Green EK, Pahwa JS, Ferreira MA, Purcell SM, Sklar P, et al. Gene ontology analysis of GWA study data sets provides insights into the biology of bipolar disorder. Am J Hum Genet. 2009;85(1):13–24.
28. Polderman TJ, Benyamin B, de Leeuw CA, Sullivan PF, van Bochoven A, Visscher PM, et al. Meta-analysis of the heritability of human traits based on fifty years of twin studies. Nat Genet. 2015;47(7):702–9.
29. Dick DM, Pagan JL, Viken R, Purcell S, Kaprio J, Pulkkinen L, et al. Changing environmental influences on substance use across development. Twin Res Hum Genet. 2007;10(2):315–26.
30. Wacholder S, Silverman DT, McLaughlin JK, Mandel JS. Selection of controls in case-control studies: II. Types of controls. Am J Epidemiol. 1992;135(9):1029–41.
31. Wacholder S, McLaughlin JK, Silverman DT, Mandel JS. Selection of controls in case-control studies: I. Principles. Am J Epidemiol. 1992;135(9):1019–28.
32. Wacholder S, Silverman DT, McLaughlin JK, Mandel JS. Selection of controls in case-control studies. III. Design options. Am J Epidemiol. 1992;135(9):1042–50.
33. Nelson EC, Agrawal A, Heath AC, Bogdan R, Sherva R, Zhang B, et al. Evidence of CNIH3 involvement in opioid dependence. Mol Psychiatry. 2016;21(5):608–14.
34. True WR, Heath AC, Scherrer JF, Waterman B, Goldberg J, Lin N, et al. Genetic and environmental contributions to smoking. Addiction. 1997;92(10):1277–87.
35. Vanyukov MM, Tarter RE, Conway KP, Kirillova GP, Chandler RK, Daley DC. Risk and resistance perspectives in translation-oriented etiology research. Transl Behav Med. 2016;6:45–54.
36. Maher BS, Latendresse S, Vanyukov MM. Informing prevention and intervention policy using genetic studies of resistance. Prev Sci. 2018;19(1):49–57.
37. International Human Genome Sequencing Consortium. Initial sequencing and analysis of the human genome. Nature. 2001;409(6822):860–921.
38. Koob GF, Volkow ND. Neurobiology of addiction: a neurocircuitry analysis. Lancet Psychiatry. 2016;3(8):760–73.
39. Wise RA. Brain reward circuitry: insights from unsensed incentives. Neuron. 2002;36(2):229–40.
40. Hodge CW, Samson HH, Chappelle AM. Alcohol self-administration: further examination of the role of dopamine receptors in the nucleus accumbens. Alcohol Clin Exp Res. 1997;21(6):1083–91.
41. Volkow ND, Wang GJ, Fowler JS, Logan J, Gatley SJ, Wong C, et al. Reinforcing effects of psychostimulants in humans are associated with increases in brain dopamine and occupancy of D(2) receptors. J Pharmacol Exp Ther. 1999;291(1):409–15.
42. Di Chiara G, Imperato A. Drugs abused by humans preferentially increase synaptic dopamine concentrations in the mesolimbic system of freely moving rats. Proc Natl Acad Sci U S A. 1988;85(14):5274–8.
43. Boileau I, Assaad JM, Pihl RO, Benkelfat C, Leyton M, Diksic M, et al. Alcohol promotes dopamine release in the human nucleus accumbens. Synapse. 2003;49(4):226–31.
44. Barrett SP, Boileau I, Okker J, Pihl RO, Dagher A. The hedonic response to cigarette smoking is proportional to dopamine release in the human striatum as measured by positron emission tomography and [11C]raclopride. Synapse. 2004;54(2):65–71.
45. Tunbridge EM, Narajos M, Harrison CH, Beresford C, Cipriani A, Harrison PJ. Which dopamine polymorphisms are functional? Systematic review and meta-analysis of COMT, DAT, DBH, DDC, DRD1-5, MAOA, MAOB, TH, VMAT1, and VMAT2. Biol Psychiatry. 2019;86(8):608–20.
46. Goldman D, Urbanek M, Guenther D, Robin R, Long JC. Linkage and association of a functional DRD2 variant [Ser311Cys] and DRD2 markers to alcoholism, substance abuse and schizophrenia in Southwestern American Indians. Am J Med Genet. 1997;74(4):386–94.
47. Comings DE, Rosenthal RJ, Lesieur HR, Rugle LJ, Muhleman D, Chiu C, et al. A study of the dopamine D2 receptor gene in pathological gambling. Pharmacogenetics. 1996;6(3):223–34.
48. Volkow ND, Wang GJ, Fowler JS, Logan J, Gatley SJ, Gifford A, et al. Prediction of reinforcing responses to psychostimulants in humans by brain dopamine D2 receptor levels. Am J Psychiatry. 1999;156(9):1440–3.
49. Swanson JM, Lerner M, Williams L. More frequent diagnosis of attention deficit-hyperactivity disorder. N Engl J Med. 1995;333(14):944.
50. Cook EH, Stein MA, Krasowski MD, Cox NJ, Olkon DM, Kieffer JE, et al. Association of attention-deficit disorder and the dopamine transporter gene. Am J Hum Genet. 1995;56(4):993–8.
51. Gill M, Daly G, Heron S, Hawi Z, Fitzgerald M. Confirmation of association between attention deficit hyperactivity disorder and a dopamine transporter polymorphism. Mol Psychiatry. 1997;2(4):311–3.
52. Daly G, Hawi Z, Fitzgerald M, Gill M. Mapping susceptibility loci in attention deficit hyperactivity disorder: preferential transmission of parental alleles at DAT1, DBH and DRD5 to affected children. Mol Psychiatry. 1999;4(2):192–6.

53. Waldman ID, Rowe DC, Abramowitz A, Kozel ST, Mohr JH, Sherman SL, et al. Association and linkage of the dopamine transporter gene and attention-deficit hyperactivity disorder in children: heterogeneity owing to diagnostic subtype and severity. Am J Hum Genet. 1998;63(6):1767–76.
54. Maher BS, Marazita ML, Ferrell RE, Vanyukov MM. Dopamine system genes and attention deficit hyperactivity disorder: a meta-analysis. Psychiatr Genet. 2002;12(4):207–15.
55. Ebstein RP, Novick O, Umansky R, Priel B, Osher Y, Blaine D, et al. Dopamine D4 receptor (D4DR) exon III polymorphism associated with the human personality trait of Novelty Seeking. Nat Genet. 1996;12(1):78–80.
56. LaHoste GJ, Swanson JM, Wigal SB, Glabe C, Wigal T, King N, et al. Dopamine D4 receptor gene polymorphism is associated with attention deficit hyperactivity disorder. Mol Psychiatry. 1996;1(2):121–4.
57. Sunohara GA, Roberts W, Malone M, Schachar RJ, Tannock R, Basile VS, et al. Linkage of the dopamine D4 receptor gene and attention-deficit/hyperactivity disorder. J Am Acad Child Adolesc Psychiatry. 2000;39(12):1537–42.
58. Swanson JM, Sunohara GA, Kennedy JL, Regino R, Fineberg E, Wigal T, et al. Association of the dopamine receptor D4 (DRD4) gene with a refined phenotype of attention deficit hyperactivity disorder (ADHD): a family-based approach. Mol Psychiatry. 1998;3(1):38–41.
59. Benjamin J, Li L, Patterson C, Greenberg BD, Murphy DL, Hamer DH. Population and familial association between the D4 dopamine receptor gene and measures of Novelty Seeking. Nat Genet. 1996;12(1):81–4.
60. Smalley SL, Bailey JN, Palmer CG, Cantwell DP, McGough JJ, Del\'92Homme MA, et al. Evidence that the dopamine D4 receptor is a susceptibility gene in attention deficit hyperactivity disorder. Mol Psychiatry. 1998;3(5):427–30.
61. Rowe DC, Stever C, Giedinghagen LN, Gard JM, Cleveland HH, Terris ST, et al. Dopamine DRD4 receptor polymorphism and attention deficit hyperactivity disorder. Mol Psychiatry. 1998;3(5):419–26.
62. Faraone SV, Biederman J, Weiffenbach B, Keith T, Chu MP, Weaver A, et al. Dopamine D4 gene 7-repeat allele and attention deficit hyperactivity disorder. Am J Psychiatry. 1999;156(5):768–70.
63. Comings DE, Gonzalez N, Wu S, Gade R, Muhleman D, Saucier G, et al. Studies of the 48 bp repeat polymorphism of the DRD4 gene in impulsive, compulsive, addictive behaviors: Tourette syndrome, ADHD, pathological gambling, and substance abuse. Am J Med Genet. 1999;88(4):358–68.
64. Bonvicini C, Faraone SV, Scassellati C. Attention-deficit hyperactivity disorder in adults: a systematic review and meta-analysis of genetic, pharmacogenetic and biochemical studies. Mol Psychiatry. 2016;21(11):1643.
65. Munafo MR, Yalcin B, Willis-Owen SA, Flint J. Association of the dopamine D4 receptor (DRD4) gene and approach-related personality traits: meta-analysis and new data. Biol Psychiatry. 2008;63(2):197–206.
66. Daurio AM, Deschaine SL, Modabbernia A, Leggio L. Parsing out the role of dopamine D4 receptor gene (DRD4) on alcohol-related phenotypes: a meta-analysis and systematic review. Addict Biol. 2020;25(3):e12770.
67. Kang P, Luo L, Peng X, Wang Y. Association of Val158Met polymorphism in COMT gene with attention-deficit hyperactive disorder: An updated meta-analysis. Medicine (Baltimore). 2020;99(48):e23400.
68. Forero DA, Lopez-Leon S, Shin HD, Park BL, Kim D-J. Meta-analysis of six genes (BDNF, DRD1, DRD3, DRD4, GRIN2B and MAOA) involved in neuroplasticity and the risk for alcohol dependence. Drug Alcohol Depend. 2015;149:259–63.
69. Vanyukov MM, Moss HB, Gioio AE, Hughes HB, Kaplan BB, Tarter RE. An association between a microsatellite polymorphism at the DRD5 gene and the liability to substance abuse: pilot study. Behav Genet. 1998;28(2):75–82.
70. Vanyukov MM, Moss HB, Kaplan BB, Kirillova GP, Tarter RE. Antisociality, substance dependence, and the DRD5 gene: a preliminary study. Am J Med Genet. 2000;96(5):654–8.
71. Munafo MR, Timpson NJ, David SP, Ebrahim S, Lawlor DA. Association of the DRD2 gene Taq1A polymorphism and smoking behavior: a meta-analysis and new data. Nicotine Tob Res. 2009;11(1):64–76.
72. Deng XD, Jiang H, Ma Y, Gao Q, Zhang B, Mu B, et al. Association between DRD2/ANKK1 TaqIA polymorphism and common illicit drug dependence: evidence from a meta-analysis. Hum Immunol. 2015;76(1):42–51.
73. Wang F, Simen A, Arias A, Lu Q-W, Zhang H. A large-scale meta-analysis of the association between the ANKK1/DRD2 Taq1A polymorphism and alcohol dependence. Hum Genet. 2013;132(3):347–58.
74. Ma Y, Wang M, Yuan W, Su K, Li MD. The significant association of Taq1A genotypes in DRD2/ANKK1 with smoking cessation in a large-scale meta-analysis of Caucasian populations. Transl Psychiatry. 2015;5:e686.
75. Olmstead MC. Animal models of drug addiction: where do we go from here? Q J Exp Psychol. 2006 Apr;59(4):625–53.
76. Müller CP, Homberg JR. The role of serotonin in drug use and addiction. Behav Brain Res. 2015;277:146–92.
77. Kirby LG, Zeeb FD, Winstanley CA. Contributions of serotonin in addiction vulnerability. Neuropharmacology. 2011;61(3):421–32.

78. Matsumoto RR. GABA receptors: are cellular differences reflected in function? Brain Res Rev. 1989;14(3):203–25.
79. Jones KA, Borowsky B, Tamm JA, Craig DA, Durkin MM, Dai M, et al. GABA B receptors function as a heteromeric assembly of the subunits GABA B R1 and GABA B R2. Nature. 1998;396(6712):674–9.
80. Schofield PR, Darlison MG, Fujita N, Burt DR, Stephenson FA, Rodriguez H, et al. Sequence and functional expression of the GABA a receptor shows a ligand-gated receptor super-family. Nature. 1987;328(6127):221–7.
81. Fonnum F. Glutamate: a neurotransmitter in mammalian brain. J Neurochem. 1984;42(1):1–11.
82. Naaijen J, Bralten J, Poelmans G, Glennon JC, Franke B, Buitelaar JK. Glutamatergic and GABAergic gene sets in attention-deficit/hyperactivity disorder: association to overlapping traits in ADHD and autism. Translational. Psychiatry. 2017;7, (1):e999.
83. Duncan LE, Keller MC. A critical review of the first 10 years of candidate gene-by-environment interaction research in psychiatry. Am J Psychiatr. 2011;168(10):1041–9.
84. Devlin B, Roeder K. Genomic control for association studies. Biometrics. 1999;55:997–1004.
85. Price AL, Patterson NJ, Plenge RM, Weinblatt ME, Shadick NA, Reich D. Principal components analysis corrects for stratification in genome-wide association studies. Nat Genet. 2006;38(8):904–9.
86. Marchitti SA, Brocker C, Stagos D, Vasiliou V. Non-P450 aldehyde oxidizing enzymes: the aldehyde dehydrogenase superfamily. Expert Opin Drug Metab Toxicol. 2008;4(6):697–720.
87. Edenberg HJ, Xuei X, Chen H-J, Tian H, Wetherill LF, Dick DM, et al. Association of alcohol dehydrogenase genes with alcohol dependence: a comprehensive analysis. Hum Mol Genet. 2006;15(9):1539–49.
88. Edenberg HJ, McClintick JN. Alcohol dehydrogenases, aldehyde dehydrogenases, and alcohol use disorders: a critical review. Alcohol Clin Exp Res. 2018;42(12):2281–97.
89. Davidoff RA. Alcohol and presynaptic inhibition in an isolated spinal cord preparation. Arch Neurol. 1973;28(1):60–3.
90. Allan AM, Spuhler KP, Harris RA. gamma-Aminobutyric acid-activated chloride channels: relationship to genetic differences in ethanol sensitivity. J Pharmacol Exp Ther. 1988;244(3):866–70.
91. Allan AM, Harris RA. Gamma-aminobutyric acid and alcohol actions: neurochemical studies of long sleep and short sleep mice. Life Sci. 1986;39(21):2005–15.
92. Reich T, Edenberg HJ, Goate A, Williams JT, Rice JP, Van Eerdewegh P, et al. Genome-wide search for genes affecting the risk for alcohol dependence. Am J Med Genet. 1998;81(3):207–15.
93. Long JC, Knowler WC, Hanson RL, Robin RW, Urbanek M, Moore E, et al. Evidence for genetic linkage to alcohol dependence on chromosomes 4 and 11 from an autosome- wide scan in an American Indian population. Am J Med Genet. 1998;81(3):216–21.
94. Wilhelmsen KC, Schuckit M, Smith TL, Lee JV, Segall SK, Feiler HS, et al. The search for genes related to a low-level response to alcohol determined by alcohol challenges. Alcohol Clin Exp Res. 2003;27(7):1041–7.
95. Schuckit MA. Low level of response to alcohol as a predictor of future alcoholism. Am J Psychiatry. 1994 Feb;151(2):184–9.
96. Ehlers CL, Gilder DA, Wall TL, Phillips E, Feiler H, Wilhelmsen KC. Genomic screen for loci associated with alcohol dependence in Mission Indians. Am J Med Genet B Neuropsychiatr Genet. 2004;129B(1):110–5.
97. Prescott CA, Sullivan PF, Kuo PH, Webb BT, Vittum J, Patterson DG, et al. Genomewide linkage study in the Irish affected sib pair study of alcohol dependence: evidence for a susceptibility region for symptoms of alcohol dependence on chromosome 4. Mol Psychiatry. 2006;11:603–11.
98. Gelernter J, Kranzler HR, Panhuysen C, Weiss RD, Brady K, Poling J, et al. Dense genomewide linkage scan for alcohol dependence in African Americans: significant linkage on chromosome 10. Biol Psychiatry. 2009;65(2):111–5.
99. Bierut LJ, Goate AM, Breslau N, Johnson EO, Bertelsen S, Fox L, et al. ADH1B is associated with alcohol dependence and alcohol consumption in populations of European and African ancestry. Mol Psychiatry. 2012;17(4):445–50.
100. Li D, Zhao H, Gelernter J. Strong association of the alcohol dehydrogenase 1B gene (ADH1B) with alcohol dependence and alcohol-induced medical diseases. Biol Psychiatry. 2011;70(6): 504–12.
101. Li D, Zhao H, Gelernter J. Further clarification of the contribution of the ADH1C gene to vulnerability of alcoholism and selected liver diseases. Hum Genet. 2012;131(8):1361–74.
102. Zaso MJ, Desalu JM, Kim J, Suryadevara K, Belote JM, Park A. Interaction between the ADH1B*3 allele and drinking motives on alcohol use among Black college students. Am J Drug Alcohol Abuse. 2018;44(3):329–38.
103. Li D, Zhao H, Gelernter J. Strong protective effect of the aldehyde dehydrogenase gene (ALDH2) 504lys (*2) allele against alcoholism and alcohol-induced medical diseases in Asians. Hum Genet. 2012;131(5):725–37.
104. Li D, Sulovari A, Cheng C, Zhao H, Kranzler HR, Gelernter J. Association of gamma-aminobutyric acid a receptor alpha2 gene (GABRA2) with alcohol use disorder. Neuropsychopharmacology. 2014;39(4):907–18.
105. Cao J, Liu X, Han S, Zhang CK, Liu Z, Li D. Association of the HTR2A gene with alcohol and heroin abuse. Hum Genet. 2014;133(3):357–65.
106. Ma Y, Fan R, Li MD. Meta-analysis reveals significant association of the 3'-UTR VNTR in SLC6A3

with alcohol dependence. Alcohol Clin Exp Res. 2016;40(7):1443–53.
107. Maher BS, Riley BP, Kendler KS. Psychiatric genetics gets a boost. Nat Genet. 2008;40, (1546–1718; 9): 1042–4.
108. Schumann G, Coin LJ, Lourdusamy A, Charoen P, Berger KH, Stacey D, et al. Genome-wide association and genetic functional studies identify autism susceptibility candidate 2 gene (AUTS2) in the regulation of alcohol consumption. Proc Natl Acad Sci U S A. 2011;108(17):7119–24.
109. Schumann G, Liu C, O''Reilly P, Gao H, Song P, Xu B, et al. KLB is associated with alcohol drinking, and its gene product beta-Klotho is necessary for FGF21 regulation of alcohol preference. Proc Natl Acad Sci USA. 2016;113(50):14372–7.
110. Walters RK, Polimanti R, Johnson EC, McClintick JN, Adams MJ, Adkins AE, et al. Transancestral GWAS of alcohol dependence reveals common genetic underpinnings with psychiatric disorders. Nat Neurosci. 2018;21(12):1656–69.
111. Zhou H, Sealock JM, Sanchez-Roige S, Clarke TK, Levey DF, Cheng Z, Li B, Polimanti R, Kember RL, Smith RV, Thygesen JH. Genome-wide meta-analysis of problematic alcohol use in 435,563 individuals yields insights into biology and relationships with other traits. Nat Neurosci. 2020;23(7):809–18.
112. Adkins DE, Clark SL, Copeland WE, Kennedy M, Conway K, Angold A, et al. Genome-wide meta-analysis of longitudinal alcohol consumption across youth and early adulthood. Twin Res Hum Genet. 2015;18(4):335–47.
113. Jorgenson E, Thai KK, Hoffmann TJ, Sakoda LC, Kvale MN, Banda Y, et al. Genetic contributors to variation in alcohol consumption vary by race/ethnicity in a large multi-ethnic genome-wide association study. Mol Psychiatry. 2017;22(9):1359–67.
114. Sanchez-Roige S, Fontanillas P, Elson SL, Team 23andMe Research, Gray JC, de Wit H, et al. Genome-wide association study of alcohol use disorder identification test (AUDIT) scores in 20 328 research participants of European ancestry. Addict Biol. 2019;24(1):121–31.
115. Sanchez-Roige S, Palmer AA, Fontanillas P, Elson SL, 23andMe Research Team the SUDWG of the PGC, Adams MJ, et al. Genome-wide association study meta-analysis of the Alcohol Use Disorders Identification Test (AUDIT) in two population-based cohorts. Am J Psychiatry. 2019;176(2):107–18.
116. Liu M, Jiang Y, Wedow R, Li Y, Brazel DM, Chen F, et al. Association studies of up to 1.2 million individuals yield new insights into the genetic etiology of tobacco and alcohol use. Nat Genet. 2019;51(2):237–44.
117. Kranzler HR, Zhou H, Kember RL, Smith RV, Justice AC, Damrauer S, et al. Genome-wide association study of alcohol consumption and use disorder in 274,424 individuals from multiple populations. Nat Commun. 2019;10(1):1–11.
118. Smith GD, Ebrahim S. Mendelian randomization: prospects, potentials, and limitations. Int J Epidemiol. 2004;33(1):30–42.
119. Linnér RK, Biroli P, Kong E, Meddens SF, Wedow R, Fontana MA, Lebreton M, Tino SP, Abdellaoui A, Hammerschlag AR, Nivard MG. Genome-wide association analyses of risk tolerance and risky behaviors in over 1 million individuals identify hundreds of loci and shared genetic influences. Nat Genet. 2019 Feb;51(2):245–57.
120. Gotti C, Clementi F. Neuronal nicotinic receptors: from structure to pathology. Prog Neurobiol. 2004;74(6):363–96.
121. Schaaf CP. Nicotinic acetylcholine receptors in human genetic disease. Genet Med. 2014;16(9):649–56.
122. Ware JJ, van den Bree MB, Munafo MR. Association of the CHRNA5-A3-B4 gene cluster with heaviness of smoking: a meta-analysis. Nicotine Tob Res. 2011;13(12):1167–75.
123. Olfson E, Saccone NL, Johnson EO, Chen LS, Culverhouse R, Doheny K, et al. Rare, low frequency and common coding variants in CHRNA5 and their contribution to nicotine dependence in European and African Americans. Mol Psychiatry. 2016;21(5):601–7.
124. Pan L, Yang X, Li S, Jia C. Association of CYP2A6 gene polymorphisms with cigarette consumption: a meta-analysis. Drug Alcohol Depend. 2015;149:268–71.
125. Jackson KJ, Chen X, Miles MF, Harenza J, Damaj MI. The neuropeptide galanin and variants in the GalR1 gene are associated with nicotine dependence. Neuropsychopharmacology. 2011;36(11):2339–48.
126. Macare C, Ducci F, Zhang Y, Ruggeri B, Jia T, Kaakinen M, et al. A neurobiological pathway to smoking in adolescence: TTC12-ANKK1-DRD2 variants and reward response. Eur Neuropsychopharmacol. 2018;28(10):1103–14.
127. Munafo M, Clark T, Johnstone E, Murphy M, Walton R. The genetic basis for smoking behavior: a systematic review and meta-analysis. Nicotine Tob Res. 2004;6(4):583–97.
128. Straub RE, Sullivan PF, Ma Y, Myakishev MV, Harris-Kerr C, Wormley B, et al. Susceptibility genes for nicotine dependence: a genome scan and followup in an independent sample suggest that regions on chromosomes 2, 4, 10, 16, 17 and 18 merit further study. Mol Psychiatry. 1999;4(2):129–44.
129. Vink JM, Beem AL, Posthuma D, Neale MC, Willemsen G, Kendler KS, et al. Linkage analysis of smoking initiation and quantity in Dutch sibling pairs. Pharmacogenomics. J. 2004 vol. 4, (1470–269; 4), pp. 274–282.
130. Swan GE, Hops H, Wilhelmsen KC, Lessov-Schlaggar CN, Cheng LS, Hudmon KS, et al. A genome-wide screen for nicotine dependence susceptibility loci. Am J Med Genet B Neuropsychiatr Genet. 2006;141B(4):354–60.

131. Li MD, Payne TJ, Ma JZ, Lou XY, Zhang D, Dupont RT, et al. A genomewide search finds major susceptibility loci for nicotine dependence on chromosome 10 in African Americans. Am J Hum Genet. 2006;79(4):745–51.
132. Duggirala R, Almasy L, Blangero J. Smoking behavior is under the influence of a major quantitative trait locus on human chromosome 5q. Genet Epidemiol. 1999;17(Suppl 1):139.
133. Morley KI, Medland SE, Ferreira MA, Lynskey MT, Montgomery GW, Heath AC, et al. A possible smoking susceptibility locus on chromosome 11p12: evidence from sex-limitation linkage analyses in a sample of Australian twin families. Behav Genet. 2006;36(1):87–99.
134. Gelernter J, Liu X, Hesselbrock V, Page GP, Goddard A, Zhang H. Results of a genomewide linkage scan: support for chromosomes 9 and 11 loci increasing risk for cigarette smoking. Am J Med Genet B Neuropsychiatr Genet. 2004;128B(1):94–101.
135. Bierut LJ, Rice JP, Goate A, Hinrichs AL, Saccone NL, Foroud T, et al. A genomic scan for habitual smoking in families of alcoholics: common and specific genetic factors in substance dependence. Am J Med Genet A. 2004;124A(1):19–27.
136. Bierut LJ, Madden PA, Breslau N, Johnson EO, Hatsukami D, Pomerleau OF, et al. Novel genes identified in a high-density genome wide association study for nicotine dependence. Hum Mol Genet. 2007;16(1):24–35.
137. Liu JZ, Tozzi F, Waterworth DM, Pillai SG, Muglia P, Middleton L, et al. Meta-analysis and imputation refines the association of 15q25 with smoking quantity. Nat Genet. 2010;42(5):436–40.
138. Thorgeirsson TE, Gudbjartsson DF, Surakka I, Vink JM, Amin N, Geller F, et al. Sequence variants at CHRNB3-CHRNA6 and CYP2A6 affect smoking behavior. Nat Genet. 2010;42(5):448–53.
139. Tobacco and Genetics Consortium. Genome-wide meta-analyses identify multiple loci associated with smoking behavior. Nat Genet. 2010;42(5):441–7.
140. Hancock DB, Reginsson GW, Gaddis NC, Chen X, Saccone NL, Lutz SM, et al. Genome-wide meta-analysis reveals common splice site acceptor variant in CHRNA4 associated with nicotine dependence. Trans Psychiatry. 2015;5(10):e651.
141. Chen J, Loukola A, Gillespie NA, Peterson R, Jia P, Riley B, et al. Genome-wide meta-analyses of FTND and TTFC phenotypes. Nicotine Tob Res. 2020;22(6):900–9.
142. Buchwald J, Chenoweth MJ, Palviainen T, Zhu G, Benner C, Gordon S, Korhonen T, Ripatti S, Madden PA, Lehtimäki T, Raitakari OT. Genome-wide association meta-analysis of nicotine metabolism and cigarette consumption measures in smokers of European descent. Mol Psychiatry. 2020 Mar;10:1–2.
143. Hancock DB, Guo Y, Reginsson GW, Gaddis NC, Lutz SM, Sherva R, et al. Genome-wide association study across European and African American ancestries identifies a SNP in DNMT3B contributing to nicotine dependence. Mol Psychiatry. 2018;23(9):1911–9.
144. Ehlers CL, Gizer IR, Vieten C, Wilhelmsen KC. Linkage analyses of cannabis dependence, craving, and withdrawal in the San Francisco family study. Am J Med Genet B Neuropsychiatr Genet. 2010;153B(3):802–11.
145. Hopfer CJ, Lessem JM, Hartman CA, Stallings MC, Cherny SS, Corley RP, et al. A genome-wide scan for loci influencing adolescent cannabis dependence symptoms: evidence for linkage on chromosomes 3 and 9. Drug Alcohol Depend. 2007;89(1):34–41.
146. Ehlers CL, Gilder DA, Gizer IR, Wilhelmsen KC. Heritability and a genome-wide linkage analysis of a Type II/B cluster construct for cannabis dependence in an American Indian community. Addict Biol. 2009;14(3):338–48.
147. Agrawal A, Lynskey MT, Hinrichs A, Grucza R, Saccone SF, Krueger R, et al. A genome\uc0\u8208 wide association study of DSM-IV cannabis dependence. Addict Biol. 2011;16(3):514–8.
148. Sherva R, Wang Q, Kranzler H, Zhao H, Koesterer R, Herman A, et al. Genome-wide association study of cannabis dependence severity, novel risk variants, and shared genetic risks. JAMA Psychiat. 2016;73(5):472–80.
149. Demontis D, Rajagopal VM, Thorgeirsson TE, Als TD, Grove J, Leppala K, et al. Genome-wide association study implicates CHRNA2 in cannabis use disorder. Nat Neurosci. 2019;22(7):1066–74.
150. Stringer S, Minic CC, Verweij KJ, Mbarek H, Bernard M, Derringer J, et al. Genome-wide association study of lifetime cannabis use based on a large meta-analytic sample of 32,330 subjects from the International Cannabis Consortium. Trans Psychiatry. 2016;6(3):e769.
151. Pasman JA, Verweij KJH, Gerring Z, Stringer S, Sanchez-Roige S, Treur JL, et al. GWAS of lifetime cannabis use reveals new risk loci, genetic overlap with psychiatric traits, and a causal influence of schizophrenia. Nat Neurosci. 2018;21(9):1161–70.
152. Johnson EC, Demontis D, Thorgeirsson TE, Walters RK, Polimanti R, Hatoum AS, et al. A large-scale genome-wide association study meta-analysis of cannabis use disorder. Lancet Psychiatry. 2020;7(12):1032–45.
153. Haerian BS. BDNF rs6265 polymorphism and drug addiction: a systematic review and meta-analysis. Pharmacogenomics. 2013;14(16):2055–65.
154. Chen D, Liu F, Shang Q, Song X, Miao X, Wang Z. Association between polymorphisms of DRD2 and DRD4 and opioid dependence: evidence from the current studies. Am J Med Genet B Neuropsychiatr Genet. 2011;156B(6):661–70.
155. Zhang J, Yan P, Li Y, Cai X, Yang Z, Miao X, et al. A 35.8 kilobases haplotype spanning ANKK1 and DRD2 is associated with heroin dependence in Han Chinese males. Brain Res. 2018;1688:54–64.

156. Hancock DB, Levy JL, Gaddis NC, Glasheen C, Saccone NL, Page GP, et al. Replication of ZNF804A gene variant associations with risk of heroin addiction. Genes Brain Behav. 2015;14(8):635–40.
157. Gelernter J, Panhuysen C, Wilcox M, Hesselbrock V, Rounsaville B, Poling J, et al. Genomewide linkage scan for opioid dependence and related traits. Am J Hum Genet. 2006;78(5):759–69.
158. Lachman HM, Fann CS, Bartzis M, Evgrafov OV, Rosenthal RN, Nunes EV, et al. Genomewide suggestive linkage of opioid dependence to chromosome 14q. Hum Mol Genet. 2007;16(11):1327–34.
159. Glatt SJ, Lasky-Su JA, Zhu SC, Zhang R, Zhang B, Li J, et al. Genome-wide linkage analysis of heroin dependence in Han Chinese: results from wave two of a multi-stage study. Drug Alcohol Depend. 2008;98(1–2):30–4.
160. Nielsen DA, Ji F, Yuferov V, Ho A, Chen A, Levran O, et al. Genotype patterns that contribute to increased risk for or protection from developing heroin addiction. Mol Psychiatry. 2008;13(4):417–28.
161. Gelernter J, Kranzler HR, Sherva R, Koesterer R, Almasy L, Zhao H, et al. Genome-wide association study of opioid dependence: multiple associations mapped to calcium and potassium pathways. Biol Psychiatry. 2014;76(1):66–74.
162. Kalsi G, Euesden J, Coleman JR, Ducci F, Aliev F, Newhouse SJ, et al. Genome-wide association of heroin dependence in Han Chinese. PLoS One. 2016;11(12):e0167388.
163. Polimanti R, Walters RK, Johnson EC, McClintick JN, Adkins AE, Adkins DE, et al. Leveraging genome-wide data to investigate differences between opioid use vs. opioid dependence in 41,176 individuals from the Psychiatric Genomics Consortium. Mol Psychiatry. 2020;25(8):1673–87.
164. Zhou H, Rentsch CT, Cheng Z, Kember RL, Nunez YZ, Sherva RM, et al. Association of OPRM1 functional coding variant with opioid use disorder: a genome-wide association study. JAMA Psychiat. 2020;77(10):1072–80.
165. Song W, Kossowsky J, Torous J, Chen CY, Huang H, Mukamal KJ, Berde CB, Bates DW, Wright A. Genome-wide association analysis of opioid use disorder: a novel approach using clinical data. Drug Alcohol Depend. 2020;1(217):108276.
166. Gelernter J, Panhuysen C, Weiss R, Brady K, Hesselbrock V, Rounsaville B, et al. Genomewide linkage scan for cocaine dependence and related traits: significant linkages for a cocaine-related trait and cocaine-induced paranoia. Am J Med Genet B Neuropsychiatr Genet. 2005;136B(1):45–52.
167. Gelernter J, Sherva R, Koesterer R, Almasy L, Zhao H, Kranzler HR, et al. Genome-wide association study of cocaine dependence and related traits: FAM53B identified as a risk gene. Mol Psychiatry. 2014;19(6):717–23.
168. Schwantes-An T-H, Zhang J, Chen L-S, Hartz SM, Culverhouse RC, Chen X, et al. Association of the OPRM1 variant rs1799971 (A118G) with non-specific liability to substance dependence in a collaborative de novo meta-analysis of European-ancestry cohorts. Behav Genet. 2015;46:151–69.
169. McGue M, Zhang Y, Miller MB, Basu S, Vrieze S, Hicks B, et al. A genome-wide association study of behavioral disinhibition. Behav Genet. 2013;43(5):363–73.
170. Johnson EO, Hancock DB, Levy JL, Gaddis NC, Page GP, Glasheen C, et al. KAT2B polymorphism identified for drug abuse in African Americans with regulatory links to drug abuse pathways in human prefrontal cortex. Addict Biol. 2016;21(6):1217–32.
171. Wetherill L, Agrawal A, Kapoor M, Bertelsen S, Bierut LJ, Brooks A, et al. Association of substance dependence phenotypes in the COGA sample. Addict Biol. 2015;20(3):617–27.
172. Sullivan P. Don't give up on GWAS. Mol Psychiatry. 2012;17(1):2–3.
173. Kendler KS, Jacobson KC, Gardner CO, Gillespie N, Aggen SA, Prescott CA. Creating a social world: a developmental twin study of peer-group deviance. Arch Gen Psychiatry. 2007;64(8):958–65.
174. Kendler KS, Baker JH. Genetic influences on measures of the environment: a systematic review. Psychol Med. 2007;37(5):615–26.
175. Maher BS, Vladimirov VI, Latendresse SJ, Thiselton DL, McNamee R, Kang M, et al. The AVPR1A gene and substance use disorders: association, replication, and functional evidence. Biol Psychiatry. 2011;70(6):519–27.

8 Epigenomic Studies of Substance Use

Elad Lax, Moshe Szyf, and Gal Yadid

Introduction

Drug addiction or drug abuse is defined by compulsive-like drug intake despite negative outcomes for the individual [1]. Biologically, drug addiction is a neurobehavioral disorder characterized by a long-term alterations in synaptic plasticity [2, 3], neuronal plasticity [4, 5], and neuronal ensembles activity [6, 7], in reward-related and decision-making brain regions such as the ventral tegmental area (VTA), nucleus accumbens (NAc), and prefrontal cortex (PFC), following repeated exposure to drugs of abuse [8–11]. These neuronal plasticity alterations require de novo protein synthesis [12, 13] and therefore reprogramming of gene-expression patterns [14–18].

Gene expression is regulated through several epigenetic mechanisms including histone modifications, DNA methylation, hydroxy methylation, and further oxidations and long and short non-coding RNA (lncRNA and miRNA, respectively). Each of these mechanisms can be altered as a response to both internal signaling and external stimuli such as drug exposure. Most of the studies relating to epigenetic mechanisms of drug addiction were done on animal models [19–22]. We therefore review in this chapter mostly basic preclinical work as well as a smaller number of human studies.

Histone Modifications

Histones are positively charged proteins, which ensemble octameric structures known as nucleosomes. DNA is tightly wrapped around the nucleosomes, which keeps the DNA in a condensed form. Histones have N-terminal tails, which contain multiple potential positions for several types of posttranscriptional modifications such as acetylation, methylation, phosphorylation, and ubiquitination [23, 24]. These modifications alter nucleosome structure and interaction with the DNA. Histone-DNA interactions have diverse functional consequences, mostly switching genomic regions between a dense chromatin state (heterochromatin), which represses gene expression to a relaxed chromatin state (euchromatin), a permissive state enabling increased gene expression.

E. Lax (✉)
Department of Molecular Biology, Ariel University, Ariel, Israel
e-mail: eladl@ariel.ac.il

M. Szyf
Department of Pharmacology and Therapeutics, McGill University, Montreal, QC, Canada
e-mail: moshe.szyf@mcgill.ca

G. Yadid
Faculty of Life Sciences & The Gonda Brain Research Center, Bar-Ilan University, Ramat-Gan, Israel

M. M. Vanyukov (ed.), *Genetics of Substance Use*, https://doi.org/10.1007/978-3-030-95350-8_8

Histone Methylation

Histone methylation occurs on lysine or arginine residues. A family of enzymes known as histone methyltransferases adds mono-, di-, or trimethyl groups on lysine and arginine residues located along the histone tails [25–27]. Histone methylation is associated with activation or repression of gene expression. The effects of histone methylation depend on the methylated residue in histone tails and the number of methyl groups bound to the residue (mono-, di-, or trimethylation) [24, 28–31]. Several permissive histone methylation marks, including H3K4me1, H3K4me2, H3K4me3, and H3K36me3 as well as repressive histone marks (H3K9me2, H3K9me3 [32–36]), were implicated in drug addiction. Methamphetamine conditioned place preference (CPP) training increased H3K4me2 and H3K4me3 protein levels in the nucleus accumbens and increased H3K4me3 binding to the promoter of oxytocin receptor [32]. On the other hand, methamphetamine self-administration did not increase H3K4me3 binding to promoters of several genes implicated in drug addiction [34, 35]. This discrepancy can be explained by using animal models of contingent vs. noncontingent drug infusions (self-administration vs. CPP, respectively) and different species (mice and rats). A comprehensive analysis of several histone methylation marks and gene expression following repeated cocaine injections found altered peak enrichment for these marks. Furthermore, repressive histone mark (H3K9me2, H3K9me3, H3K27me3) peaks were correlated to downregulated genes, and permissive histone mark (H3K4me1, H3K4me3, H3K36me3) peaks were correlated to upregulated genes [33]. Other studies on repeated cocaine exposure found a global decrease of H3K9me2 due to repression of the lysine dimethyltransferase G9a, which specifically dimethylates H39K residues [36]. H3K9me3 showed a different pattern of changes following cocaine exposure, while acute cocaine administration leads to short-term increase in H3K9me3 levels. Repeated cocaine exposure resulted in a short-term increase and a long-term decrease in global H3K9me3 levels [37]. Similarly, H3K9me2 levels were decreased following chronic morphine administration [38]. Upregulation of H3K4me2 levels at FosB promoter in the striatum of chronically stressed rats promoted morphine-CPP [39], while the knockdown of dimethyltransferase G9a in the nucleus accumbens shell reduced cocaine self-administration [40].

Histone deacetylases (HDACs) are enzymes that remove acetyl groups from histone, and histone methyltransferases (HMTs) are enzymes that add methyl groups onto histones. Together, these two groups of enzymes promote histone condensation through reduced acetylation and increased methylation. Indeed, several studies successfully manipulated the levels of these enzymes providing evidence for the causal effects of histone methylation in drug addiction and suggesting future tools for intervention. Aguilar-Valles et al. [32] showed that NAc-specific knockdown of the histone lysine (K)-specific demethylase KDM5c reduced methamphetamine CPP through an increase in H3K4me3. Inhibition of histone methyltransferase G9a increased cocaine- and morphine-CPP, while overexpression of G9a opposed these effects [36, 38]. Overexpression of G9a in the NAc shell also increased cocaine self-administration and reinstatement [41]. Histone arginine methylation is less studied in the context of drug addiction. However, at least one paper [42] showed decreased histone arginine methylation in the nucleus accumbens following repeated cocaine injections in mice and in cocaine-addicted humans. This was due to the reduced levels of protein-R (arginine)-methyltransferase-6 (PRMT6) in medium spiny neurons expressing dopamine D2 receptors.

Histone Acetylation

Histone acetylation is a histone mark on lysine residues generally associated with euchromatin, which is a more relaxed and open form of DNA compared to heterochromatin. Acetylated histones are read by acetylated lysine "readers" from the BET protein family [43], mostly BRD4 in the brain, which promotes neuronal gene expression, neuronal plasticity, and memory, including cocaine-induced memory [44, 45]. The open DNA regions enable the binding of various transcription factors, the RNA polymerase II machinery, and increased gene expression [24, 30, 31]. Different classes of drugs of abuse were shown to alter histone acetylation, mostly in reward-related brain regions. Repeated exposure to drugs increased histone acetylation and gene expression. Many of these genes have functions related to neuronal activity and synaptic plasticity. These findings were observed for psychostimulants such as cocaine [46] and methamphetamine [47], for nicotine [48, 49], and also for opioids such as morphine [50–52] and heroin [53]. Histone acetylation enrichment often occurs in tandem with histone methylation (H3K4me3), which is associated with active transcription of neighboring genes. One such finding is an enrichment for both H3K27ac and H3K4me3 as well as the transcription factor Nr4a1 on the promoter of *CARTPT* (encoding cocaine- and amphetamine-regulated transcript protein) following repeated cocaine administration [54]. Other studies found that "gateway" substances such as nicotine [48, 55] and alcohol [56] promote histone 3 and histone 4 acetylation and reduce HDAC expression to ultimately prime and potentiate cocaine-seeking behaviors. Additionally, chronic cocaine reduced the binding of the histone deacetylate Sirt1 to gene-coding regions in the nucleus accumbens and increased H4K16 acetylation of downstream deacetylation targets of Sirt1 [57]. Cocaine self-administration also has cross-generational effects: male rats trained to self-administer cocaine showed elevated histone 3 acetylation, and their male offspring showed reduced cocaine intake [58]. Male offspring also showed impaired spatial memory, synaptic plasticity deficits, and enrichment of histone acetylation and permissive histone methylation marks [59]. Also, early exposure to synthetic cannabinoids in adulthood leads to cross-sensitization to cocaine, which includes hyper-acetylation of histones and reduced levels of HDAC6 in rats [60]. However, other studies demonstrated reduced levels of histone acetylation and increased levels of histone deacetylase enzymes that remove acetyl groups from the chromatin upon drug administration. Martin et al. [61] described reduced histone 3 acetylation at the promoter of the actin-binding protein drebrin (encoded by *Dbn1*) along with an increase of HDAC2 following heroin or morphine administration. Li et al. [62] found that HDAC5 levels bidirectionally regulate methamphetamine-seeking behaviors after long-term forced abstinence (known as "incubation of craving"). Overexpression of HDAC5 in the dorsal striatum increased methamphetamine seeking, while HDAC5 downregulation decreased it. Repeated systemic injections of sodium butyrate, an HDAC class I inhibitor, during cocaine-conditioned place preference (CPP) extinction training facilitated extinction and attenuated drug-induced CPP reinstatement [63]. Also, the selective HDAC3 inhibitor RGFP966 enhanced the extinction of cocaine-seeking behaviors [64]. Altogether, these findings suggest that deacetylation promotes persistence of drug-related memories.

Additional Histone Modifications

Other histone modifications and histone variations besides histone methylation and histone acetylation have been studied in less detail. It has been shown, nevertheless, that chromatin poly-ADP ribosylation by PARP1 in the central amygdala is necessary for the retrieval of cocaine-related memories, and PARP inhibition was sufficient to block cocaine CPP and to facilitate cocaine-seeking extinction in a self-administration model [65]. Similarly, others have found increased poly-ADP ribosylation following cocaine exposure [66, 67]. Overexpression of PARG (poly(ADP-ribose) glycohydrolase), which catabolyze poly-ADP ribose chains in the nucleus accumbens, reduced cocaine-seeking [66]. In line with these observations, chronic systemic treatment with nicotinamide, an endogenous inhibitor of PARP1 activation [68], attenuated cue-induced cocaine-seeking in male rats following self-administration in a dose-dependent manner [69].

The incorporation of histone variants into the chromatin can stably modify transcriptional programming. One postmortem study found increased mRNA levels of H3F3B (histone variant of histone 3) in the midbrain of cocaine abusers. H3F3B is a replication-independent histone variant and probably acts as an epigenetic imprint of active chromatin regions [70]. More recently, cocaine self-administration has been shown to lead to neuron-specific accumulation of the H3.3 histone variant in the nucleus accumbens; this variant is involved in neuronal plasticity [71] and depressive-like behaviors [72]. This accumulation was enriched with gene promoters and correlated with elevated expression of genes associated with neuronal plasticity. These findings suggest that H3.3 variant accumulation contributes to cocaine-induced transcriptional reprogramming in the nucleus accumbens [73].

DNA Methylation

DNA methylation, an addition of a methyl group onto cytosine bases of the DNA, is a major epigenetic modification. DNA methylation happens in mammals mostly on cytosine residues that reside next to guanine (a CpG dinucleotide) [74, 75], although non-CpG methylation (often known as CpH dinucleotide) also occurs, especially in non-dividing cells such as neurons [76]. DNA methylation regulates gene expression through several mechanisms. First, it inhibits transcription factor binding [77]. Furthermore, methyl marks on the DNA attract a family of proteins known to preferentially bind methylated DNA. This family includes the methyl-CpG-binding protein 2 (Mecp2) and the methyl-CpG-binding domain (MBD) family (MBD1–4). These proteins, in turn, recruit transcriptional regulatory complexes to regulate gene expression. DNA methylation, through gene-expression regulation, maintains many neuronal functions and behavioral phenotypes such as learning and memory [78, 79], reward [80], and stress [81, 82].

Methyl groups can be added to or removed from the DNA, resulting in hypermethylation or hypomethylation, respectively. A group of three mammalian enzymes, called DNA methyltransferases (DNMTs), which includes DNMT1, DNMT3a, and DNMT3b, can attach methyl groups onto cytosine in DNA [31, 83], using S-adenosylmethionine (SAM) as a methyl donor. Another group of enzymes, called Tet methylcytosine dioxygenases (TETs), which include TET1, TET2, and TET3, catalyzes oxidation of methylated cytosines, making the DNA hydroxy-methylated [84, 85]. Next, further oxidation by TET enzymes might result in demethylation [86–88]. Of note, hydroxy-methylated DNA, as well as further oxidation of the methyl residue, are thought to be involved in epigenetic regulation of gene expression [86], especially in the central nervous system [89–92].

Accumulating evidence linked DNA methylation alterations in several brain regions, such as the nucleus accumbens and prefrontal cortex, to drug intake and drug-seeking behaviors [93]. Several classes of drugs, including cocaine [94–101], amphetamine, and methamphetamine [34, 102–104], nicotine [105–108], alcohol [109–113], and opiates such as morphine [114], heroin [115, 116], and oxycodone [117, 118], were associated with DNA methylation alterations in relevant brain regions as well as peripheral white blood cells.

Several studies found global and site-specific reduction in methylation levels within the nucleus accumbens and prefrontal cortex of rats and mice following repeated cocaine administration. For example, in mice, Tian et al. found demethylation of a c-MYB binding site upstream of Bdnf IV in the nucleus accumbens in cocaine-conditioned place preference [95]. Others have found that DNA methylation changes in the nucleus accumbens following chronic cocaine are regulated mostly through Dnmt3a [97], and later findings suggested that Dnmt3a2 isoform specifically plays a major role in cue-induced cocaine-seeking after reinstatement [119], [120]. In line with these results, restoration of DNA methylation levels through systemic supplementation of methionine, a precursor of the methyl donor S-adenosylmethionine (SAM), or directly treating with SAM, reversed several cocaine-seeking behaviors, including CPP [99] and drug-primed reinstatement to cocaine self-administration [94]. The promoters of *Pp1c* and

Fosb, two genes known to participate in cocaine-induced neuroadaptations [121, 122], were tested for alterations in DNA methylation. Pp1c was hypermethylated and FosB was hypomethylated after acute and repeated cocaine injections [96]. Supplementation of SAM increased cocaine-induced locomotor sensitization and normalized both hypo- and hypermethylation in the nucleus accumbens [123].

The "incubation of craving" model recapitulates the period of abstinence after first exposure to a drug and thus reflects a common situation in humans where an initial exposure is followed by a period without drug before a second exposure or a period of detoxification that is commonly used in treatment, followed by re-exposure. The animal model reveals that the extent of craving is amplified rather than reduced following the incubation period [124, 125]. This finding is in line with reports in human addicts [126]. This raises the question of whether this effect is mediated by epigenetic reprogramming of gene expression. Massart et al. [98] used the incubation-of-craving model in rats trained to self-administer cocaine. This study has delineated large genome expression changes in the nucleus accumbens not only following direct exposure but also following a long period of cocaine incubation. Importantly, numerous changes in DNA methylation, including genes known to be involved in addiction, were discovered, consistent with a mechanism involving DNA methylation.

While associations do not prove causation, epigenetic manipulations test the feasibility of an epigenetic mechanism as well as point to the possibility of using epigenetic therapy to "cure" addiction, particularly where long periods of abstinence might have aggravated the craving as in the animal model. Importantly, in contrast to traditional pharmacotherapy targeting receptors by agonists and antagonists, which requires continuous administration of the drug to maintain the effect, the reversal of epigenetic reprogramming that was induced by a complex set of behaviors erases the defective epigenetic program encoded in DNA methylation underpinning the behavior, and the effect should be persistent. Thus, it is expected that epigenetic remodulation should bring about a "cure" rather than symptomatic relief. A single intra-NAc SAM infusion was sufficient to increase cocaine-seeking in the incubation-of-craving model, while inhibition of Dnmt enzymes with a specific inhibitor RG108 decreased cocaine-seeking in this model [98]. Importantly, the effect remained stable for additional 30 days even after a single administration of either RG108 or SAM. Two proteins demethylated by RG108, the estrogen receptor 1 (ESR1), which was activated by RG108, and cyclin-dependent kinase 5 (CDK5), which was inhibited by RG108 (demethylation was in the gene that is associated with silencing), were targeted to test whether DNA methylation mediates addiction through changes in the expression of critical genes. Treatment with an intra-NAc injection of the ESR1 agonist propylpyrazoletriol (10 nm) or the CDK5 inhibitor roscovitine (28 μM) on day 30 of withdrawal significantly decreased cue-induced cocaine-seeking [98].

Altogether, the findings suggest that DNA methylation is involved in the different effects of cocaine on downstream behaviors, and these effects might entail different behavioral consequences, consistent with the hypothesis that DNA methylation is a mediator of these effects. Notably, DNA methylation modulators used in those different models provide evidence for a causal role. Therefore, these data point towards a new avenue for therapeutic interventions that may result in a persistent reduction in craving by removing the underlying epigenomic cause of the behavioral change.

Animal studies offer an insight into fundamental brain mechanisms, dissecting different modalities of their behavioral consequences, such as the differences between immediate exposure and long-term abstinence. The great advantage of animal models is by offering us the possibility of examining the relevant brain regions, since DNA methylation is important in setting up cell-type-specific DNA methylation profiles. In living humans, we are limited to peripheral tissues, which are not expected to reflect accurately the exquisite cell-type-specific DNA methylation dynamics taking place in the brain. However, any future utility of DNA methylation in predicting, diagnosing, or treating addiction will necessitate peripheral markers. Surprisingly, in contrast to the common wisdom that it is futile to search for behaviorally relevant DNA methylation markers in the blood, several studies have associated behavioral and neuropsychiatric conditions with peripheral DNA methylation markers. Changes were reported in brain-relevant genes such as *BDNF* [127], oxytocin receptor [128], and serotonin transporter *SLC6A4* [129], in stress-related genes such as *FKBP5* and the glucocorticoid receptor *NR3C1* [130, 131], as well as in genes relevant to inflammation and immune function [132, 133]. A few studies have examined genome-wide DNA methylation association with drug addiction. A study that profiled methylation levels in the peripheral blood of individuals with the ICD-10 diagnosis of cocaine dependence found mostly hypomethylated CpG sites as compared to healthy controls [134]. A gene network analyses found an enrichment for genes related to transcription and chromatin regulation and to cellular signaling pathway (61 hypermethylated CpGs vs. 125 hypomethylated CpGs). A similar trend of mostly hypomethylated CpGs was also found for a cohort of multi drug abusers [135].

DNA Methylation and Exposure to Other Stimulants

DNA methylation alterations are not limited to cocaine exposures. Repeated administration of other stimulants such as amphetamine and methamphetamine resulted in altered DNA methylation as well. A global hypermethylation was observed in the medial prefrontal cortex of mice repeatedly injected with methamphetamine, while no effect was observed for modafinil [103]. In another study in mice, chronic methamphetamine led to decreased expression of several immediate early genes (*Arc*, *Egr2*, *Fos*, *Klf10*, and *Nr4a1*) in both the prefrontal cortex and hippocampus. Altered DNA methylation in several CpGs annotated to *Fos* and *Arc* genes was found in the prefrontal cortex, and several CpGs were differentially methylated at the genes *Klf10* and *Nr4a1* in the hippocampus [104]. A genome-wide study found differentially hydroxymethylated regions in genes encoding both calcium- and voltage-dependent potassium channels in the rat nucleus accumbens [136]. Also, several targeted analyses for specific genes have been conducted. For example, an analysis of gene promoter methylation of AMPA (α-amino-3-hydroxy-5-methyl-4-isoxazolepropionic acid) receptor subunits in the striatum following chronic methamphetamine found reduced methylation and hydroxymethylation of *GluA1* (glutamate receptor 1) and *GluA2* (glutamate receptor 2) [137]. Additionally, acute methamphetamine produced a long-term accumbal hypomethylation at sites near the *Crh* gene (encoding for corticotropin-releasing hormone) and in the gene body of *Avp* (encoding for arginine vasopressin) coupled with increased hydroxymethylation at the *Crh* gene transcription start site and the *Avp* gene body. Both the *Crh* and *Avp* peptides are known to participate in stress response and acute reaction to psychostimulants in several brain regions, including the nucleus accumbens. These effects were mediated through the 5-methylcytosine oxygenases *Tet1* and *Tet3* (but not *Tet2*) [138]. Parental methamphetamine during pregnancy in mice showed enhanced response to cocaine and hyperlocomotion in male offspring accompanied by altered DNA methylation in the hippocampus [102].

DNA methylation alterations are not limited to psychostimulant exposure. Nicotine was found to decrease the expression of Dnmt1 mRNA and protein, reduced DNA methylation levels of the *Gad67* promoter, and increased *Gad67* expression in GABAergic interneurons [106]. Also, since nicotine is widely used and is legal almost globally, several human studies linking DNA methylation and nicotine or tobacco exposure have been conducted. DNA methylation was found as a potential long-term biomarker for tobacco exposure [105, 139, 140]; however, others have found that changes in DNA methylation following nicotine use are partly reversible after smoking cessation, although levels were not completely restored to those of nonsmokers [141].

Additional studies examined the effects of in utero nicotine exposure to maternal smoking. Altered DNA methylation, reduced neuronal content, and impaired neuronal differentiation were found in the dorsolateral prefrontal cortex of fetuses [142]. The effects of in utero nicotine on DNA methylation are not restricted to brain development as lung and placental tissues also showed alterations in methylation landscape [143]; however, further research is required in order to find out if these observations are linked to heightened risk of addiction in the offspring.

Alcohol intake is also associated with DNA methylation differences both in the brain and in the peripheral tissues (blood, saliva). Rats chronically exposed to alcohol showed global increase in methylation levels both in the prefrontal cortex and the nucleus accumbens and increased neuronal DNMT1 protein. Intracerebroventricular infusion of the DNMT inhibitor RG108 reduced alcohol intake and prevented gene-expression changes induced by alcohol suggesting a causal role for DNMT1 and DNA methylation in programming gene-expression changes involved in alcohol intake [144]. A possible mechanism was illustrated in a rat animal model: alcohol intake was associated with a dynamic change in DNA methylation, which correlated with changes in expression at the promoter regions of *Gdnf* (glial cell-derived neurotrophic factor), a key gene influencing alcohol intake. In the nucleus accumbens, the core promoter of *Gdnf* was hypomethylated following alcohol intake, and mRNA levels were higher in the withdrawal group. In the ventral tegmental area, there was reduced methylation of negative regulatory element upstream of the *Gdnf* and reduced gene mRNA levels after withdrawal [113]. These findings are in line with previous work demonstrating the protective effects of *Gdnf* against excessive alcohol intake [145].

In humans, an epigenome-wide study in the blood found a set of 144 differentially methylated CpGs, which together could serve a biomarker of heavy alcohol consumption [110]. Another large-scale study, which included several replications, found that differentially methylated regions in glucocorticoid signaling and inflammation-related genes were associated with alcohol use behaviors, with the top hit at the long non-coding RNA *Gas5* that is implicated in the regulation of glucocorticoid receptor mRNA levels [146]. Another study found an association between methylation of the protein phosphatase gene (*PPM1G)* and alcohol use and brain activity [109]. DNA methylation of the *LEP* gene (encoding for leptin) was associated with alcohol craving during withdrawal [111]. This finding is in line with previous evidence linking leptin serum levels and alcohol intake [147]. A recent meta-analysis found very little evidence for individual CpGs or differentially methylated regions in offspring with history of maternal alcohol drinking [148]. In contrast, a few studies did find DNA methylation in offspring associated with in utero nicotine exposure (reviewed by Mandal et al. [149]).

Few studies reported cross-generational effects of opiates and cannabis (or THC) use on DNA methylation. Watson et al. [150] found differentially methylated regions in nucleus accumbens from rats with parental THC exposure, which suggests cross-generational effects of cannabis on DNA methylation. Along these lines, Murphy et al. [151] found altered DNA methylation in the sperm of both rats and humans following THC, with enrichment for genes related to pathways in cancer. They also found that parental THC in rats affects the offspring behavior in an attentional performance task [152]; however, the mechanism that potentially links aberrant sperm DNA methylation to impaired attention is yet to be explored. Based on the knowledge of genetic associations between the *DRD4* gene (encoding the dopamine D4 receptor) and several neuropsychiatric disorders including addiction [153, 154], another study on women using cannabis during pregnancy did not find significant changes in methylation levels at the *DRD4* gene in the offsprings [155].

Barrow et al. analyzed the effects of acute and chronic morphine administration on the methylation of a few candidate genes in ten rat brain regions and found highly localized effects [114]. Another group found that oxytocin can reverse the effects of oxycodone CPP [117] and that the effect of oxytocin was at least partially mediated by global hypomethylation, hypomethylation of the *Syn* and *PSD95* genes (encoding synaptophysin and postsynaptic density protein 95, respectively), downregulation of *Dnmt1,* and upregulation of *Tet1–3* [118].

A recent study found that in the dorsal hippocampus of rats trained to self-administer heroin, *Dnmt3a* was degraded through E2 ubiquitin-conjugating enzyme Ube2b-mediated ubiquitination, leading to hypomethylation and increased expression of *CaMKK1* (calcium–/calmodulin-dependent protein kinase kinase 1) gene promoter, and this, in turn, affected actin polymerization and heroin-induced behavior [156]. In humans, an epigenome-wide study on postmortem orbitofrontal cortex (OFC) of heroin users, suicide completers, and controls found hundreds of CpGs differentially methylated between heroin users and controls. Hypermethylated CpGs were enriched for genes specific to glutamatergic neurons, axonogenesis, and synapses, while hypomethylated CpGs were enriched for genes encoding transcription factors and gene-expression regulatory mechanisms [115].

The DNA methylation reader Mecp2 binds to methylated CpG and CpH and controls chromatin state and gene expression [157–159]. Mecp2 is highly expressed in neurons and is essential to neuronal functions [160, 161], and Mecp2 mutations are the main cause of the Rett syndrome [162]. Activity-dependent Mecp2 phosphorylation modulates its activity and downstream neuronal development and function [160, 163–165]. Therefore, the involvement of MeCP2 in the effects of drugs of abuse on neuronal activity and drug-seeking behaviors is very plausible. Indeed, previous studies found that Mecp2 in the nucleus accumbens acts to limit the rewarding effect and neuronal plasticity induced by psychostimulants like cocaine and amphetamine. Nucleus accumbens-targeted viral overexpression and downregulation of Mecp2, as well as genetic manipulations of Mecp2, bidirectionally affect cocaine- and amphetamine-seeking behaviors and neuronal plasticity in mice, providing strong evidence for a critical role of Mecp2 in psychostimulant-seeking behaviors [166, 167]. Another study found a negative correlation between cocaine intake and Mecp2 immunoreactivity levels in the nucleus accumbens, consistent with an inhibitory role in cocaine-seeking [168]. Mecp2 expression was increased in the dorsal striatum and decreased in the prefrontal cortex following long access to cocaine [169]. Also, investigator-administered cocaine increases MeCP2 (and also MBD1) expression in several brain regions while reducing histone 3 acetylation [170]. These studies might suggest that MeCp2 plays an adaptive role to cocaine-seeking as a negative feedback regulator of cocaine intake. The effects of Mecp2 on cocaine are brain-region and drug-intake-course dependent [171].

Conclusions and Future Directions

Research findings, mostly from recent years, provided us with ample evidences clearly pointing towards a major contribution of epigenetics to drug addiction and abuse. These lines of evidence are based mostly on animal model studies but also on some human studies and encompass different drug classes. The findings suggest that both histone modifications and DNA methylation play a role in drug addiction through long-term regulation of gene-expression programs and ultimately neuronal plasticity and brain function, playing a causal and important role in precipitating drug addiction. An individual in a drug-free state is still far from being considered a fully rehabilitated one [172–174]. Therefore, advanced management is needed to attenuate the major problem of treatment: the high rates of relapse to drug use after periods of forced or self-imposed abstinence. The inability to break the cycle of drug use that leads to drug-seeking behavior after withdrawal presents a major challenge to mental health and social services.

To address this challenge, we must tackle the critical questions of how to predict which potential treatment will benefit the individual addict and how to identify subjects who are at a higher risk of relapse. Solutions to these issues would provide important opportunities for generating and delivering therapeutic interventions that could have a profound impact on society.

One approach to matching treatment involves developing specific and accurate biological biomarkers that can be correlated to social/cognitive characteristics. Since epigenetic alterations, unlike genetic ones, are dynamic and strongly depend on the environment and social habits, it is intriguing to think that rehabilitation of an addict in a therapeutic center having an enriched environment will urge rehabilitation. Hence, therapeutic centers that do not use a relapse therapy but suggest strong social programs [175] may lead to a reprogrammed DNA methylation that will result in changes that lead to cure.

Also, if indeed DNA methylation plays a causal role in addiction, pharmacological DNA modulators might be used to reverse epigenetic programming and the addictive state. Epigenetic therapy that reverses drug-triggered epigenetic reprogramming could potentially result in a cure rather than relief in symptoms. An animal study suggests that a single administration of a DNA methylation inhibitor resulted in a lasting change in drug craving [98].

However, there are still gaps and apparent disagreements between animal studies. It is highly likely that the epigenetic effects observed following a drug regimen are drug-, time-, and brain-region-specific, as well as characteristic of the particular animal model used in preclinical studies. Side-by-side comprehensive analyses of several epigenetic modifications across several key brain regions within the same animal study could reconcile earlier observations.

Human studies are mostly underpowered and limited to peripheral white blood cells; thus, the understanding of DNA methylation's association with addiction in the human brain is very limited. There is a need for more large-scale epigenome-wide human studies for both peripheral epigenetic effects (also as potential biomarkers) and postmortem brain studies. Such studies would potentially identify predictive and diagnostic markers of drug addiction that could inspire early intervention. Human and animal studies with epigenetic modulators could move the field to the development of potential new therapeutics for drug addiction.

References

1. American Psychiatric Association. Diagnostic and statistical manual of mental disorders (5th ed.). Arlington, VA: Author; 2013.
2. Kauer JA, Malenka RC. Synaptic plasticity and addiction. Nat Rev Neurosci. 2007;8(11):844–58.
3. Wolf ME. Synaptic mechanisms underlying persistent cocaine craving. Nat Rev Neurosci. 2016;17(6):351–65.
4. Kourrich S, Calu DJ, Bonci A. Intrinsic plasticity: an emerging player in addiction. Nat Rev Neurosci. 2015;16(3):173–84.
5. Hyman SE, Malenka RC, Nestler EJ. Neural mechanisms of addiction: the role of reward-related learning and memory. Annu Rev Neurosci. 2006;29:565–98.
6. Cruz FC, Koya E, Guez-Barber DH, Bossert JM, Lupica CR, Shaham Y, et al. New technologies for examining the role of neuronal ensembles in drug addiction and fear. Nat Rev Neurosci. 2013;14(11):743–54.
7. Bobadilla AC, Heinsbroek JA, Gipson CD, Griffin WC, Fowler CD, Kenny PJ, et al. Corticostriatal plasticity, neuronal ensembles, and regulation of drug-seeking behavior. Prog Brain Res. 2017;235:93–112.
8. Kalivas PW, Volkow ND. The neural basis of addiction: a pathology of motivation and choice. Am J Psychiatry. 2005;162(8):1403–13.
9. Luscher C. The emergence of a circuit model for addiction. Annu Rev Neurosci. 2016;39:257–76.
10. Nestler EJ. Molecular basis of long-term plasticity underlying addiction. Nat Rev Neurosci. 2001;2(2):119–28.
11. Ostroumov A, Dani JA. Inhibitory plasticity of Mesocorticolimbic circuits in addiction and mental illness. Trends Neurosci. 2018;41(12):898–910.
12. Dunbar AB, Taylor JR. Inhibition of protein synthesis but not beta-adrenergic receptors blocks reconsolidation of a cocaine-associated cue memory. Learn Mem. 2016;23(8):391–8.
13. Younts TJ, Monday HR, Dudok B, Klein ME, Jordan BA, Katona I, et al. Presynaptic protein synthesis is required for long-term plasticity of GABA release. Neuron. 2016;92(2):479–92.
14. West AE, Greenberg ME. Neuronal activity-regulated gene transcription in synapse development and cognitive function. Cold Spring Harb Perspect Biol. 2011;3(6):a005744.
15. Schiltz CA, Kelley AE, Landry CF. Acute stress and nicotine cues interact to unveil locomotor arousal and activity-dependent gene expression in the prefrontal cortex. Biol Psychiatry. 2007;61(1):127–35.
16. Chen LF, Zhou AS, West AE. Transcribing the connectome: roles for transcription factors and chromatin regulators in activity-dependent synapse development. J Neurophysiol. 2017;118(2):755–70.
17. Friedman A, Frankel M, Flaumenhaft Y, Merenlender A, Pinhasov A, Feder Y, et al.

Programmed acute electrical stimulation of ventral tegmental area alleviates depressive-like behavior. Neuropsychopharmacology. 2009; 34(4):1057–66.
18. Bruchim-Samuel M, Lax E, Gazit T, Friedman A, Ahdoot H, Bairachnaya M, et al. Electrical stimulation of the vmPFC serves as a remote control to affect VTA activity and improve depressive-like behavior. Exp Neurol. 2016;283(Pt A):255–63.
19. Walker DM, Nestler EJ. Neuroepigenetics and addiction. Handb Clin Neurol. 2018;148:747–65.
20. Robison AJ, Nestler EJ. Transcriptional and epigenetic mechanisms of addiction. Nat Rev Neurosci. 2011;12(11):623–37.
21. Campbell RR, Wood MA. How the epigenome integrates information and reshapes the synapse. Nat Rev Neurosci. 2019;20(3):133–47.
22. Anderson EM, Penrod RD, Barry SM, Hughes BW, Taniguchi M, Cowan CW. It is a complex issue: emerging connections between epigenetic regulators in drug addiction. Eur J Neurosci. 2019;50(3):2477–91.
23. Rothbart SB, Strahl BD. Interpreting the language of histone and DNA modifications. Biochim Biophys Acta. 2014;1839(8):627–43.
24. Jenuwein T, Allis CD. Translating the histone code. Science. 2001;293(5532):1074–80.
25. Jambhekar A, Dhall A, Shi Y. Roles and regulation of histone methylation in animal development. Nat Rev Mol Cell Biol. 2019;20(10):625–41.
26. Husmann D, Gozani O. Histone lysine methyltransferases in biology and disease. Nat Struct Mol Biol. 2019;26(10):880–9.
27. Fulton MD, Brown T, Zheng YG. Mechanisms and inhibitors of histone arginine methylation. Chem Rec. 2018;18(12):1792–807.
28. Hyun K, Jeon J, Park K, Kim J. Writing, erasing and reading histone lysine methylations. Exp Mol Med. 2017;49(4):e324.
29. Cholewa-Waclaw J, Bird A, von Schimmelmann M, Schaefer A, Yu H, Song H, et al. The role of epigenetic mechanisms in the regulation of gene expression in the nervous system. J Neurosci. 2016;36(45):11427–34.
30. Rice JC, Allis CD. Histone methylation versus histone acetylation: new insights into epigenetic regulation. Curr Opin Cell Biol. 2001;13(3):263–73.
31. Jaenisch R, Bird A. Epigenetic regulation of gene expression: how the genome integrates intrinsic and environmental signals. Nat Genet. 2003;33(Suppl):245–54.
32. Aguilar-Valles A, Vaissiere T, Griggs EM, Mikaelsson MA, Takacs IF, Young EJ, et al. Methamphetamine-associated memory is regulated by a writer and an eraser of permissive histone methylation. Biol Psychiatry. 2014;76(1):57–65.
33. Feng J, Wilkinson M, Liu X, Purushothaman I, Ferguson D, Vialou V, et al. Chronic cocaine-regulated epigenomic changes in mouse nucleus accumbens. Genome Biol. 2014;15(4):R65.
34. Godino A, Jayanthi S, Cadet JL. Epigenetic landscape of amphetamine and methamphetamine addiction in rodents. Epigenetics. 2015;10(7):574–80.
35. Krasnova IN, Chiflikyan M, Justinova Z, McCoy MT, Ladenheim B, Jayanthi S, et al. CREB phosphorylation regulates striatal transcriptional responses in the self-administration model of methamphetamine addiction in the rat. Neurobiol Dis. 2013;58:132–43.
36. Maze I, Covington HE 3rd, Dietz DM, LaPlant Q, Renthal W, Russo SJ, et al. Essential role of the histone methyltransferase G9a in cocaine-induced plasticity. Science. 2010;327(5962):213–6.
37. Maze I, Feng J, Wilkinson MB, Sun H, Shen L, Nestler EJ. Cocaine dynamically regulates heterochromatin and repetitive element unsilencing in nucleus accumbens. Proc Natl Acad Sci U S A. 2011;108(7):3035–40.
38. Sun H, Maze I, Dietz DM, Scobie KN, Kennedy PJ, Damez-Werno D, et al. Morphine epigenomically regulates behavior through alterations in histone H3 lysine 9 dimethylation in the nucleus accumbens. J Neurosci. 2012;32(48):17454–64.
39. Chen M, Zhang X, Hao W. H3K4 dimethylation at FosB promoter in the striatum of chronic stressed rats promotes morphine-induced conditioned place preference. PLoS One. 2019;14(8):e0221506.
40. Anderson EM, Sun H, Guzman D, Taniguchi M, Cowan CW, Maze I, et al. Knockdown of the histone di-methyltransferase G9a in nucleus accumbens shell decreases cocaine self-administration, stress-induced reinstatement, and anxiety. Neuropsychopharmacology. 2019;44(8):1370–6.
41. Anderson EM, Larson EB, Guzman D, Wissman AM, Neve RL, Nestler EJ, et al. Overexpression of the histone Dimethyltransferase G9a in nucleus Accumbens Shell increases cocaine self-administration, stress-induced reinstatement, and anxiety. J Neurosci. 2018;38(4):803–13.
42. Damez-Werno DM, Sun H, Scobie KN, Shao N, Rabkin J, Dias C, et al. Histone arginine methylation in cocaine action in the nucleus accumbens. Proc Natl Acad Sci U S A. 2016;113(34):9623–8.
43. Marmorstein R, Zhou MM. Writers and readers of histone acetylation: structure, mechanism, and inhibition. Cold Spring Harb Perspect Biol. 2014;6(7):a018762.
44. Sartor GC, Powell SK, Brothers SP, Wahlestedt C. Epigenetic readers of lysine acetylation regulate cocaine-induced plasticity. J Neurosci. 2015;35(45):15062–72.
45. Korb E, Herre M, Zucker-Scharff I, Darnell RB, Allis CD. BET protein Brd4 activates transcription in neurons and BET inhibitor Jq1 blocks memory in mice. Nat Neurosci. 2015;18(10):1464–73.
46. Rogge GA, Wood MA. The role of histone acetylation in cocaine-induced neural plasticity and behavior. Neuropsychopharmacology. 2013;38(1):94–110.

47. Harkness JH, Hitzemann RJ, Edmunds S, Phillips TJ. Effects of sodium butyrate on methamphetamine-sensitized locomotor activity. Behav Brain Res. 2013;239:139–47.
48. Levine A, Huang Y, Drisaldi B, Griffin EA, Jr., Pollak DD, Xu S, et al. Molecular mechanism for a gateway drug: epigenetic changes initiated by nicotine prime gene expression by cocaine. Sci Transl Med. 2011;3(107):107ra9.
49. Gozen O, Balkan B, Yildirim E, Koylu EO, Pogun S. The epigenetic effect of nicotine on dopamine D1 receptor expression in rat prefrontal cortex. Synapse. 2013;67(9):545–52.
50. Wei L, Zhu YM, Zhang YX, Liang F, Barry DM, Gao HY, et al. Microinjection of histone deacetylase inhibitor into the ventrolateral orbital cortex potentiates morphine induced behavioral sensitization. Brain Res. 1646;2016:418–25.
51. Wang Y, Lai J, Cui H, Zhu Y, Zhao B, Wang W, et al. Inhibition of histone deacetylase in the basolateral amygdala facilitates morphine context-associated memory formation in rats. J Mol Neurosci. 2015;55(1):269–78.
52. Mashayekhi FJ, Rasti M, Rahvar M, Mokarram P, Namavar MR, Owji AA. Expression levels of the BDNF gene and histone modifications around its promoters in the ventral tegmental area and locus ceruleus of rats during forced abstinence from morphine. Neurochem Res. 2012;37(7):1517–23.
53. Chen WS, Xu WJ, Zhu HQ, Gao L, Lai MJ, Zhang FQ, et al. Effects of histone deacetylase inhibitor sodium butyrate on heroin seeking behavior in the nucleus accumbens in rats. Brain Res. 1652;2016:151–7.
54. Carpenter MD, Hu Q, Bond AM, Lombroso SI, Czarnecki KS, Lim CJ, et al. Nr4a1 suppresses cocaine-induced behavior via epigenetic regulation of homeostatic target genes. Nat Commun. 2020;11(1):504.
55. Kandel ER, Kandel DB. Shattuck lecture. A molecular basis for nicotine as a gateway drug. N Engl J Med. 2014;371(10):932–43.
56. Griffin EA Jr, Melas PA, Zhou R, Li Y, Mercado P, Kempadoo KA, et al. Prior alcohol use enhances vulnerability to compulsive cocaine self-administration by promoting degradation of HDAC4 and HDAC5. Sci Adv. 2017;3(11):e1701682.
57. Ferguson D, Shao N, Heller E, Feng J, Neve R, Kim HD, et al. SIRT1-FOXO3a regulate cocaine actions in the nucleus accumbens. J Neurosci. 2015;35(7):3100–11.
58. Vassoler FM, White SL, Schmidt HD, Sadri-Vakili G, Pierce RC. Epigenetic inheritance of a cocaine-resistance phenotype. Nat Neurosci. 2013;16(1):42–7.
59. Wimmer ME, Briand LA, Fant B, Guercio LA, Arreola AC, Schmidt HD, et al. Paternal cocaine taking elicits epigenetic remodeling and memory deficits in male progeny. Mol Psychiatry. 2017;22(11):1641–50.
60. Scherma M, Qvist JS, Asok A, Huang SC, Masia P, Deidda M, et al. Cannabinoid exposure in rat adolescence reprograms the initial behavioral, molecular, and epigenetic response to cocaine. Proc Natl Acad Sci USA. 2020;117(18):9991–10002.
61. Martin JA, Werner CT, Mitra S, Zhong P, Wang ZJ, Gobira PH, et al. A novel role for the actin-binding protein drebrin in regulating opiate addiction. Nat Commun. 2019;10(1):4140.
62. Li X, Carreria MB, Witonsky KR, Zeric T, Lofaro OM, Bossert JM, et al. Role of dorsal striatum histone deacetylase 5 in incubation of methamphetamine craving. Biol Psychiatry. 2018;84(3):213–22.
63. Malvaez M, Sanchis-Segura C, Vo D, Lattal KM, Wood MA. Modulation of chromatin modification facilitates extinction of cocaine-induced conditioned place preference. Biol Psychiatry. 2010;67(1):36–43.
64. Malvaez M, McQuown SC, Rogge GA, Astarabadi M, Jacques V, Carreiro S, et al. HDAC3-selective inhibitor enhances extinction of cocaine-seeking behavior in a persistent manner. Proc Natl Acad Sci U S A. 2013;110(7):2647–52.
65. Lax E, Friedman A, Massart R, Barnea R, Abraham L, Cheishvili D, et al. PARP-1 is required for retrieval of cocaine-associated memory by binding to the promoter of a novel gene encoding a putative transposase inhibitor. Mol Psychiatry. 2017;22(4):570–9.
66. Scobie KN, Damez-Werno D, Sun H, Shao N, Gancarz A, Panganiban CH, et al. Essential role of poly(ADP-ribosyl)ation in cocaine action. Proc Natl Acad Sci U S A. 2014;111(5):2005–10.
67. Dash S, Balasubramaniam M, Rana T, Godino A, Peck EG, Goodwin JS, et al. Poly (ADP-Ribose) Polymerase-1 (PARP-1) induction by cocaine is post-transcriptionally regulated by miR-125b. eNeuro. 2017;4(4):ENEURO.0089-17.2017.
68. Suzuki E, Okuda H, Nishida K, Fujimoto S, Nagasawa K. Protective effect of nicotinamide against poly(ADP-ribose) polymerase-1-mediated astrocyte death depends on its transporter-mediated uptake. Life Sci. 2010;86(17–18):676–82.
69. Witt EA, Reissner KJ. The effects of nicotinamide on reinstatement to cocaine seeking in male and female Sprague Dawley rats. Psychopharmacology. 2020;237(3):669–80.
70. Bannon MJ, Savonen CL, Hartley ZJ, Johnson MM, Schmidt CJ. Investigating the potential influence of cause of death and cocaine levels on the differential expression of genes associated with cocaine abuse. PLoS One. 2015;10(2):e0117580.
71. Maze I, Wenderski W, Noh KM, Bagot RC, Tzavaras N, Purushothaman I, et al. Critical role of histone turnover in neuronal transcription and plasticity. Neuron. 2015;87(1):77–94.
72. Lepack AE, Bagot RC, Pena CJ, Loh YE, Farrelly LA, Lu Y, et al. Aberrant H3.3 dynamics in NAc promote vulnerability to depressive-like behavior. Proc Natl Acad Sci U S A. 2016;113(44):12562–7.
73. Wimmer ME, Fant B, Swinford-Jackson SE, Testino A, Van Nest D, Abel T, et al. H3.3 barcoding of

nucleus Accumbens transcriptional activity identifies novel molecular cascades associated with cocaine self-administration in mice. J Neurosci. 2019;39(27):5247–54.
74. Cedar H, Razin A. DNA methylation and development. Biochim Biophys Acta. 1990;1049(1):1–8.
75. Razin A, Cedar H. DNA methylation and genomic imprinting. Cell. 1994;77(4):473–6.
76. Guo JU, Su Y, Shin JH, Shin J, Li H, Xie B, et al. Distribution, recognition and regulation of non-CpG methylation in the adult mammalian brain. Nat Neurosci. 2014;17(2):215–22.
77. Moore LD, Le T, Fan G. DNA methylation and its basic function. Neuropsychopharmacology. 2013;38(1):23–38.
78. Halder R, Hennion M, Vidal RO, Shomroni O, Rahman RU, Rajput A, et al. DNA methylation changes in plasticity genes accompany the formation and maintenance of memory. Nat Neurosci. 2016;19(1):102–10.
79. Miller CA, Gavin CF, White JA, Parrish RR, Honasoge A, Yancey CR, et al. Cortical DNA methylation maintains remote memory. Nat Neurosci. 2010;13(6):664–6.
80. Day JJ, Childs D, Guzman-Karlsson MC, Kibe M, Moulden J, Song E, et al. DNA methylation regulates associative reward learning. Nat Neurosci. 2013;16(10):1445–52.
81. Labonte B, Suderman M, Maussion G, Navaro L, Yerko V, Mahar I, et al. Genome-wide epigenetic regulation by early-life trauma. Arch Gen Psychiatry. 2012;69(7):722–31.
82. Suderman M, McGowan PO, Sasaki A, Huang TC, Hallett MT, Meaney MJ, et al. Conserved epigenetic sensitivity to early life experience in the rat and human hippocampus. Proc Natl Acad Sci U S A. 2012;109(Suppl 2):17266–72.
83. Szyf M, Detich N. Regulation of the DNA methylation machinery and its role in cellular transformation. Prog Nucleic Acid Res Mol Biol. 2001;69:47–79.
84. Tahiliani M, Koh KP, Shen Y, Pastor WA, Bandukwala H, Brudno Y, et al. Conversion of 5-methylcytosine to 5-hydroxymethylcytosine in mammalian DNA by MLL partner TET1. Science. 2009;324(5929):930–5.
85. Ito S, Shen L, Dai Q, Wu SC, Collins LB, Swenberg JA, et al. Tet proteins can convert 5-methylcytosine to 5-formylcytosine and 5-carboxylcytosine. Science. 2011;333(6047):1300–3.
86. Szyf M. The elusive role of 5′-hydroxymethylcytosine. Epigenomics. 2016;8(11):1539–51.
87. Melamed P, Yosefzon Y, David C, Tsukerman A, Pnueli L. Tet enzymes, variants, and differential effects on function. Front Cell Dev Biol. 2018;6:22.
88. Kohli RM, Zhang Y. TET enzymes, TDG and the dynamics of DNA demethylation. Nature. 2013;502(7472):472–9.
89. Massart R, Suderman M, Provencal N, Yi C, Bennett AJ, Suomi S, et al. Hydroxymethylation and DNA methylation profiles in the prefrontal cortex of the non-human primate rhesus macaque and the impact of maternal deprivation on hydroxymethylation. Neuroscience. 2014;268:139–48.
90. Massart R, Freyburger M, Suderman M, Paquet J, El Helou J, Belanger-Nelson E, et al. The genome-wide landscape of DNA methylation and hydroxymethylation in response to sleep deprivation impacts on synaptic plasticity genes. Transl Psychiatry. 2014;4:e347.
91. Kriaucionis S, Heintz N. The nuclear DNA base 5-hydroxymethylcytosine is present in Purkinje neurons and the brain. Science. 2009;324(5929):929–30.
92. Kozlenkov A, Li J, Apontes P, Hurd YL, Byne WM, Koonin EV, et al. A unique role for DNA (hydroxy) methylation in epigenetic regulation of human inhibitory neurons. Sci Adv. 2018;4(9):eaau6190.
93. Lax E, Szyf M. The role of DNA methylation in drug addiction: implications for diagnostic and therapeutics. Prog Mol Biol Transl Sci. 2018;157:93–104.
94. Wright KN, Hollis F, Duclot F, Dossat AM, Strong CE, Francis TC, et al. Methyl supplementation attenuates cocaine-seeking behaviors and cocaine-induced c-Fos activation in a DNA methylation-dependent manner. J Neurosci. 2015;35(23):8948–58.
95. Tian W, Wang J, Zhang K, Teng H, Li C, Szyf M, et al. Demethylation of c-MYB binding site mediates upregulation of Bdnf IV in cocaine-conditioned place preference. Sci Rep. 2016;6:22087.
96. Anier K, Malinovskaja K, Aonurm-Helm A, Zharkovsky A, Kalda A. DNA methylation regulates cocaine-induced behavioral sensitization in mice. Neuropsychopharmacology. 2010;35(12):2450–61.
97. LaPlant Q, Vialou V, Covington HE 3rd, Dumitriu D, Feng J, Warren BL, et al. Dnmt3a regulates emotional behavior and spine plasticity in the nucleus accumbens. Nat Neurosci. 2010;13(9):1137–43.
98. Massart R, Barnea R, Dikshtein Y, Suderman M, Meir O, Hallett M, et al. Role of DNA methylation in the nucleus accumbens in incubation of cocaine craving. J Neurosci. 2015;35(21):8042–58.
99. Tian W, Zhao M, Li M, Song T, Zhang M, Quan L, et al. Reversal of cocaine-conditioned place preference through methyl supplementation in mice: altering global DNA methylation in the prefrontal cortex. PLoS One. 2012;7(3):e33435.
100. Fonteneau M, Filliol D, Anglard P, Befort K, Romieu P, Zwiller J. Inhibition of DNA methyltransferases regulates cocaine self-administration by rats: a genome-wide DNA methylation study. Genes Brain Behav. 2017;16(3):313–27.
101. Vaillancourt K, Ernst C, Mash D, Turecki G. DNA methylation dynamics and cocaine in the brain: progress and prospects. Genes (Basel). 2017;8(5).
102. Itzhak Y, Ergui I, Young JI. Long-term parental methamphetamine exposure of mice influences behavior and hippocampal DNA methylation of the offspring. Mol Psychiatry. 2015;20(2):232–9.
103. Gonzalez B, Jayanthi S, Gomez N, Torres OV, Sosa MH, Bernardi A, et al. Repeated methamphet-

amine and modafinil induce differential cognitive effects and specific histone acetylation and DNA methylation profiles in the mouse medial prefrontal cortex. Prog Neuro-Psychopharmacol Biol Psychiatry. 2018;82:1–11.
104. Cheng MC, Hsu SH, Chen CH. Chronic methamphetamine treatment reduces the expression of synaptic plasticity genes and changes their DNA methylation status in the mouse brain. Brain Res. 1629;2015:126–34.
105. Shenker NS, Ueland PM, Polidoro S, van Veldhoven K, Ricceri F, Brown R, et al. DNA methylation as a long-term biomarker of exposure to tobacco smoke. Epidemiology. 2013;24(5):712–6.
106. Satta R, Maloku E, Zhubi A, Pibiri F, Hajos M, Costa E, et al. Nicotine decreases DNA methyltransferase 1 expression and glutamic acid decarboxylase 67 promoter methylation in GABAergic interneurons. Proc Natl Acad Sci U S A. 2008;105(42):16356–61.
107. Hancock DB, Wang JC, Gaddis NC, Levy JL, Saccone NL, Stitzel JA, et al. A multiancestry study identifies novel genetic associations with CHRNA5 methylation in human brain and risk of nicotine dependence. Hum Mol Genet. 2015;24(20):5940–54.
108. Buck JM, Sanders KN, Wageman CR, Knopik VS, Stitzel JA, O'Neill HC. Developmental nicotine exposure precipitates multigenerational maternal transmission of nicotine preference and ADHD-like behavioral, rhythmometric, neuropharmacological, and epigenetic anomalies in adolescent mice. Neuropharmacology. 2019;149:66–82.
109. Ruggeri B, Nymberg C, Vuoksimaa E, Lourdusamy A, Wong CP, Carvalho FM, et al. Association of protein phosphatase PPM1G with alcohol use disorder and brain activity during behavioral control in a genome-wide methylation analysis. Am J Psychiatry. 2015;172(6):543–52.
110. Liu C, Marioni RE, Hedman AK, Pfeiffer L, Tsai PC, Reynolds LM, et al. A DNA methylation biomarker of alcohol consumption. Mol Psychiatry. 2018;23(2):422–33.
111. Hillemacher T, Weinland C, Lenz B, Kraus T, Heberlein A, Glahn A, et al. DNA methylation of the LEP gene is associated with craving during alcohol withdrawal. Psychoneuroendocrinology. 2015;51:371–7.
112. Philibert R, Dogan M, Noel A, Miller S, Krukow B, Papworth E, et al. Genome-wide and digital polymerase chain reaction epigenetic assessments of alcohol consumption. Am J Med Genet B Neuropsychiatr Genet. 2018;177(5):479–88.
113. Maier HB, Neyazi M, Neyazi A, Hillemacher T, Pathak H, Rhein M, et al. Alcohol consumption alters Gdnf promoter methylation and expression in rats. J Psychiatr Res. 2020;121:1–9.
114. Barrow TM, Byun HM, Li X, Smart C, Wang YX, Zhang Y, et al. The effect of morphine upon DNA methylation in ten regions of the rat brain. Epigenetics. 2017;12(12):1038–47.
115. Kozlenkov A, Jaffe AE, Timashpolsky A, Apontes P, Rudchenko S, Barbu M, et al. DNA methylation profiling of human prefrontal cortex neurons in heroin users shows significant difference between genomic contexts of hyper- and hypomethylation and a younger epigenetic age. Genes (Basel). 2017;8(6):152.
116. Fragou D, Zanos P, Kouidou S, Njau S, Kitchen I, Bailey A, et al. Effect of chronic heroin and cocaine administration on global DNA methylation in brain and liver. Toxicol Lett. 2013;218(3):260–5.
117. Fan XY, Shi G, Zhao P. Reversal of oxycodone conditioned place preference by oxytocin: promoting global DNA methylation in the hippocampus. Neuropharmacology. 2019;160:107778.
118. Fan XY, Shi G, Zhao P. Methylation in Syn and Psd95 genes underlie the inhibitory effect of oxytocin on oxycodone-induced conditioned place preference. Eur Neuropsychopharmacol. 2019;29(12):1464–75.
119. Cannella N, Oliveira AMM, Hemstedt T, Lissek T, Buechler E, Bading H, et al. Dnmt3a2 in the nucleus Accumbens shell is required for reinstatement of cocaine seeking. J Neurosci. 2018;38(34):7516–28.
120. Lax E, Sapozhnikov DM. Dnmt3a2 in the nucleus Accumbens shell mediates Cue-induced cocaine-seeking behavior. J Neurosci. 2019;39(14):2574–6.
121. Pol Bodetto S, Carouge D, Fonteneau M, Dietrich JB, Zwiller J, Anglard P. Cocaine represses protein phosphatase-1Cbeta through DNA methylation and methyl-CpG binding protein-2 recruitment in adult rat brain. Neuropharmacology. 2013;73:31–40.
122. Nestler EJ. FosB: a transcriptional regulator of stress and antidepressant responses. Eur J Pharmacol. 2015;753:66–72.
123. Anier K, Zharkovsky A, Kalda A. S-adenosylmethionine modifies cocaine-induced DNA methylation and increases locomotor sensitization in mice. Int J Neuropsychopharmacol. 2013;16(9):2053–66.
124. Grimm JW, Hope BT, Wise RA, Shaham Y. Neuroadaptation. Incubation of cocaine craving after withdrawal. Nature. 2001;412(6843):141–2.
125. Pickens CL, Airavaara M, Theberge F, Fanous S, Hope BT, Shaham Y. Neurobiology of the incubation of drug craving. Trends Neurosci. 2011;34(8):411–20.
126. Gawin FH, Kleber HD. Abstinence symptomatology and psychiatric diagnosis in cocaine abusers. Clin Observ Arch Gen Psychiatry. 1986;43(2):107–13.
127. Kundakovic M, Gudsnuk K, Herbstman JB, Tang D, Perera FP, Champagne FA. DNA methylation of BDNF as a biomarker of early-life adversity. Proc Natl Acad Sci U S A. 2015;112(22):6807–13.
128. Kimmel M, Clive M, Gispen F, Guintivano J, Brown T, Cox O, et al. Oxytocin receptor DNA methylation in postpartum depression. Psychoneuroendocrinology. 2016;69:150–60.

129. Wang D, Szyf M, Benkelfat C, Provencal N, Turecki G, Caramaschi D, et al. Peripheral SLC6A4 DNA methylation is associated with in vivo measures of human brain serotonin synthesis and childhood physical aggression. PLoS One. 2012;7(6):e39501.
130. Tozzi L, Farrell C, Booij L, Doolin K, Nemoda Z, Szyf M, et al. Epigenetic changes of FKBP5 as a link connecting genetic and environmental risk factors with structural and functional brain changes in major depression. Neuropsychopharmacology. 2018;43(5):1138–45.
131. Di Sante J, Ismaylova E, Nemoda Z, Gouin JP, Yu WJ, Caldwell W, et al. Peripheral DNA methylation of HPA axis-related genes in humans: cross-tissue convergence, two-year stability and behavioural and neural correlates. Psychoneuroendocrinology. 2018;97:196–205.
132. Steiger H, Booij L, Kahan, McGregor K, Thaler L, Fletcher E, et al. A longitudinal, epigenome-wide study of DNA methylation in anorexia nervosa: results in actively ill, partially weight-restored, long-term remitted and non-eating-disordered women. J Psychiatry Neurosci. 2019;44(3):205–13.
133. Nemoda Z, Massart R, Suderman M, Hallett M, Li T, Coote M, et al. Maternal depression is associated with DNA methylation changes in cord blood T lymphocytes and adult hippocampi. Transl Psychiatry. 2015;5:e545.
134. Camilo C, Maschietto M, Vieira HC, Tahira AC, Gouveia GR, Feio Dos Santos AC, et al. Genome-wide DNA methylation profile in the peripheral blood of cocaine and crack dependents. Braz J Psychiatry. 2019;41(6):485–93.
135. Lax E, Warhaftig G, Ohana D, Maayan R, Delayahu Y, Roska P, et al. A DNA methylation signature of addiction in T cells and its reversal with DHEA intervention. Front Mol Neurosci. 2018;11:322.
136. Cadet JL, Brannock C, Krasnova IN, Jayanthi S, Ladenheim B, McCoy MT, et al. Genome-wide DNA hydroxymethylation identifies potassium channels in the nucleus accumbens as discriminators of methamphetamine addiction and abstinence. Mol Psychiatry. 2017;22(8):1196–204.
137. Jayanthi S, McCoy MT, Chen B, Britt JP, Kourrich S, Yau HJ, et al. Methamphetamine downregulates striatal glutamate receptors via diverse epigenetic mechanisms. Biol Psychiatry. 2014; 76(1):47–56.
138. Jayanthi S, Gonzalez B, McCoy MT, Ladenheim B, Bisagno V, Cadet JL. Methamphetamine induces TET1- and TET3-dependent DNA hydroxymethylation of Crh and Avp genes in the rat nucleus Accumbens. Mol Neurobiol. 2018;55(6):5154–66.
139. Reynolds LM, Magid HS, Chi GC, Lohman K, Barr RG, Kaufman JD, et al. Secondhand tobacco smoke exposure associations with DNA methylation of the aryl hydrocarbon receptor repressor. Nicotine Tob Res. 2017;19(4):442–51.
140. Dawes K, Andersen A, Vercande K, Papworth E, Philibert W, Beach SRH, et al. Saliva DNA methylation detects nascent smoking in adolescents. J Child Adolesc Psychopharmacol. 2019;29(7):535–44.
141. Tsaprouni LG, Yang TP, Bell J, Dick KJ, Kanoni S, Nisbet J, et al. Cigarette smoking reduces DNA methylation levels at multiple genomic loci but the effect is partially reversible upon cessation. Epigenetics. 2014;9(10):1382–96.
142. Chatterton Z, Hartley BJ, Seok MH, Mendelev N, Chen S, Milekic M, et al. In utero exposure to maternal smoking is associated with DNA methylation alterations and reduced neuronal content in the developing fetal brain. Epigenetics Chromatin. 2017;10:4.
143. Chhabra D, Sharma S, Kho AT, Gaedigk R, Vyhlidal CA, Leeder JS, et al. Fetal lung and placental methylation is associated with in utero nicotine exposure. Epigenetics. 2014;9(11):1473–84.
144. Barbier E, Tapocik JD, Juergens N, Pitcairn C, Borich A, Schank JR, et al. DNA methylation in the medial prefrontal cortex regulates alcohol-induced behavior and plasticity. J Neurosci. 2015;35(15):6153–64.
145. Barak S, Carnicella S, Yowell QV, Ron D. Glial cell line-derived neurotrophic factor reverses alcohol-induced allostasis of the mesolimbic dopaminergic system: implications for alcohol reward and seeking. J Neurosci. 2011;31(27):9885–94.
146. Lohoff FW, Roy A, Jung J, Longley M, Rosoff DB, Luo A, et al. Epigenome-wide association study and multi-tissue replication of individuals with alcohol use disorder: evidence for abnormal glucocorticoid signaling pathway gene regulation. Mol Psychiatry. 2020;87:S113.
147. Roth MJ, Baer DJ, Albert PS, Castonguay TW, Dorgan JF, Dawsey SM, et al. Relationship between serum leptin levels and alcohol consumption in a controlled feeding and alcohol ingestion study. J Natl Cancer Inst. 2003;95(22):1722–5.
148. Sharp GC, Arathimos R, Reese SE, Page CM, Felix J, Kupers LK, et al. Maternal alcohol consumption and offspring DNA methylation: findings from six general population-based birth cohorts. Epigenomics. 2018;10(1):27–42.
149. Mandal C, Halder D, Jung KH, Chai YG. Gestational alcohol exposure altered DNA methylation status in the developing fetus. Int J Mol Sci. 2017;18(7).
150. Watson CT, Szutorisz H, Garg P, Martin Q, Landry JA, Sharp AJ, et al. Genome-wide DNA methylation profiling reveals epigenetic changes in the rat nucleus Accumbens associated with cross-generational effects of adolescent THC exposure. Neuropsychopharmacology. 2015;40(13):2993–3005.
151. Murphy SK, Itchon-Ramos N, Visco Z, Huang Z, Grenier C, Schrott R, et al. Cannabinoid exposure and altered DNA methylation in rat and human sperm. Epigenetics. 2018;13(12):1208–21.
152. Levin ED, Hawkey AB, Hall BJ, Cauley M, Slade S, Yazdani E, et al. Paternal THC exposure in rats causes long-lasting neurobehavioral effects in the offspring. Neurotoxicol Teratol. 2019;74:106806.

153. McGeary J. The DRD4 exon 3 VNTR polymorphism and addiction-related phenotypes: a review. Pharmacol Biochem Behav. 2009;93(3):222–9.
154. Lai JH, Zhu YS, Huo ZH, Sun RF, Yu B, Wang YP, et al. Association study of polymorphisms in the promoter region of DRD4 with schizophrenia, depression, and heroin addiction. Brain Res. 2010;1359:227–32.
155. Fransquet PD, Hutchinson D, Olsson CA, Allsop S, Elliott EJ, Burns L, et al. Cannabis use by women during pregnancy does not influence infant DNA methylation of the dopamine receptor DRD4. Am J Drug Alcohol Abuse. 2017;43(6):671–7.
156. Chen ZG, Wang YJ, Chen RS, Geng F, Gan CL, Wang WS, et al. Ube2b-dependent degradation of DNMT3a relieves a transcriptional brake on opiate-induced synaptic and behavioral plasticity. Mol Psychiatry. 2019;
157. Guy J, Cheval H, Selfridge J, Bird A. The role of MeCP2 in the brain. Annu Rev Cell Dev Biol. 2011;27:631–52.
158. Lewis JD, Meehan RR, Henzel WJ, Maurer-Fogy I, Jeppesen P, Klein F, et al. Purification, sequence, and cellular localization of a novel chromosomal protein that binds to methylated DNA. Cell. 1992;69(6):905–14.
159. Mellen M, Ayata P, Dewell S, Kriaucionis S, Heintz N. MeCP2 binds to 5hmC enriched within active genes and accessible chromatin in the nervous system. Cell. 2012;151(7):1417–30.
160. Cohen S, Gabel HW, Hemberg M, Hutchinson AN, Sadacca LA, Ebert DH, et al. Genome-wide activity-dependent MeCP2 phosphorylation regulates nervous system development and function. Neuron. 2011;72(1):72–85.
161. Kinde B, Gabel HW, Gilbert CS, Griffith EC, Greenberg ME. Reading the unique DNA methylation landscape of the brain: non-CpG methylation, hydroxymethylation, and MeCP2. Proc Natl Acad Sci U S A. 2015;112(22):6800–6.
162. Amir RE, Van den Veyver IB, Wan M, Tran CQ, Francke U, Zoghbi HY. Rett syndrome is caused by mutations in X-linked MECP2, encoding methyl-CpG-binding protein 2. Nat Genet. 1999;23(2):185–8.
163. Ebert DH, Gabel HW, Robinson ND, Kastan NR, Hu LS, Cohen S, et al. Activity-dependent phosphorylation of MeCP2 threonine 308 regulates interaction with NCoR. Nature. 2013; 499(7458):341–5.
164. Zhou Z, Hong EJ, Cohen S, Zhao WN, Ho HY, Schmidt L, et al. Brain-specific phosphorylation of MeCP2 regulates activity-dependent Bdnf transcription, dendritic growth, and spine maturation. Neuron. 2006;52(2):255–69.
165. Stefanelli G, Gandaglia A, Costa M, Cheema MS, Di Marino D, Barbiero I, et al. Brain phosphorylation of MeCP2 at serine 164 is developmentally regulated and globally alters its chromatin association. Sci Rep. 2016;6:28295.
166. Deng JV, Wan Y, Wang X, Cohen S, Wetsel WC, Greenberg ME, et al. MeCP2 phosphorylation limits psychostimulant-induced behavioral and neuronal plasticity. J Neurosci. 2014;34(13):4519–27.
167. Deng JV, Rodriguiz RM, Hutchinson AN, Kim IH, Wetsel WC, West AE. MeCP2 in the nucleus accumbens contributes to neural and behavioral responses to psychostimulants. Nat Neurosci. 2010;13(9):1128–36.
168. Lewis CR, Staudinger K, Scheck L, Olive MF. The effects of maternal separation on adult methamphetamine self-administration, extinction, reinstatement, and MeCP2 immunoreactivity in the nucleus Accumbens. Front Psych. 2013;4:55.
169. Im HI, Hollander JA, Bali P, Kenny PJ. MeCP2 controls BDNF expression and cocaine intake through homeostatic interactions with microRNA-212. Nat Neurosci. 2010;13(9):1120–7.
170. Cassel S, Carouge D, Gensburger C, Anglard P, Burgun C, Dietrich JB, et al. Fluoxetine and cocaine induce the epigenetic factors MeCP2 and MBD1 in adult rat brain. Mol Pharmacol. 2006;70(2):487–92.
171. Feng J, Nestler EJ. MeCP2 and drug addiction. Nat Neurosci. 2010;13(9):1039–41.
172. Prangley T, Pit SW, Rees T, Nealon J. Factors influencing early withdrawal from a drug and alcohol treatment program and client perceptions of successful recovery and employment: a qualitative study. BMC Psychiatry. 2018;18(1):301.
173. Perfas FB, Spross S. Why the concept-based therapeutic community can no longer be called drug-free. J Psychoactive Drugs. 2007;39(1):69–79.
174. McCusker J, Stoddard A, Frost R, Zorn M. Planned versus actual duration of drug abuse treatment. Reconciling observational and experimental evidence. J Nerv Ment Dis. 1996;184(8):482–9.
175. Vanderplasschen W, Colpaert K, Autrique M, Rapp RC, Pearce S, Broekaert E, et al. Therapeutic communities for addictions: a review of their effectiveness from a recovery-oriented perspective. ScientificWorldJournal. 2013;2013:427817.

Index

M. M. Vanyukov (ed.), *Genetics of Substance Use*, https://doi.org/10.1007/978-3-030-95350-8

D

MIX
Papier aus verantwortungsvollen Quellen
Paper from responsible sources
FSC® C105338

If you have any concerns about our products,
you can contact us on
ProductSafety@springernature.com

In case Publisher is established outside the EU,
the EU authorized representative is:
Springer Nature Customer Service Center GmbH
Europaplatz 3, 69115 Heidelberg, Germany

Printed by Libri Plureos GmbH
in Hamburg, Germany